MEDICINE IN CHINA
A History of Pharmaceutics

MEDICINE IN CHINA
A History of Pharmaceutics

PAUL U. UNSCHULD

UNIVERSITY OF CALIFORNIA PRESS
Berkeley   Los Angeles   London

Illustration opposite title page

The conclusion of the scroll fragment found in Tun-huang containing the *Shen-nung pen-ts'ao ching chi-chu* and the T'ang Period date 718.

University of California Press
Berkeley and Los Angeles, California

University of California Press, Ltd.
London, England

Library of Congress Cataloging in Publication Data

Unschuld, Paul Ulrich, 1943–
    Medicine in China.

    (Comparative studies in health systems and medical care)
    Bibliography: p.
    Includes indexes.
    1. Pharmacy—China—History.   2. Materia medica—
China—History.   I. Title.   II. Series.   [DNLM: 1. Med-
icine, Oriental—History—China.   2. Pharmacy—History—
China.   3. Drugs—History—China.   WZ 70 JC6 U5mb]
RS67.C6U57 1984   615'.1'0951   83-4937
ISBN 0-520-05025-8

Printed in the United States of America
1   2   3   4   5   6   7   8

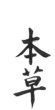

Contents

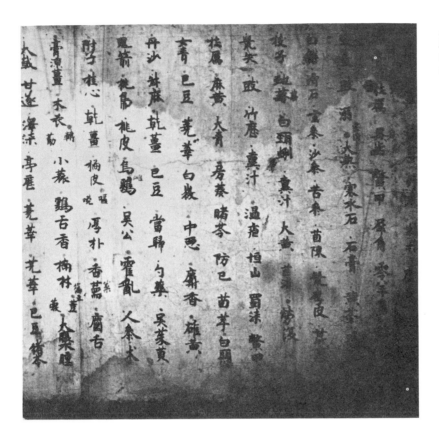

A portion of the Tun-huang fragment of the *Shen-nung pen-ts'ao ching chi-chu* illustrating the differentiation of drug properties by means of red and black dots.

Illustrations and Supplementary Material

A NOTE ON THE ILLUSTRATIONS

Numerous illustrations complement the text of this book. They have been taken from various Chinese pharmaceutical works dating from the 13th through the 19th centuries. The selection was made so as to provide illustrations from the animal, plant, and mineral domains. Some motifs were intentionally repeated to allow a comparison of *Pen-ts'ao* works from various centuries. In general, Chinese pharmaceutical literature adopted illustrations of the original plant, animal, or mineral from which the drug was obtained. The depiction of crude drugs is somewhat rare. The abundance of illustrative material reproduced here enables an extensive comparison with the development of illustrations in botanical, zoological, and mineral works from other cultures.

The captions to the illustrations generally provide the most familiar terms for the depicted original material—material from which the drugs were produced—and, in parentheses, a transliteration of the respective Chinese termini. The captions also include the source of the illustrations. Further information on these works can be found in the text by consulting the appropriate title in the index. The specific editions used and the libraries which gave their kind permission for the reproduction of material are presented below:

Shen-nung pen-ts'ao ching chi-chu—Tun-huang fragment—Ryugoku University, Kyoto, Japan

Hsin-hsiu pen-ts'ao—Tun-huang fragment—British Museum, London, England

Shih-liao pen-ts'ao—Tun-huang fragment—British Museum, London, England

Ta-kuan pen-ts'ao—facsimile of the edition of 1208—library of the author

Shao-hsing pen-ts'ao—facsimile of the fragments found in Japanese libraries, date uncertain—library of the author

Ch'ung-hsiu cheng-ho pen-ts'ao—facsimile of the edition of 1249—library of the author

Hsin-pien lei-yao t'u-chu pen-ts'ao—Yüan edition—Library of the Imperial Household, Tokyo, Japan

Yin-shan cheng-yao—facsimile of the Ming edition—library of the author

Pen-ts'ao p'in-hui ching-yao—18th century manuscript copy of the edition of 1505—Staatsbibliothek Berlin, Stiftung Preussischer Kulturbesitz, Berlin

Pen-ts'ao kang mu—Chiang-hsi edition of 1603—Staatsbibliothek Berlin, Stiftung Preussischer Kulturbesitz—Berlin

Pen-ts'ao hui—Ch'ing edition—Library of the Botanical Gardens, Kyoto, Japan

Pen-ts'ao hui-yen—Ch'ing edition—Ryugoku University, Kyoto, Japan

T'u-hsiang pen-ts'ao meng-ch'üan—edition of 1628—Ryugoku University, Kyoto, Japan

Chiu-huang-yeh p'u—Ch'ing edition—Library of parliament, Tokyo, Japan

Chih-wu ming-shih-t'u k'ao—facsimile of the illustrations of 1848—library of the author

Acknowledgments

This book is a revised and expanded version of *Pen-ts'ao.
2000 Jahre traditionelle pharmazeutische Literatur Chinas,*
published by H. Moos, Munich, in 1973. A major part
of the German original was translated into English by Frank
and Waltraut Lehmann. The amended script has been read by
Dr. Akira Akahori. I am most grateful for his valuable suggestions.

A. Introduction

1. GENERAL APPROACH

Chinese civilization has, over the past two thousand years, developed an abundance of information on the use of natural substances and manmade chemicals for therapeutic purposes. Today this knowledge is neither obsolete nor forgotten, in spite of the introduction of modern Western-type drug therapy more than a century ago. Innumerable Chinese healers prescribe remedies based on formulas that were elaborated many centuries, if not millennia, ago. In addition to a continuing lively tradition of teacher-apprentice instruction in ancient Chinese pharmaceutical knowledge, a wealth of literary sources is available today, enabling the historian, as an outsider, to assess the development of pharmaceutics in China. It is a central task of this book to provide, through a description and analysis of the structure and contents of traditional Chinese pharmaceutical literature, detailed information on the history of pharmaceutics in China. Obviously, a number of constraints limit the achievement of this task. The information gathered and published in the pharmaceutical literature represents only a fraction of the drug therapy in China. Individuals who compiled works on drugs had to choose between focusing on but one single plant or describing thousands of herbal, mineral, and animal substances. As members of a literate, educated elite in society, they had varying degrees of access to the actual practice of drug therapy. Some authors appear to have extracted all their wisdom from earlier literary sources while others took great pains to visit, over many decades, different geographic regions and to talk to peasants, laborers, and scholars alike in order to accumulate the most accurate information available on drugs and their properties. The historian has to select too; not all drug works written and published in earlier centuries are available to him and, even with respect to those at hand, an economic choice has to be made as to which ones should be included in an analysis. Some of the works under consideration are very short; others are extremely voluminous and would require many months, if not years, to translate in full. Therefore, additional choices have to be made regarding which aspect of the available literature an analysis should focus on in order to present a faithful account of at least the more important facets of the history of Chinese pharmaceutics as far as they are documented in print. Therefore, despite its wide scope in terms of both the historical period covered and the number of works described, the present book cannot claim comprehensiveness and must, out of necessity, leave many questions unanswered; its basic approach and its contribution to our understanding of Chinese culture in general and of Chinese science in particular may be outlined as follows.

The traditional medical and pharmaceutical literature of China is a genre of impressive size. The *Isekiko* of 1819 by the Japanese scholar Tamba Mototane—published in China, in 1936, under the title *Chung-kuo i-chi k'ao*, as the hitherto most comprehensive bibliography of Chinese medicine—lists no fewer then 2,605 titles for the period from the Han dynasty to the nineteenth century. For the shorter time span from the Han dynasty through the Sung period, Okanishi Tameto's bibliography *Sung-i-ch'ien i-chi k'ao* (1969) mentions approximately 1,975 medical works. This vast complex of Chinese medical literature can be divided roughly into three genres: the literature of medical theory, that of prescriptions, and the pharmaceutical literature. The term *pharmaceutical literature* needs further explanation to distinguish it from the other two genres. By pharmaceutical literature I mean all works meant to impart knowledge about individual drugs. This genre comprises not only views (obtained by theoretical deduction or by practical experience) about the medicinal effectiveness of drugs but also descriptions of the partial or complete process by which a raw drug progresses from breeding, cultivation, or manufacture to a state of medicinal applicability. This may involve a plant, part of a plant, an animal or a part or product of an animal, a mineral, a chemical substance, an object from everyday life, or a substance from the human body.

Not every pharmaceutical work need treat all of the above-mentioned areas in a similar manner; there are comprehensive, encyclopedic works which leave hardly a question unanswered as well as specialized works devoted to a single problem.

Numerous references to pharmaceutical activities are also found in the prescription literature. For example, directions for the preparation of drugs and for the production of suitable forms of medication are often appended to the list of ingredients for the prescriptions. To differentiate pharmaceutical literature from prescription literature, however, we should keep in mind that the former, basically, always deals with an individual drug, whereas in the latter it is the composition of drugs, and especially the diseases to be treated with these drugs, that form the starting point for almost all discussions.

In the two bibliographies mentioned above, the ratio of pharmaceutical works to medical works is, in general, approximately the same. In the *Sung-i-ch'ien i-chi k'ao* (approximately 270 titles) it is 13.7 percent; in the *Chung-kuo i-chi k'ao* (370 titles), 14.2 percent. Some 260 titles are given in a third bibliography, the *Hsien-ts'un pen-ts'ao shu-lu* by Lung Po-chien, which lists, as the title indicates, only those pharmaceutical works of two millennia of traditional Chinese medical literature that arc still extant today.

The pharmaceutical literature is especially well suited for the first analysis of a segment of traditional Chinese medical literature in a Western language. Because of its small percentage within the impressive total of medical literature, it is easier to survey than other genres. Its development can be traced from its origins during the Western

Han dynasty (206 B.C.–A.D. 8) to the twentieth century, and such an examination makes possible interesting conclusions about other areas of Chinese history of science, since pharmaceutics—even more than medicine—is anchored in all the natural sciences.

Original Chinese works that I could obtain in the United States, in Europe, and above all in East Asia, as well as a reasonable number of secondary works, provide the source for this description and analysis of traditional Chinese pharmaceutical literature.

From each of the various traditions of thought expressed in the traditional pharmaceutical literature, I have chosen a number of representative works whose descriptions form the core of the present study. The factors determining the choice were the originality of the works and their representativeness of various traditions in Chinese pharmaceutical literature. The descriptions of approximately 100 works chosen according to these criteria are based on the individual author, his motives for writing the work, and the contents of the work itself. I have recorded here, on the one hand, characteristics such as classification systems and numbers of drugs described. On the other hand, I have translated and rendered numerous prefaces, introductions, and drug monographs in their entirety or in excerpts, in order to clarify the contents of the individual works.

The choice of excerpts to be translated was determined first of all by the availability of the texts. It certainly would have been very interesting, for example, to translate and examine the first Chinese monograph on a single drug that was published as an individual work. Though mentioned in early bibliographies, this text has long been lost, and the wish cannot be realized.

Most of the translations are texts of prefaces or introductions in which the authors attempted to explain the purpose of their works. Not every preface, however, is suited for translation, either in whole or in part, for they often do not contain a statement concerning the work and its contents, or of the author and his intentions.

I have selected and translated various drug descriptions (so-called monographs) from individual works. My aim was to trace the description of one drug from the earliest time through several schools and traditions of pharmaceutical literature in order to make comparisons between periods in historical development and also between different contemporary attitudes.

Moreover, I have rendered excerpts that exemplify the works from which they are taken and which would be of potential value for a later comparison with corresponding features in the development of pharmaceutical literature in the West.

2. THE SOCIAL CONTEXT OF CHINESE PHARMACEUTICAL LITERATURE

From the Han period on, there exists documented evidence of court officials and public employees whose special tasks apparently included pharmaceutics. Moreover, from the eleventh century to the beginning of the Ming dynasty (and possibly even longer), there existed a system

of apothecary shops under governmental supervision. Beyond these
beginnings, however, one cannot claim that any of the groups practicing pharmaceutical activities had been institutionalized, organized
as a class, or even considered important by the government, especially
with respect to comprehensive regulation. As I have shown elsewhere,
the "professional" physician, selling his medical knowledge and skills
for money, was not socially respected in premodern China.[1] This was
even more true for the apothecary who specialized in selling drugs
and in whose hands plants, minerals, or animal products were nothing
but merchandise.

The socially insignificant role of all groups practicing medicine or
pharmaceutics for a living, however, must not lead us to rash conclusions concerning the respect for health care per se during the two
millennia of the Chinese Empire discussed here. The hesitation of
traditional Chinese society to advance the medical and pharmaceutical
ranks was probably grounded in a general characteristic of Confucian
policy not to allow any experts with a specialized expert knowledge
to rise socially as a group, because this might have led to social tensions, crises, and even restructuring. Instead, it was postulated that
every individual had to possess sufficient medical, including pharmaceutical, knowledge, so that he could help his fellow men—that is,
the members of his family.

This general attitude may have contributed to the fact that, while
a detailed malpractice legislation was elaborated from T'ang times on,
no comprehensive governmental regulation of the vocational practice
of health care and, above all, almost no supervision of the qualifica-
tions of the physicians and pharmacists as a whole were introduced
during the Imperial age. A training system for medical practitioners
in government service and for Confucian medical scholars, the origins
of which are discernible from the second century B.C. onward, was
adapted into an examination system for regular state officials during
the T'ang period and was further developed during the Sung period.[2]
However, because it comprised only a relatively small number of practicing physicians, and because there was corruption and periodic administrative disinterest, the impact of governmentally supervised
training and qualifying examinations on the actual practice of medicine
and pharmaceutics may have been negligible.

Along with the absence of general governmental regulation of
"professional" health care was the lack of a legally binding pharmacopoeia. These never existed in the traditional medical system in
China. In Chinese literature, I have occasionally read the claim that
the T'ang pen-ts'ao ("T'ang materia medica," see C, I, 3.2) had been
the first "pharmacopoeia" in the world, because this herbal was compiled and published on governmental order by a commission set up
by the government.[3] In such claims, comparisons are made with the
earliest "pharmacopoeia" in Europe, compiled by Valerius Cordus of
Nuremberg in 1546. But such a comparison is incorrect, and the
attribution "first pharmacopoeia in the world" for the T'ang pen-ts'ao
is erroneous in two respects.

Various authors of Western pharmaceutical history have examined
the question of what is actually meant by a "pharmacopoeia." The

term *pharmacopoeia* was introduced in Central Europe in the sixteenth century, at first only as a component of titles, meaning "the making of drugs." Later, the term became independent as a title for works with pharmaceutical contents, that is, for books on medications in general.[4]

In addition, the term has been used to specify a special type of pharmaceutical literature. "It describes a selected series of medications, for which the way of production, the quality, and the analytic methods of testing have been determined, while the book as a whole has the force of law thus subjecting the drug trade to its rules."[5] The *Dispensatorium* by Valerius Cordus of Nuremberg, as well as a long series of later European and American drug works (including a series of *United States Pharmacopoeias*) belong to this type of pharmacopoeia, which is legally binding.

The *T'ang pen-ts'ao* neither was the first book on medications in China or in the world, nor can it be considered an official pharmacopoeia in the indicated narrower sense. Its contents, like the contents of all earlier and subsequent herbals of traditional Chinese pharmaceutics before the twentieth century, written upon governmental or private initiative, were not binding for any vocational group.

The term *pharmacopoeia* has become so ambiguous, so closely associated with the European (and American) development of pharmaceutics since the sixteenth century, that it should not be used for traditional Chinese herbals compiled and published during the Imperial age.

3. AUTHORSHIP AND SCOPE OF CONTENTS

The great majority of all traditional Chinese pharmaceutical works were written and published by private citizens at their own initiative. These could be practicing physicians or members of the imperial family. High officials, who had the opportunity, on their long travels, to become acquainted with the plants, animals, and minerals of other countries and provinces and their medicinal uses, wrote pharmaceutical books, as did Taoists living in solitude, who wrote down their insights and experiences on how to achieve a long life without aging. Sons recorded their mothers' advice; textual critics published drug works which they considered a contribution to the revelation of the true origin of pharmaceutics. In short, the authors came from every possible level or group of the population able to write, and I do not know of any case where such a work was criticized as having been written by nonexperts. Pharmaceutics was part of a general education, and, consequently, everybody had the authority to publish such a work.

Only a few titles out of the entire field of traditional Chinese pharmaceutical literature were compiled and published as a result of governmental orders and aid. Interestingly enough, with the definite exception of the *T'ang pen-ts'ao,* it appears to be a common characteristic of the government sponsored herbals that they were the least suited for actual everyday medical and pharmaceutical practice; that is, these works, as I will show, did not correspond closely to the needs of any vocational group of health care practitioners. Throughout the three centuries of the two Sung dynasties (960–1279), as well as during Ming and Ch'ing times, large committees called together by the administration, as well as a small number of dedicated individuals, created voluminous herbals of an encyclopedic nature. These compilations offered a comprehensive view of current thought and knowledge about animals, plants, and minerals, and their medicinal use. The reader could find information about external and inherent peculiarities and characteristics of the individual drugs. He could also obtain information concerning their original materials, their places of origin, the times of collection, the medicinally usable parts of the original plants, animals, and so on, the compatibility, contraindications and incompatibilities, the possibilities of adulteration, the criteria for the genuineness of the drugs, as well as the processing and preparation of prescriptions from several individual drugs. Some of these works contained theoretical treatises, and most of them, detailed information on the indications and modes of effect of the drugs. This spectrum of pharmaceutical information was certainly broad enough to satisfy all requirements of drug therapy, and yet, with the exception of the famous *Pen-ts'ao kang mu* by Li Shih-chen (1596; see C, III, 2.1.2.4), the encyclopedic works gave little concrete assistance for actual medical and pharmaceutical practice. They were, in many respects, far too long-winded, voluminous, and expensive for such a purpose. To the outside observer and modern historian of science, though, the encyclopedic works seem to be the most valuable sources for various investigations, precisely because of these characteristics. As a consequence, it is this segment of traditional Chinese pharmaceutical literature whose reputation and fame first reached the West.

It was a very different type of pharmaceutical literature, however, that achieved widest circulation among everyday practitioners. The selected contents, convenient structure, and handy size of those pharmaceutical works described below as "eclectic tradition" (see C, IV, 1–6) won highest esteem among Chinese practitioners. On the Chinese mainland, the dominance of eclectic works appears at present to have been somewhat weakened by the availability of a large number of useful contemporary manuals for traditional drug therapy. In Chinese communities outside of the People's Republic, though, these Ming and, mostly, Ch'ing works continue to be widely distributed. Because the modern historian finds it difficult to consider the eclectic tradition as the best or most attractive product of traditional Chinese pharmaceutical literature, a bias may be introduced into analyses of premodern Chinese drug therapy of which a reader should be made aware.

4. ILLUSTRATIONS, DRUG CLASSIFICATION, AND THE ISSUE OF PROGRESS IN TRADITIONAL CHINESE PHARMACEUTICAL LITERATURE

Traditional Chinese pharmaceutical literature contains important information concerning progress and conservativism in traditional Chinese science. The data gathered in this book provide ample evidence of the dynamics of the Chinese interpretation of nature; there is hardly one aspect in the broad field of pharmaceutical knowledge that has succumbed to stagnation over an extended period of time. And yet, it would be inaccurate to apply a notion of steady progress, shared by many, from speculation to observation, from belief to truth, to the history of pharmaceutics in China. The dynamics of pharmaceutical knowledge during the Imperial era were characterized, first, by an emergence of a number of distinct traditions coinciding with major sociopolitical currents, and, second, by the absence of a social institution that could have supported the development of a standardized knowledge commonly accepted by a majority of "scientists" and practitioners. The nature of illustrations and the structural patterns discernible in the herbals may serve here as preliminary justification for such a statement; it will be further corroborated in the main part of this book where the contents of these works are described.

Because the herbalists had available only a limited number of appropriate criteria for testing, the advice published in the herbals concerning examinations for the genuineness of individual drugs could never be very detailed or perhaps even totally unequivocal. Nevertheless, the emphasis on the illustrations, especially useful for making distinctions between individual plants, varies strikingly from herbal to herbal. A peak in the artistic execution of the drug illustrations is undoubtedly found in the paintings of the *Pen-ts'ao p'in-hui ching-yao* (see pp. 139–140). They were, however, never published. A number of works contain very precise, true-to-nature illustrations—for example, the *Chih-wu ming-shih-t'u k'ao* (see p. 258)—which can hardly be distinguished from the modern drawings in our botanical texts. The illustrations in the great pharmaceutical works of the Sung period were also already of high quality. By contrast, other works, including even the first and second editions of the famous *Pen-ts'ao kang mu* (see C, III, 2.3.1), were provided with rather rough sketches, poorly suited for botanical definitions. Many herbals did not contain any illustrations. Frequently, one and the same drawing of a drug or a plant was reproduced by subsequent works for centuries, even though illustrations of better quality had long since been prepared and could have served as models. No continuous development is discernible here.

The prevailing structural principle of Chinese traditional pharmaceutical literature consisted primarily in the arrangement of the materia medica according to the natural origin of the drugs—that is, from minerals, animals, or plants. Exceptions to this include the oldest pharmaceutical text known, the *Pen-ching* (see B, 1.1.2), and the *Pen-ts'ao ch'iu-chen* of the eighteenth century (see C, IV, 5). In the former, the overall structure was determined by a three-class division based on a macrocosmic concept of heaven, man, and earth; in the *Pen-ts'ao ch'iu-chen*, the author organized the individual monographs according to similarities in the therapeutic indications of the drugs. But such attempts remained the exceptions. It appears to be more important to investigate the development of the structure based upon the natural origin of drugs.

The earliest example of this structure available to us is found in the *Pen-ching*. Within the three classes of drugs corresponding to heaven, man, and earth, the drugs were grouped according to mineral, plant, and animal origin; these, in turn, were followed by foodstuffs. One might point out that a progression is discernible in this arrangement: from dead matter, to living but immobile plants, and, finally, to living creatures capable of motion.

T'ao Hung-ching (452–536) provided an important impetus to this structural pattern when he placed it above the three classes. While the *Pen-ching* had arranged the animal drugs as follows—quadrupeds, fowl, worms, fish—T'ao Hung-ching changed the order to reptiles, fish, fowl, quadrupeds. He gave no reason for the change, but it may be considered another step towards the evaluation scale of Li Shih-chen (1518–1593), the author of the *Pen-ts'ao kang mu*, who proceeded "from the small to the large" when he established the sequence of waters, fires, soils, metals, minerals, herbs, grains, vegetables, fruits, trees, and "ascended from the low to the sublime" in the arrangement of worms, scaly animals, crustaceans, fowl, quadrupeds, and man (see C, III).

Within these groups, which were expanded from ten in the *Pen-ching* to sixteen in the *Pen-ts'ao kang mu*, the designation "related types" appeared in the eleventh century in the *Chia-yu pen-ts'ao* (see C, I, 5.4). Because it proved impossible to arrange newly introduced descriptions into one of the three macrocosmic categories, which had been retained for so long as subdivisions, the authors of that time were forced to seek new possibilities for the division of drugs within the groups of natural origin. The result was that similar things were placed together. These related types often corresponded to the later, well-defined subgroups in the *Pen-ts'ao kang mu*. Within these subgroups, Li Shih-chen then arranged entries according to—in modern terms—families or species, using a binominal system of designation.

Surprisingly for the modern historian and without any obvious reason, this interesting development was not carried any further. The structural pattern of the *Pen-ts'ao kang mu*, which seems to anticipate Darwin's natural sequence of species as well as elements of Linne's systematic botany, remained an individual achievement of Li Shih-chen. None of the succeeding authors of herbals appears to have noticed the importance which we ascribe to this pattern. It lacked the powers to rouse subsequent writers. Indeed, the structure was adopted by just a few authors, apparently only because they considered the *Pen-ts'ao kang mu* as a whole a great and exemplary work. Others followed arbitrary variations of its structural pattern, preferring at one time this sequence, and, at another time, that. Finally, during the eighteenth and nineteenth centuries some authors even resumed the three-class division. Many an individual achievement by prominent Chinese naturalists, whose early greatness surprises us and exacts our admiration, is characterized, like Li Shih-chen's structural pattern, by the fact that it fell into oblivion or at least did not become common cultural property.

We are frequently tempted, as Western historians, to search in ancient Chinese sources for a mirror image of our own history of science; we focus on and point out specific events and developments in China that appear to be closely related to the kind of "truth" we have discovered when in fact they were of insignificant importance in

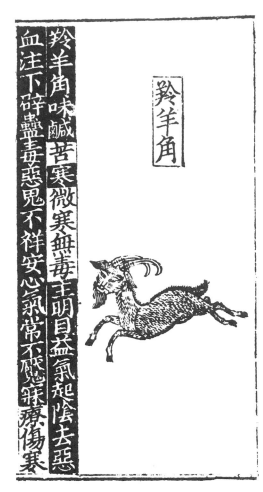

antelope horn *(ling-yang-chiao)*—*Ch'ung-hsiu cheng-ho pen-ts'ao*

the context of traditional Chinese culture. Yielding to this temptation may easily lead one to present a distorted reality of Chinese science which then, in turn, may give rise to ill-founded evaluations and comparisons. To resist this approach, though, does not imply that we should disregard even the most isolated thoughts published by an ancient Chinese author that resemble certain achievements in Western history of science. On the contrary, such discoveries should stimulate us to consider thoroughly the differences and similarities between Chinese and Western interpretations of nature and to study social and cultural factors that may have contributed to the prominence and continuous development of some insights and concepts in one civilization and to their neglect in another.

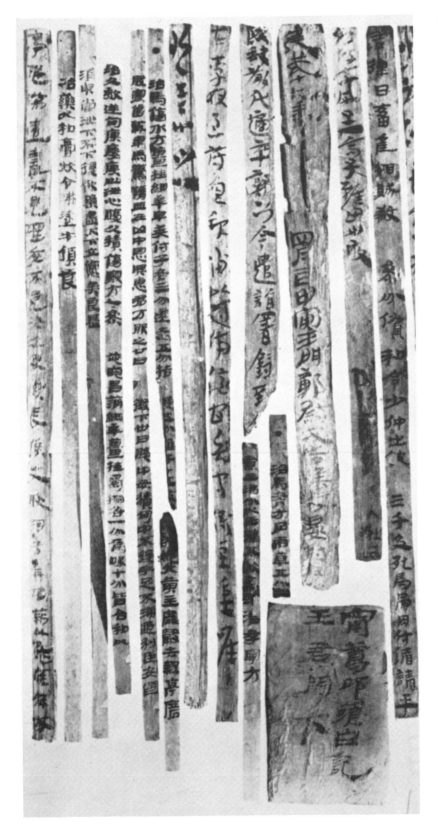

Wood strips containing prescriptions and pharmaceutical information, 5th–1st centuries B.C.

B. Shen-nung, *Pen-ts'ao*, and the Origins of Pharmaceutical Literature in China

Closely associated with the entire complex of traditional Chinese pharmaceutics and pharmaceutical literature is Shen-nung, a deity which lent its name to some of the earliest herbals documented in ancient Chinese bibliographies. Shen-nung ("Divine Peasant") is mentioned by Mencius (372–289 B.C.) as the model of a certain group, whose members—probably through philosophical motivation—were concerned with agriculture and with the simple life in the country. The "Great Commentary" (*Ta-chuan*) on the "Book of Changes" (*I-ching*), written at approximately the same time as the works of Mencius, ascribed the invention of the plow and the founding of markets to Shen-nung. The first reference to a connection between this legendary culture hero and pharmaceutics, a reference upon which all later similar statements are based, is found in the *Huai-nan tzu*, a work compiled by scholars from the circle of Liu An (died 122 B.C.), who is known to have leaned toward Taoism:

> The people of Antiquity consumed herbs and drank water. They gathered the fruits of the trees and ate the flesh of the clams. They frequently suffered from illnesses and poisonings. Then Shen-nung taught the people for the first time how to sow the five kinds of grains, and to observe whether the land was dry or moist, fertile or stony, located on hills or in the lowland. He tried the tastes of all herbs and [examined] the springs, whether they were sweet or bitter. Thus he informed the people of what they ought to avoid and where they could go. At that time [Shen-nung] encountered on one day seventy [herbs, liquids, etc.] with medicinal effectiveness (*tu*).[1,2]

The first title of a book mentioning Shen-nung in connection with a therapeutic subject dates from the first century A.D. and is found in the bibliographical section *I-wen-chih* of the history of the Western Han dynasty (*Han-shu*). The work is the *Shen-nung Huang-ti shih-chin* (see D, I, 1). Although the contents are unknown, the title indicates that it must have been a manual for dietetics.

Another book title that contains the name of Shen-nung—the *Shen-nung ching*—is cited in various works by physicians and Taoists of the Chin period; these include the *Yang-sheng lun* ("On the Preservation of Life") by Chi K'ang (223–262), the *Po-wu chih* ("Notes on the Examination of Things") by Chang Hua (232–300), and the *Pao-p'u tzu* ("Book about the Master Who Maintained Solidarity") by Ko

11

Hung (281–341).[3] A book entitled *Shen-nung ching* from this time has not been preserved, and one cannot draw any conclusions about the contents from the neutral title itself, "Shen-nung's Classic." The fact, however, that the works in which it is mentioned deal with medical problems, such as the "art of prolonging life," clearly points to the book's connection with this subject matter.

Beyond the description in Liu An's *Huai-nan tzu* of the legendary emperor as the founder of pharmaceutics itself, the fact that Shen-nung was also considered the author of the first Chinese special work on pharmaceutics is underlined by book titles containing the phrase *Shen-nung pen-ts'ao.* These titles are first mentioned by the Taoist scholar T'ao Hung-ching (452–536) and were later recorded in the bibliographies of the official Sui and T'ang histories (*Sui-shu, T'ang-shu*). T'ao Hung-ching explains the legend in the preface to an herbal which he compiled in the year 500:

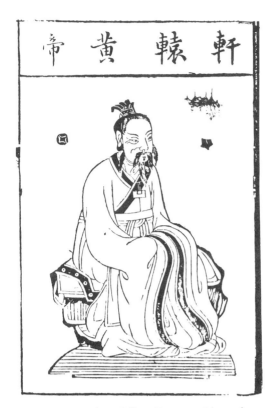

Hsüan Yüan, the "Yellow Emperor," legendary ruler of antiquity—*T'u-hsiang pen-ts'ao meng-ch'üan*

Pien Ch'io, semilegendary physician of the 5th century B.C.—*T'u-hsiang pen-ts'ao meng-ch'üan*

> In old accounts it is always said that Shen-nung [composed the] *Pen [-ts'ao] ching.* I agree with this opinion. However, when Shen-nung governed the empire in ancient times, he drew the eight trigrams for an understanding of the nature of demons and spirits. He introduced agriculture, in order to stop the unfortunate destruction of life. He effected the widespread use of medications and the curing of illnesses, in order to preserve [humanity] from the fate of early death and the harms of injuries. These three principles were further extended and carried on by all the exemplary men of later times. Out of the eight trigrams King Wen created the 64 symbols. Confucius supplied these with verbal explanations. Thus, both furthered a deep understanding of Man and nature. Hou Chi and I Yin called [the people's] attention to the kinds of grain, giving this grace to the whole of humanity. Ch'i [Po], Huang [-ti], P'eng [-tsu] and Pien [Ch'io] carried on this work; they helped and guided mankind. The grace [of Shen-nung] has thus been handed down and was kept alive. Three thousand years have passed and the people still require it. There was, however, no written tradition before Hsüan Yüan; the six oracle signs, for example, were handed down by signs made with the fingers. In order to pass on knowledge about agriculture illustrations were used. Only in this manner could objects leave traces. The knowledge about the medical effectiveness of drugs was passed on consecutively from one expert to the next; how else could one have obtained it? Only from the time in which T'ung [-chün] and Lei [-kung] lived were the [traditions preserved on] bamboo slabs.[4]

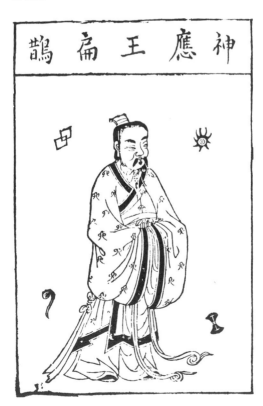

We will still often find in commentaries of later centuries the opinion that Shen-nung himself wrote the work on drugs that was named after him. But T'ao Hung-ching, while recognizing the legendary emperor's creation of pharmaceutics, ascribed to him only an indirect authorship of the work *Shen-nung pen-ts'ao ching.*

The tradition of Chinese pharmaceutical literature is also inseparably connected with *pen-ts'ao*, a term that is often used for its name in general and forms part of the title in a large number of pharmaceutical works. The original meaning of the two characters pen-ts'ao has been explained in various ways through the course of centuries and has not yet been clearly identified. Before I quote various opinions on the meaning of the concept, I will describe the context of its earliest known appearance in Chinese literature.

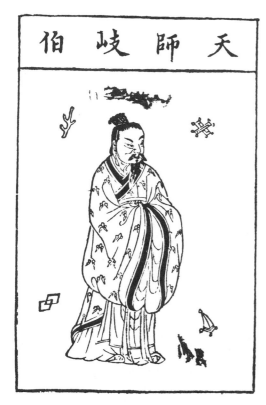

Ch'i Po, the "supernal teacher," legendary Minister of the Yellow Emperor and knowledgeable in medicine—*T'u-hsiang pen-ts'ao meng-ch'üan*

Shen-nung, the "divine farmer," legendary ruler of antiquity—*T'u-hsiang pen-ts'ao meng-ch'üan*

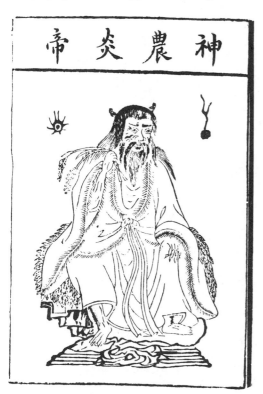

Since the time of the Warring States, magicians, alchemists, and similar practitioners had been able to impress the rulers and the educated with their theories and abilities. The first emperor of the short-lived Ch'in dynasty, Shih Huang-ti (259–210 B.C.), is supposed to have had great confidence in the efforts to attain the Taoist ideal of "long life without aging." He sent Hsü Fu, together with a large following of virgins and young men, eastward to the sea to obtain a suitable elixir from the islands of the sages. Emperor Wu-ti, the ruler of the Western Han dynasty from 140 to 86 B.C., had similar notions. Under his reign, a large number of officials were occupied solely with evaluating the numerous theories and drugs presumed suitable for the preparation of an immortality elixir. Similar efforts were continued with varying intensity until the year 31 B.C. At that time, the officials K'uang Heng and Chang T'an appealed to the emperor Ch'eng-ti (46–45 B.C.), who had assumed the throne one year before, to give up all such attempts, since the fulfillment of the idea of immortality was impossible. In a description in the *Han-shu* of the measures taken after this petition, we find, among the names given to the dismissed specialists, the term *pen-ts'ao* for the first time: "More than seventy prescription masters, aides, assistants and pen-ts'ao officials were sent home."[5]

A few decades later, a great literary congress was held in the capital. Among the invited participants were pen-ts'ao specialists, as indicated by a note in the official historical account:

> Called to the court were all experts on lost classics, old records, astronomy, the calendar, bell pitch, minor studies, historical writings, prescription techniques, and pen-ts'ao as well as teachers of the five classics, of the *Lun-yü*, the *Hsiao-ching*, and the *Erh-ya*. They were sent to the capital from their respective places of living by horse-drawn carriages. Several thousand men arrived.[6]

In both quotations, the use of the term *pen-ts'ao* does not yet allow its restriction to one specific literary work. Its usage points to a whole area of knowledge, probably to pharmaceutics. This assumption is also supported by the following, third mention of the term *pen-ts'ao*, which is found in the *Hou-Han-shu*, the official history of the Eastern Han dynasty:

> Lou Hu, whose *tzu*-name was Chün-ching, came from Ch'i. In his father's family, medical abilities had been transmitted for centuries. At an early age, [Lou Hu] followed his father to Ch'ang-an, where the latter wanted to practice medicine. Both made frequent visits to homes of the imperial family. Hu had mastered the medical classics, the *pen-ts'ao*, and alchemy, a total of several 100,000 words.[7]

Various facts and legends played a role in the attempts of Chinese authors to clarify the original meaning of the character combination pen-ts'ao. Han Pao-sheng (ca. 950) expressed the following view in his herbal *Ch'ung-kuang ying-kung pen-ts'ao*: "Among the drugs there are precious stones, minerals, trees, fowl, quadrupeds, reptiles/worms, and fish. Thus we speak of pen-ts'ao because among all the drugs the class of herbs [ts'ao] is the largest."[8]

In this sense, the term *pen-ts'ao* would mean approximately "[pharmaceutics whose] basis [*pen*] [is] herbs [*ts'ao*]." This is in agreement with the definition of the character *yao* ("drug," "medication") in the *Shuo-wen chieh-tzu,* the earliest Chinese etymological dictionary (ca. A.D. 100): "*Yao* are herbs used to treat illnesses."[9]

本草

藥

In the Sung period, the author of the *Chia-yu pu-chu Shen-nung pen-ts'ao,* Chang Yü-hsi (992–1068), wrote: "Since there were no characters in former times, [knowledge about drugs] was transmitted [orally] from teacher to student. This was called *pen-ts'ao* [that is, 'knowledge based (*pen*) upon familiarity with the drugs (*ts'ao*) themselves']."[10]

In the Ming period, Hsieh Chao-chi referred to the statement in the *Huai-nan tzu,* quoted here in an earlier paragraph already: "Shen-nung experimented with the herbs in order to heal sickness. Therefore [his] book [on drugs] is called *pen-ts'ao* [that is, 'which is based on herbs']."[11]

Proceeding from the first usage of this character combination, we may conclude from its context that the dismissed pen-ts'ao specialists were practitioners of the art of prolonging life who used herbs—in the sense of drugs—in their effort. *Pen* would thus be understood as a verb. Possibly, the expression became independent in the course of time and assumed the general meaning of "pharmaceutics." It has been used in this sense ever since. A title such as the above-mentioned *Shen-nung pen-ts'ao ching* might therefore be translated accurately as "Shen-nung's Classic of Pharmaceutics" or as "Shen-nung's Classic on Materia Medica."

Although the *Shen-nung pen-ts'ao ching* represents the oldest known Chinese pharmaceutical work in the sense defined in the preceding chapter, it is not the first Chinese written source on pharmaceutical data available today. The oldest written evidence for an effort to cure illnesses in China dates from the second millennium B.C. Since the end of the past century, archaeologists based in the An-yang district of the province Honan have discovered more than 150,000 bone fragments and tortoise shells from the Shang dynasty, on which numerous characters had been scratched for oracles. Among these characters, the names of fourteen different illnesses have been identified in a therapeutic context which elsewhere I have called "ancestral healing."[12] However, medical drugs are not mentioned, as far as we know.[13] Other archaeological finds from the beginning of the twentieth century and in more recent years have brought to light, though, prescription texts from the late Chou (third century B.C.) through the early Eastern Han period (first century A.D.) with rich information on numerous drugs and their usage. The oldest records of this kind were found most recently. In 1973, the so-called Han Grave No. 3 of the Ma-wang-tui site near Ch'ang-sha yielded various medical silk manuscripts, four of them containing data on materia medica.[14] Of these, the most valuable for today's historian is a fragmentary text that contemporary Chinese scholars call *Wu-shih-erh ping fang* ("Prescriptions Against 52 Illnesses") because of the number of health care issues listed in it.[15] The *Wu-shih-erh ping fang* mentions, in 170 different prescriptions, various therapeutic techniques, including moxa-cauterization, petty surgery, pressure with stones, massage, cupping, steaming, spells, and, dominating the text, the application of a total of about 247 drugs. Detailed instructions are often provided on pharmaceutical preparation and dosage forms of substances originating from mineral, herbal, animal, and human sources, as well as from the realm of commodities, such as "clothes of the dead" or "a female's first menstruation towel." The drugs are recommended for internal or external use either in their natural state or after having been processed in different ways into a broad range of preparations. These include powders (ground either from dried or variously roasted substances), pills (with wine, vinegar, and animal fat as excipients; honey and date pulp were not yet employed in the *Wu-shih-erh ping fang* but in two other, possibly younger texts also discovered at Ma-wang-tui), aqueous preparations (common solutions, decoctions, steam preparations and suspensions), medical wines (pure wines, as well as solutions and decoctions of drugs in wine), medical vinegars (vinegar solutions or decoctions of drugs), ointments from fats or oil, and dietetic preparations.[16]

It is quite legitimate to regard the data provided by the *Wu-shih-erh ping fang* as part of a pharmaceutical tradition which was later systematized in the pen-ts'ao literature. Approximately one half of the substances mentioned in this text are listed also in the first of the pen-ts'ao herbals, that is, in the *Shen-nung pen-ts'ao ching*.

The *Wu-shih-erh ping fang* does not contain any explicit references to theoretical foundations for using specific drugs against particular illnesses; yet, from the context of the prescriptions it is obvious that notions of magic correspondence and demonology have played a significant role in determining the selection of substances. The majority of therapeutic indications in the *Wu-shih-erh ping fang*, however, do not provide any clues at all on a conceptual relationship between health problems and drugs recommended, a fact already pointing to the characteristic pragmatism of Chinese materia medica literature during the entire first millennium A.D.

Less rich in their contents but historically closer to the origins of systematized pharmaceutical literature are collections of texts written on narrow wooden or bamboo slabs, unearthed in West and Northwest China in 1908 through 1916 (partly by the British archaeologist Stein),[17] in 1930 (the Chü-yen finds from the O-chi-na River region), and in 1972 (in a Han grave in Wu-wei County, Kansu).[18] The last discovery was the most extensive, yielding ninety-two slabs with a total of thirty prescriptions listing one hundred drugs. As modern analysts agree, these texts appear to have been written during the early Eastern Han period.[19] In contrast to the *Wu-shih-erh ping fang* and also to the *Shen-nung pen-ts'ao ching*, no human substances are recommended for medication. However, the therapeutic indications of the individual drugs conform closer to those of the *Shen-nung pen-ts'ao ching* than is the case with the *Wu-shih-erh ping fang*. Also, a higher proportion of the drugs noted in the Wu-wei texts (69 percent) also appear in the *Shen-nung pen-ts'ao ching*. The Wu-wei prescriptions are, like those of the *Wu-shih-erh ping fang*, mostly complex, combining from three to fifteen different substances for a single treatment. In addition to preparations already proposed in the *Wu-shih-*

erh ping fang, the Wu-wei texts advocate drops and suppositories. The range of excipients includes honey, lard, milk, and cheese prepared from camel's milk.

As we may assume from these ancient records, the literary knowledge on pharmaceutics was embedded originally in texts on prescriptions. As the silk fragments from Ma-wang-tui and the bamboo slabs from Wu-wei indicate, centuries of familiarity with the internal and external use of therapeutic substances led to the development of a rather sophisticated materia medica which, at one point in time, virtually demanded the formation of a specialized literary genre. This step appears to have been carried out with the compilation of the classic of traditional Chinese materia medica, the *Shen-nung pen-ts'ao ching*.

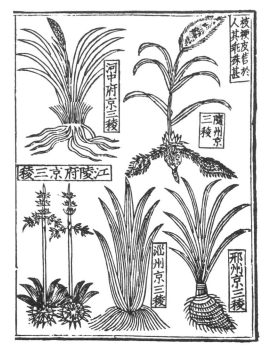

clubrush stem tubers *(ching-san-leng)*—*Ch'ung-hsiu cheng-ho pen-ts'ao*

C. The Pen-ts'ao Literature with Comprehensive Contents

I. THE MAIN TRADITION OF PEN-TS'AO LITERATURE

1. Early pen-ts'ao Works before T'ao Hung-ching

Shen-nung pen-ts'ao ching
"Shen-nung's Classic of Pharmaceutics"
Short titles: *Shen-nung pen-ching; Pen-ching; Shen-nung pen-ts'ao*
3 chapters / 365 drug descriptions
Author: unknown
Written: later Han period

Lei-kung chi-chu Shen-nung pen-ts'ao
"Shen-nung's Materia Medica, Compiled and Annotated by Lei-kung"
Short titles: *Pen-ching; Shen-nung pen-ching; Shen-nung pen-ts'ao; Shen-nung pen-ts'ao ching*
4 chapters // 595/431/319 drug descriptions
Authors: Wu P'u (?–250), Li Tang-chih (?–250), and others responsible for various revisions
Written: ca. 200–250

T'ao Hung-ching (456–536), whom I have already mentioned, was probably the first to express the view that the knowledge of pharmaceutics transmitted orally from Shen-nung's time must have been written down during the Eastern Han dynasty. This opinion was based upon the fact that the names used for the places of origin of the drugs in the various pen-ts'ao works of T'ao's time were common to the later Han period.

Not all of the early pharmaceutical works written before T'ao Hung-ching used the term *pen-ts'ao* in their titles. Yet we can count them as part of the so-called pen-ts'ao literature because the contents are the deciding factor. At that time, as in later centuries, some of these works were given phrases such as *yao-lu* ("Notes on Drugs"), *yao-mu* ("List of Drugs"), *yao-tui* ("Comparison of Drugs") or *yao-ching* ("Drug Classic") as a distinguishing part of their titles. A first comprehensive—though perhaps not complete—list of the pen-ts'ao works before T'ao Hung-ching can be found in the bibliographical section of the history of the Sui dynasty; this list is partly based upon the *Ch'i-lu,* a long-lost catalogue of literature of the Liang period. All pharmaceutical works recorded in this catalogue have been lost. Part of what is known about their contents today is to be found in scattered quotes in encyclopedias or other sources.[1] Also, the main branch of the following pen-ts'ao tradition, whose characteristics will be defined below, has transmitted at least the contents of those early pen-ts'ao writings that T'ao Hung-ching used as a basis for his own pharmaceutical works.

In a preface, T'ao Hung-ching mentions the *T'ung-chün ts'ai-yao lu* ("Mr. T'ung's Notes on the Gathering of Drugs"), the *(Lei-kung) yao-tui* ("Lei-kung's Comparison of Drugs"), and different editions of a *Shen-nung pen-ts'ao ching* as writings on which he has based his own work (see p. 31). He also mentions a Mr. T'ung (legendary), Chang Chi (142–220?), Hua T'o (190–265), Wu P'u (died 250), and Li Tang-chih (died 250) as authors who before him had been occupied with the revision of earlier versions of the *Shen-nung pen-ts'ao ching* or with the compilation of independent works on drugs. It can no longer be proved whether there was, in fact, ever a specific, original work entitled *Shen-nung pen-ts'ao ching,* or whether various pharmaceutical collections of the Han period were written with this or a similar title.

The above-mentioned bibliographical section of the Sui history, in which the pharmaceutical works of T'ao Hung-ching are already included, lists, among others, the following early pen-ts'ao works, which seem connected, at least by title, to the presumed first *Shen-nung pen-ts'ao ching:*

1. *Shen-nung pen-ts'ao,* 8 chapters
2. *Shen-nung pen-ts'ao,* 5 chapters
3. *Shen-nung pen-ts'ao shu-wu,* 2 chapters
4. *Shen-nung ming-t'ang t'u,* 1 chapter
5. *T'ao Yin-chü pen-ts'ao,* 10 chapters
6. *T'ao Hung-ching Shen-nung pen-ts'ao ching chi-chu,* 7 chapters
7. *Shen-nung pen-ts'ao,* 4 chapters
8. *Shen-nung pen-ts'ao ching,* 3 chapters

Only two of these titles are named in the older history of the T'ang dynasty (*Chiu T'ang-shu*):

Shen-nung pen-ts'ao, 3 chapters
Pen-ts'ao chi-chu, 7 chapters

These two works probably correspond to the above-mentioned titles 8 and 6 and were written by T'ao Hung-ching.

After considering the data quoted here and a remark by T'ao Hung-ching in the preface of his own work that he had used an edition with four chapters, Okanishi explained the multiplicity of the pen-ts'ao works listed in the *Sui-shu* and *Chiu-T'ang-shu* in the following manner: title 5 represents a combined edition of the works 6 and 8, works written by T'ao Hung-ching himself; title 1 may have represented a combined version of 2, 3, and 4. One can thus conclude that the works 1, 2, 3, and 7 were handed down during the time of T'ao Hung-ching.[2]

1.1. Structure and content of the *Pen-ching*

The work of T'ao Hung-ching, as well as the *Shen-nung pen-ts'ao ching* (referred to from now on as *Pen-ching*—"Original Classic") on which it is largely based, form the recognizable beginnings of the subsequent main tradition of pen-ts'ao literature, and for the reaction, starting in the seventeenth century, against the innovations in drug literature introduced in the twelfth and thirteenth centuries that deviated from the original tradition. For many centuries, the *Pen-ching* influenced the contents and structure of works on drugs. Therefore it seems useful to give here a detailed description of this work, for only in comparison can the characteristics and aims of the four most important epochs in the development of Chinese drug literature be weighed correctly against one another.

The first of the four chapters of the *Pen-ching* contains ten general essays; the remaining three chapters consist of the individual drug monographs.

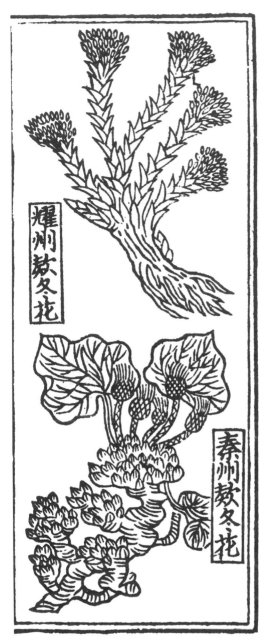

coltsfoot blossoms *(k'uan-tung-hua)—Ch'ung-hsiu cheng-ho pen-ts'ao*

[5] Drugs may be processed into the following medicinal forms, in accord with [their respective effectiveness]: pills, powders, aqueous decoctions, saturations in wine, and pastes. Sometimes a drug is also suited for several medicinal forms, or there are drugs which must not be immersed in hot water or wine. The characteristic effects of the drugs must always be considered; they must never be ignored.[7]

[6] In order to cure illnesses, the origin and progress [of the illness] should first be examined. If the five depots of the body (wu-tsang)[8] are not yet affected by depletions (hsü), if the six palaces (liu-fu)[9] are not yet exhausted, if the blood vessels are not yet out of order, and if [one's] subtle matter and spirit have not yet passed away, then medications will certainly be effective. If the illness, however, has broken out already, a cure can still be achieved in 50 percent of the cases. If the influence of the illness has progressed too far, it will be difficult to restore [the respective patient's] existence.[10]

五藏
虛 六府

[7] In treating illnesses with drugs of a strongly medicinal effectiveness, one should first start with a dosage the size of a millet seed. If the illness is cured [with that], administration of the drug should be halted immediately. If the illness persists, the amount of the dosage should be doubled. If the illness continues even then, the dosage should be increased ten times. The cure [of the illness] should mark the limit [of the treatment].[11]

[8] [Illnesses due to the influence of] cold [in the body] should be treated with drugs of a hot [thermo-influence]. [Illnesses due to the influence of] heat [in the body] should be treated with drugs of a cold [thermo-influence]. If the digestion of food and drink ceases, emetics and laxatives should be used. Against demonic possessions and the poison of the ku,[12] drugs with powerful effectiveness should be used. For boils, swellings, bumps, and tumors, abscess-drugs should be taken. [Illnesses caused by the influences of] wind and moisture should be treated with wind and moisture drugs. In each case one should follow a suitable course.[13]

蠱

[9] In the case of illnesses located above the diaphragm, the medications should be taken after meals. For illnesses situated below the diaphragm, medications should be taken before meals. If the illness is located in the four limbs or in the blood vessels, the medications ought to be taken in the morning on an empty stomach. If the illness is in the bones, the medication should be taken at night after eating.[14]

[10] The most important kinds of serious illnesses [are the following]: being hit by wind (chung-feng); illnesses caused by cold (shang-han); succession of hot and cold fits (han-je); malaria fevers (wen-yao);[15] being hit by the malevolent (chung-o); sudden [intestinal] chaos (huo-luan); abdominal swelling (ta-fu); edema (shui-chung); dysentery-like diarrhea (ch'ang-p'i hsia-li); urinary retention and constipation (ta hsiao pien pu t'ung); running pig [syndrome] (pen-t'un); cough (shang-ch'i k'e-ni); vomiting (ou-t'u); jaundice (huang-tan); pathological thirst (hsiao-k'e); stagnation of drinking liquids in the body (liu-yin); indigestion (p'i-shih); hardenings (chien-chi); obstructive swelling (cheng-chia); to be frightened by some evil (ching-hsieh); madness and cramps (tien-hsien); demonic possession (kuei-chu); closure of the throat (hou-pi); toothache; deafness; blindness; cuts and bruises; fractures; boils; swellings; malignant boils; hemorrhoids; throat and neck swellings; for men: the five types of fatigation and seven types of injuries, depletions, and consumption; for women: discharge, very strong menstrual flow, absence of period; sores in the female genital area; injuries through the poisons of worms, snakes and ku. This is a rough classification. Within it changes and divergences are possible as [in a system of] branches and leaves. In order to master them, beginning and end must be considered.[16]

中風   傷寒
寒熱   溫瘧
中惡   霍亂
大腹   水腫
腸澼下痢   大小便不通
賁肫   上氣欬逆
嘔吐   黃疸   消渴
留飲   癖食
堅積   癥瘕
驚邪   癲癇
鬼注   喉痺

1.1.1. The ten general sections in the first chapter of the *Pen-ching*

君
無毒

[1] The upper class of drugs comprises 120 kinds. They are the rulers (*chün*). They control the maintenance of life and correspond to heaven. They do not have a markedly medicinal effectiveness (*wu-tu*). The taking [of these drugs] in larger amounts or over a long period of time is not harmful to Man. If one wishes to take the material weight from the body, to supplement the influences [circulating in the body], and to prolong the years of life without aging, he should base [his efforts] on [drugs mentioned in] the upper [class of this] classic.

臣

The middle class of drugs comprises 120 kinds. They are the ministers (*ch'en*). They control the preservation of the human nature and correspond to Man. One part of them possesses medicinal effectiveness, another part does not. For every application, the choice of the suitable [drugs] should be considered carefully. If one wishes to prevent illnesses and to balance depletions and consumption, he should base [his efforts] on [drugs mentioned in] the middle [class of this] classic.

佐使
有毒
邪氣

The lower class of drugs comprises 125 kinds. They are the assistants (*tso*) and aides (*shih*). They control the curing of illnesses and correspond to earth. They possess a markedly medicinal effectiveness (*yu-tu*) and must not be taken over a long period of time. If one wishes to remove cold, heat, and [other] evil influences (*hsieh-ch'i*) from the body, to break constipations [of any sort], and to cure illnesses, he should base [his efforts] on [drugs mentioned in] the lower [class of this] classic.

The three classes together are composed of 365 drugs. This corresponds to 365 degrees. One degree corresponds to one day. Together that makes one year.[3]

[2] The drugs are subdivided into rulers, ministers, assistants, and aides. They should be combined according to mutual usefulness. Suitable [is the combination of] one ruler, two ministers, three assistants, and five aides. [The combination of] one ruler, three ministers, and nine assistants and aides is also possible.[4]

單行
相須
相使
相畏
相惡
相反
相殺

[3] [In prescriptions] drugs are [matched according to whether they belong to the] *yin* or *yang* [category]. There are child/mother and older/younger brother [relationships], there are also root-, stalk-, blossom-, and fruit-drugs, as well as herb-, mineral-, bone-, and flesh-drugs. There are [drugs] which prefer to act alone (*tan-hsing*), others whose effectiveness depends [on one or more other drugs] (*hsiang-hsü*). There are [drugs] which reinforce each other [in their effectiveness] (*hsiang-shih*), and those who fear each other (*hsiang-wei*). Some [drugs] hate each other in combinations (*hsiang-wu*), and others are directly opposed in their effectiveness (*hsiang-fan*). [Finally, there are drugs] which kill each other (*hsiang-sha*).

These seven emotions must be kept in mind when combining (drugs). If the application of drugs which depend upon and support each other is called for, one should by no means use those which directly oppose or hate each other. If it is necessary to combine drugs with strongly medicinal effectiveness, drugs which weaken or neutralize each other can be used. The combination [of drugs] must conform strictly to these principles.[5]

五味

四氣

[4] The drugs have the five basic tastes (*wu-wei*): sour, salty, sweet, bitter, and acrid. Furthermore, they possess four kinds of [thermo-] influence (*ssu-ch'i*): cold, hot, warm, and cool. [Some drugs] have markedly medicinal effectiveness, others none. [There are drugs which must be] dried in the shade, [others which must be] dried in the sun. The time of the collection and preparation [of drugs], whether they are raw or boiled, the place of their origin, adulteration and genuineness, as well as whether [the drugs are to be used after having been] stored or in fresh state, everything is subject to specific rules.[6]

1.1.2. The monograph section of the *Pen-ching*

Corresponding to the subdivision of the totality of drugs as explained in the general sections of the first chapter of the *Pen-ching*, the first chapter of the monograph section is devoted to the drugs of the upper class, the second chapter to the drugs of the middle class, and the third chapter to those of the lower class. In all three classes, mineral, plant, and animal substances are to be found. Their organization and approximate numerical division can be recognized in Table 1.

The totals of 141, 111, and 103 given here for the individual drug classes do not correspond to the figures 120, 120, and 125 listed in the general sections. Since the seventeenth century, several Chinese and Japanese scholars have tried to reconstruct precisely the numerical combination of the monograph section of the *Pen-ching*. These efforts produced various, more or less diverging results, and it appears that, despite much agreement, some questions can never be clearly resolved. I will not go further into these problems here, but I will return to the reconstruction attempts in detail in chapter C. sec. V., as they must be understood as part of the reaction to the changes in medical thinking in the Chin-Yüan period, a reaction which began, as noted above, in the seventeenth century.

The individual monographs in the *Pen-ching* were kept very brief. Following a short identification of the drug involved, they are limited to information about the general taste (*wei*),[17] (thermo-) influence (*ch'i*; also: *hsing*),[18] effectiveness and indications, secondary names, and the specific or general place of origin. One example is the monograph on the drug *pa-tou* ("bean from Pa"), known to Western pharmacy as the croton seed:

味
氣性

巴豆

> *Pa-tou,* taste: acrid; [thermo-influence:] warm. Controls harms caused by cold, malaria-fevers, fits of cold and heat; breaks up bowel obstructions of different kinds, hardenings; stagnation of drinking liquids, mucous congestions, abdominal swellings, edema; purges the five depots

TABLE 1

Sections	Classes			Total
	upper	middle	lower	
Precious stones, Minerals	18	14	10	42
Herbs	72	47	49	168
Trees	19	17	17	53
Man	1	0	0	1
Quadrupeds	6	7	4	17
Fowl	2	2	0	4
Worms, fish	10	17	18	45
Fruits	6	1	2	9
Vegetables	5	4	2	11
Rice, Grains	2	2	1	5
	141	111	103	365

and six palaces; opens and breaks through obstructions; it clears the
way for water and grains; removes spoiled flesh; expels poisonings
caused by demons, [removes] possessions by the *ku* and [other] evil   巴椒
things; kills worms and fish. Another name [for *pa-tou*] is *pa-chiao*
["Pa-pepper"].[19]

Pa-tou was listed in the *Pen-ching* among the lower class of drugs.
Another example for a substance considered to be "medicinally active"
and, therefore, listed in the same class is *lang-tang*, henbane, also well
known to Western pharmacy since antiquity:

> *Lang-tang,* taste: bitter; [thermo-influence:] cold. Controls toothache.
> Drives out worms, numbness of the flesh, seizures and cramps. Enables
> one to walk vigorously and to see demons. If large amounts are eaten
> they force one to walk madly. Consumed over a long time, (*lang-tang*)
> takes the material weight from the body, and in running one may reach
> a fleeing horse.[20]

The following monographs are examples from the upper class of
drugs in the *Pen-ching;* namely *shui-yin* ("quicksilver"), *jen-shen*
("ginseng"), *tse-hsieh* ("water-plantain"), and *p'u-t'ao* ("grapes").

> *Shui-yin,* taste: acrid; [thermo-influence:] cold. Controls itching, sca-
> bies, baldness. Kills worms and parasites in the skin. (Causes) miscar-
> riages. Eliminates heat. Kills poisons of gold, silver, copper, tin. Through
> melting processes it is reversible into cinnabar. Consumed over a long
> time [it changes one into] a spirit-hermit who will not die.[21]
>
> *Jen-shen,* taste: sweet; [thermo-influence:] slightly cold. Controls the
> filling of the five depots. Pacifies the spirit; fixes the *hun*- and *p'o*-souls.[22]
> Ends fright and agitation. Expels evil influences. Clears the eyes. Opens
> the heart and benefits one's wisdom. Consumed over a long time, it
> takes the material weight from the body and extends one's years of life.
> Other names are "man's bit" and "demon's cover."[23]
>
> *Tse-hsieh,* taste: sweet, [thermo-influence:] cold. Controls numbness
> [caused by] wind, cold, moisture. [Controls] difficulties in [producing]
> milk. Diminishes water. Nourishes the five depots. Benefits one's influ-
> ences and strength. Fattens and invigorates. Consumed over a long time
> it clears ears and eyes, one does not feel hungry, it extends one's years
> of life, and it takes the material weight from the body. One's face
> develops brightness and one is able to walk on water.[24]
>
> *P'u-t'ao,* taste: sweet, [thermo-influence:] neutral. Controls numbness
> [caused by] moisture in joints and bones. Benefits the influences, doubles
> one's strength, and improves one mind. Lets a man become fat and
> vigorous; [enables one] to endure hunger and to be resistant against
> wind and cold. Eaten over a long time, it takes the material weight from
> the body and one will not age. (*P'u-t'ao*) extends one's years of life.
> Can be used to produce wine.[25]

The drugs described in the *Pen-ching* come mainly from areas north
of the Yang-tzu, but there are also drugs from southern and more
distant regions, such as Ning-hsia, Sinkiang, Ch'ing-hai, Hsi-k'ang,
Vietnam, and Korea. Thus, a drug trade not limited to one region and
bridging great distances existed already in the Han period, bringing
important substances from the far west, south, and north to the central
areas of China.[26]

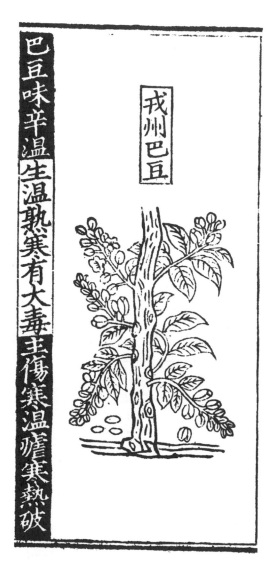

croton seeds *(pa-tou)—Ch'ung-hsiu cheng-ho pen-ts'ao*

1.2. Observations on the content of the *Pen-ching*

One of the first questions that arises from a study of the content of the *Pen-ching* is, for whom or with what intention was the work compiled and written. Was it meant for those considered to be practicing physicians or pharmacists, for Taoist practitioners or theorists, or was the work perhaps aimed at all these and related groups? Important criteria for an answer to these questions are the classification of the drugs, the contents of the monographs, and the extent of their theorization.

1.2.1. The classification of drugs in the *Pen-ching*

The drugs in the *Pen-ching* are divided according to their membership in the upper, middle, and lower classes. Among the substances in the upper class are some drugs whose inclusion seems to be based mainly upon theoretical considerations. Cinnabar, tortoise shells, or "dragon bones"[27] are examples of such drugs. Cinnabar, the only nontoxic mercury compound, and the chemical processes of its production probably attracted the interest of experimenting magicians very early. Tortoise shells, whose obvious durable qualities mean centuries of existence, are suitable as material embodiment of the principle of longevity. As some natural philosophers may have reached the conclusion that this principle must be embodied concretely within the shells, their placement as drugs of the upper class is not surprising. Similar reasoning may apply to "dragon bones" and other examples.

As the text of the *Pen-ching* shows, no direct medicinal effectiveness was expected of drugs in the upper class. The long-term application of these drugs was described as harmless. We might add that the definition of "medicinal effectiveness" (*wu-tu*; lit. "nonpoisonous"), as applied by the *Pen-ching* to the substances of the upper class, does not always correspond to modern pharmacological knowledge. Water-plantain (*tse-hsieh*), for instance, quoted above, is acknowledged by contemporary scientists as a potent diuretic.[28]

The lower class of drugs in the *Pen-ching*, in contrast, is supposed to contain those genuinely medicinal drugs, to which a more or less strongly marked effectiveness was ascribed during the Han period.

The obvious value judgment involved in the distribution of drugs into the highest and lowest classes, together with the naming of these classes according to social positions (i.e., "rulers," "ministers," "assistants," "aides") provides first clues concerning the character of the *Pen-ching* and the therapeutic thinking of its authors.

Looking back once more to what we assumed to be the original usage of the term *pen-ts'ao,* we remember that the pen-ts'ao experts were practitioners who based their efforts for a "long life without aging" on experiments with mostly herbal drugs. It is in the circles of these men that we must look for the authors of the *Shen-nung pen-ching.* Their experiments were not primarily aimed at the actual medicinal value of these drugs, but rather at their ability to strengthen

TABLE 2

Function	Class		
	upper	middle	lower
Take the material weight from the body	84	20	7
Extend the years of life	39	1	1
Eliminate aging	31	3	1
Eliminate the desire to eat and enable one to endure hunger	20	4	0
Transform one into spirit-hermits	11	1	0

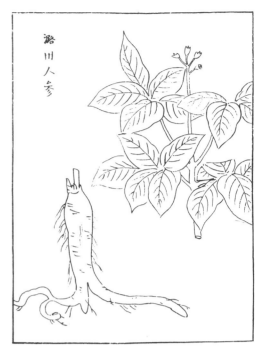

ginseng (jen-shen)—Shao-hsing pen-ts'ao

the body and protect it, over long periods of time, from health problems of all kinds. The actual therapeutic properties of drugs appear to have been regarded, at least theoretically, with only secondary interest. Accordingly, therapeutically effective drugs were assigned the lowest ranks of the drug hierarchy. I have pointed out elsewhere that the identification of drugs without medicinal effectiveness as upper class and as "rulers" signals a subtle political dimension, especially so if compared with a classification of therapeutic substances in the *Huang-ti nei-ching su-wen.*[29] The latter is the classic of the medicine of systematic correspondence, a therapeutic system supported, most of all, by Confucian-Legalist interests. Therefore, it should be of no surprise that the authors of the *Huang-ti nei-ching su-wen,* in contrast to those of the *Pen-ching,* categorized as "rulers" those drugs that actually attack an illness. The Confucian-Legalist notion of a strong government's active participation in the solving of social crises is reflected in the *Huang-ti nei-ching su-wen* on a therapeutic level. In the *Pen-ching,* however, the "ruler" is designated to create the basis for an existence free of crises, while the "assistants" and "aides" may be called upon for help in times of actual disorder. In quantitative terms, this rather Taoist orientation of the *Pen-ching* may be illustrated as follows. The percentage numbers in Table 2 indicate the proportion of drugs in a particular class presumably exerting the respective function.

plantain seeds (ch'e-ch'ien-tzu)—Shao-hsing pen-ts'ao

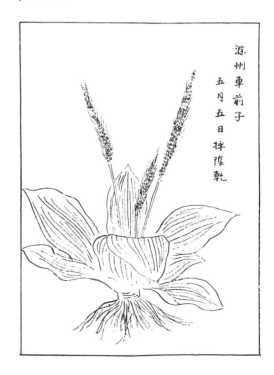

The middle class of drugs, which I have not yet discussed, also reveals the conceptual orientation of the *Pen-ching* compilers. Seen from a medical-systematic point of view, this class is superfluous for it contains by definition drugs that could also have been included in the upper class, and drugs that—because of their special effectiveness—might belong in the lower class. The establishment of a middle class could be explained by the effort to bring the division of drugs into agreement with a specific cosmological world view of the Han period, as it was expressed, for example, in the works of Tung Chung-shu (second century B.C.). Accordingly, man was positioned between heaven and earth as the third member of the cosmic unity. Just as the division of drugs into three groups corresponded to the trinity heaven–man–earth, the number of drugs in the *Pen-ching,* with 365 monographs, corresponded intentionally to the number of days in a solar year, indicating a macrobiotic orientation of the authors.

The arrangement of the individual monographs in the *Pen-ching*—according to the mineral, plant, and animal origin of the drugs as well as the group of common foodstuffs—is subordinated to the division of all drugs into the upper, middle, and lower class. This means that the ten sections, from the precious stones/minerals to the rice/grains, occur three times with the corresponding monographs within the upper, middle, and lower drug classes. The division of the drugs according to an artificial concept was, therefore, given priority over a division according to their natural origin. This pattern was already abandoned and reversed in the following revision of systematized materia medica by T'ao Hung-ching around the year 500 (see p. 42).

1.2.2. The theoretical foundations of pharmaceutical knowledge in the *Pen-ching*

At the time of the compilation of the *Pen-ching*, that is, during the first centuries A.D., at least three basic paradigms were available in Chinese culture to explain the origin of illness and to provide a theoretical basis for appropriate therapeutic intervention. These include the concepts of demonology, of magic correspondence,[30] and of systematic correspondence.[31] Demonology was based on a belief that illness may be the result of an assault by demons on a human person. Demonological therapy included, initially, spells, amulets, and talismans, and, possibly, the needling of afflicted body parts in order to chase away or kill the malevolent entities responsible for pain, swellings, or other symptoms. Beginning with the *Wu-shih-erh ping fang* of the third century B.C., we have evidence that drugs were recommended as valuable means to kill or drive out demonic intruders from the body.[32] Drugs, then, were used against demonologically defined health problems on the basis of a demonological pharmacology. That is, a theoretical relationship was discovered between some demonologically defined characteristics of a particular substance and a particular demonological illness. In addition, it appears that substances were used on empirical grounds against illnesses understood to be caused by demons. The *Pen-ching* was heavily influenced by this type of therapeutic approach. Approximately 15 percent of all 357 drug monographs listed in the version reconstructed by Mori Risshi mention the "killing" or "chasing away" of demons and the elimination of "demonic possessions" as a therapeutic indication.

For instance, in the case of "peach blossoms" (*t'ao-hua*), a substance recommended by the *Pen-ching* in its lower class of drugs, we read the following: "Kills malevolent demons by which one is possessed. Lets one have a good complexion."[33] Considering the fact that bows to shoot arrows were made from peach wood in ancient China, one may conclude that internal use of peach-tree substances was supposed to achieve the same results against demons within one's body as peach wood bows were known to achieve against external enemies. This reasoning is tied to demonology and can be termed demonological pharmacology; in addition, it is based on another paradigm accepted in China since remote antiquity: magic correspondence. In fact, a pharmacology of magic correspondence represents the second theoretical foundation of drug utilization in the *Pen-ching*; most of the animal substances listed, but also drugs of herbal or mineral origin, can be linked to the health problems they are supposed to master by means of such concepts. Further studies are needed, though, to determine the proportion of substances in the *Pen-ching* that may have found their way into materia medica owing to considerations of magic correspondence.

The third therapeutic paradigm mentioned above, that is, the paradigm of systematic correspondence, is almost completely missing in the *Pen-ching*. As we have seen, the drugs are brought into relation to yin and yang in a brief remark of the general sections of the first chapter. This categorization, however, was probably based upon primary observations rather than upon an abstract theory. The statements in the first chapter of the *Pen-ching* about the "mother/child" and "older brother/younger brother" relationships among drugs can probably be interpreted similarly. Perhaps they were meant to refer to botanical-systematical connections, an opinion advocated in the Ming period in the *Chih-yüan i-ts'ao:*

> As to the mother/child [relationships]: the peach tree produces its seeds. In this case, the peach tree represents the mother and the peach seed the child. The seed, in turn, contains small peach trees. Now, as for [the meaning of] the older brother/younger brother [relationship]: the elms encompass large-leaved and small-leaved kinds.[34]

Elsewhere, on the occasion of an attempt to reconstruct the *Pen-ching*, Lu Fu (ca. 1600) endeavored to interpret the older/younger brother relationship by pointing out a controlling and a supporting effect of two drugs in a prescription:

> Now, to [the terms] older brother/younger brother. In the spring one makes use of the fire of elm and willow. Elm and willow are both items [affecting] the liver. The elm can be the older brother [in a prescription] and the willow the younger brother; conversely, the willow can also be classified as the older and the elm as the younger brother. One must always consider which [of the two drugs] controls the illness in question; this drug should then be given quantitative priority. From this the meaning of [the term] older brother/younger brother becomes quite clear.[35]

Lu Fu's following remarks concerning the mother/child relationship of drugs, however, probably do not correspond to the original meaning in the *Pen-ching*, but may have been influenced by the thoughts of the Chin/Yüan period, which were modeled on the contents of the *Su-wen:*

> Wood nourishes fire. Thus, the liver [which corresponds to wood] nourishes the heart [which corresponds to fire]. Therefore, the drugs for the liver can be considered as mother-drugs for the heart. The drugs for the heart can act as child-drugs with respect to the liver. If one, starting from these [examples], arranges the mutual generation of all drugs according to the Five Phases and child/mother [relationships], the meaning of [the term] child/mother is as clear as the sun and the stars.[36]

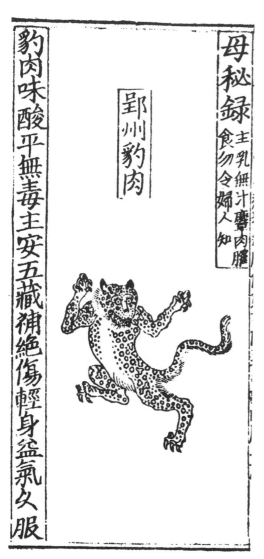

leopard flesh *(pao-jou)—Ch'ung-hsiu cheng-ho pen-ts'ao*

The thermo-influence *ch'i*—that is, the effect a drug produces in the body after it has been taken—and the taste *wei*—the sensation the drug causes in the mouth—still represent, in the *Pen-ching,* attempts to characterize the drugs based upon concrete experiences. They are not yet used as connecting links (as in the *Su-wen* and later, in the Chin/Yüan period, also in the drug literature) to integrate the drugs and their effects into the system of the Five Phases and of yinyang. In other words, there are no significant traces of a pharmacology of systematic correspondence in the *Pen-ching.*

One interesting exception is a cycle of five monographs about different forms of the drug *chih,* an aid for the prolongation of life which was held in high esteem in Taoist circles. These monographs have been adjusted precisely to the theory of the Five Phases. It may well be that there existed some tradition in early Chinese materia medica linking the use of drugs with the subtle concepts of the Five Phases and yinyang. Na Ch'i quotes from the *Yang-sheng yao-shu,* a book mentioned first in the history of the Sui dynasty, a quotation from a *Shen-nung ching* which apparently relates primary characteristics of drugs to specified therapeutic functions.[37] If this quotation is genuine, it obviously belonged to a marginal tradition which was not adopted by the mainstream of pen-ts'ao literature during the first millennium A.D. Since the authors of the pen-ts'ao works following the *Pen-ching* were well-educated men who must have been familiar with the concepts of the Five Phases and yinyang, one cannot but assume that they deliberately rejected the theoretical foundations of the *Su-wen* tradition. The reason for opposition to a scientific paradigm that provided, for instance, a theoretical rationale for acupuncture may once again be found in the ideological contrast between Confucian-Legalist interests on the one hand and Taoist interests on the other. The medical application of the yinyang and Five Phases theories was holistic in a sense that the well-being of society and individuals depended on a healthy life-style demanding adherence to, among others, specified dietetic and moral rules. Taoists in search of the norms of nature (in contrast, for instance, to those Taoist groups related to the *t'ai-p'ing* movement) rejected such moral rules as artificial and condemned them as responsible for the social ills they were supposed to cure. The pragmatic use of drugs is not tied to any standards of human morality; the belief in the curative or preventive properties of natural or man-made substances provides a basis for a life-style that is solely in accordance with one's own perceptions. The threat of becoming ill because one has violated specific moral norms is eliminated if one knows that illness can be prevented or treated by means of therapeutic substances acting independently from these norms. Pragmatic materia medica may have been understood by some circles of Chinese society as containing a dimension of social liberation. As a result, the pen-ts'ao tradition of pragmatic materia medica and the *Su-wen* tradition of theoretically legitimized prevention and therapy by means of a specified life-style and such medical techniques as acupuncture, remained separate until the sociopolitical climate of Neoconfucianism allowed for their union.

1.3. The characteristics of the main pen-ts'-ao tradition

We do not know how widely the *Pen-ching* itself was distributed. It must, however, have attained an important position as a compendium of pharmaceutics, for only thus can we understand the exceptionally long tradition established by this work. Through many centuries the *Pen-ching* was continually revised, and one can recognize the clear tendency of expansion in accordance with recent discoveries and of correction of old mistakes.

Beginning with the preparation of the "Newly Revised Materia Medica" (*Hsin-hsiu pen-ts'ao*) in the year 657, commissions were occasionally appointed by the government, and new sources from all areas of literature and human experience were drawn upon to produce more complete and comprehensive editions. The number of the drugs described and the length of their descriptions increased steadily. Thus, the main pen-ts'ao tradition was formed, marked by various characteristics that are valid for all the works included in this tradition.

Each work in the main tradition takes over nearly the entire contents of the previous pen-ts'ao. New drugs and dissenting or supplementary commentaries are not inserted instead of but are added to the old, perhaps outdated statements. All quotations from earlier pen-ts'ao works and other sources are clearly marked as such. Up until the last work of the main pen-ts'ao tradition, which appeared in the thirteenth century, the arrangement of the drugs into the upper, middle, and lower class is maintained. All works in the main tradition are based upon mostly pragmatic principles and do not show any decisive theorization.

Thus, the main pen-ts'ao tradition was not a succession of several similar drug manuals, with one taking the place of the other, but consisted of a number of editions of one and the same original work, continuously improved during the course of centuries. The steady progress in the recording of new knowledge about drugs was concealed beneath a conservative form.

In addition to the pen-ts'ao works in the main tradition, numerous other, mostly less extensive pen-ts'ao studies were written during the centuries; in these works specialized or regional peculiarities were emphasized. I refer collectively to these works as a secondary tradition, although in discussing them I will differentiate this secondary line into individual traditions and special works. The knowledge collected in the secondary pen-ts'ao tradition was frequently absorbed by one of the subsequent main works.

2.1. T'ao Hung-ching

2. The Drug Works Compiled by T'ao Hung-ching

T'ao Hung-ching and, in the sixteenth century, Li Shih-chen, are the two outstanding personalities in the long succession of pen-ts'ao authors. Through their works they gave new impulses to the drug literature; and, from the standpoint of Western natural sciences, they produced the most important pen-ts'ao works.

T'ao Hung-ching was born in 456 into a family of respected social status and learning.[38] His father and grandfather are reported to have been particularly familiar with pharmaceutical knowledge. T'ao himself attained great scholarship in a wide range of areas and served as an official in various prestigious positions during the Sung and Ch'i dynasties before he withdrew to Mao-shan to pursue philological and, later, alchemical studies. Among several minor accomplishments, such as comments on the classics, T'ao Hung-ching produced three major literary works: the *Teng-chen yin-chüeh* ("Concealed Instructions for Ascent to Perfection"), the *Chen-kao* ("Declarations of the Perfected"), and the *(Shen-nung) pen-ts'ao ching chi-chu* ("Collected Commentaries on [Shen-nung's] Classic of Materia Medica"). The first two of these compilations were related to revelations presented to a Yang Hsi and two members of a family named Hsü during the years of 364 to 370. These revelations contained, among other information, practical directives and ritual instructions enabling one to ascend to the realm of the Perfected Immortals. T'ao Hung-ching, whose interest into these matters in general and into these specific texts in particular had been aroused early, took great pains to collect the autographs of Yang Hsi and the Hsüs as far as they were still extant in his own time. In 492, at the age of thirty-six, he retired to Mao-shan, a retreat to which the younger of the Hsüs had moved some ninety years earlier, to edit and annotate the materials he had collected at different places from various hands. It appears that by the year 500 he had completed all three projects mentioned above.

The compilation and extensive annotation of the Yang-Hsü manuscripts as well as T'ao Hung-ching's alchemical studies—which preoccupied him, on imperial behest, from 504 until the end of his life in 536—made him, as M. Strickmann formulates it, "the virtual founder of Mao Shan Taoism. It was with him that the line of great Mao Shan masters, confidants of emperors, really began."[39] Mao-shan Taoism, as suggested in the Yang-Hsü manuscripts and as further elaborated by T'ao Hung-ching, was based on various insights. It was known that another world, hierarchically ordered into seven levels, existed, inhabited by gods, demons, specters, spirits of the dead, and immortals with varying ranks, functions, and abilities to communicate with the living humans. It was known further that means existed, and a great variety of them were revealed to Yang Hsi and the Hsüs, for transcending one's earthly existence and ascending to the heavens of the immortals.

One of the technical terms denoting physical death by an elixir for the purpose of achieving liberation from one's corpse and gaining acceptance in the other world should be of special interest to us: 遺帶 *i-tai*, "to abandon the waistband," that is, "to cast aside the constraining girdle of proper social *tenue*."[40] Here again we meet the dimension of social liberation inherent in Taoism. But we should not overlook the fact that the religious traditions of Taoism had already created their own "constraining girdles" by elaborating definitions of good deeds and proper moral conduct, allegedly securing access to the desired state of immortality. In the previous paragraph I hypothesized reasons for the support of pragmatic drug therapy and rejection of the yinyang and Five Phases theories of systematic correspondence by some groups in Chinese society. I offered the amoral nature of therapeutic substances as a probable answer to this question. This hypothesis is further supported by the fact that the first and most important sect of religious Taoism, namely, the Way of the Celestial Master following the revelations to Chang Tao-ling in A.D. 142, appears to have implicitly renounced the employment of drugs in therapy. That is, once this group realized the links between morality in life-style and susceptibility to illness, it also realized that therapeutic means other than natural and manmade substances were best suited to reinforce adherence to this morality and, thus, to prevent or treat illness.[41]

This therapeutic purity of religious Taoism, however, appears not to have prevailed for long, at least as far as a significant proportion of followers is concerned. Individual substances and the alchemical elixirs produced from them were obviously accepted, in the course of the third century, by leading members of the Taoist church. When T'ao Hung-ching founded Mao-shan Taoism, his religious world view with its belief in the beatifying powers of morality in life-style, on the one hand, and the practice of alchemy and of pharmacotherapy, on the other, did not seem contradictory.

2.2. The Pen-ts'ao works of T'ao Hung-ching

T'ao Hung-ching apparently compiled his version of Shen-nung's materia medica in two different sizes. At first he completed a *Shen-nung pen-ts'ao ching* in three chapters; shortly afterward he regrouped the arrangement of the material and published a *Pen-ts'ao ching chi-chu* ("Collected Commentaries on the Classic of Pharmaceutics"). The contents of both scriptures were identical; a note at the end of the preface of the latter work indicates that the former was merely rewritten into seven chapters. The number seven must have been of special significance to T'ao Hung-ching. He distinguished between seven levels of the spiritual world, and he divided his editions of the *Teng-chen yin-chüeh* and of the *Chen-kao* into seven chapters as well. Although not quite correctly, T'ao Hung-ching's pharmaceutical works are often quoted together under one title as *Shen-nung pen-ts'ao ching chi-chu*.

In the preface to his materia medica T'ao Hung-ching, whose style-name was Yin-chü ("Residing in Concealment"), explains his methods and sources.

> Mr. Yin-chü resided on the Mao-shan [mountains]. In his spare time between breathing exercises he let his thoughts roam deeply into the prescription techniques and he observed the nature of the pharmaceutical drugs. It was his intention to put the heart of an exemplary man into these [areas of knowledge]. Therefore, he pursued and discussed them. . . . The present book should in fact resemble the *Su-wen*, but later people have changed and expanded it several times. The burning

Shen-nung pen-ts'ao ching
"Shen-nung's Classic of Pharmaceutics"
Short Title: *Shen-nung pen-ts'ao*
3 chapters / 730 drug descriptions
Author: T'ao Hung-ching (452–536)
　　　tzu: T'ung-ming
　　　hao: Yin-chü, Cheng-pai
　　　from: Mo-ling in Tan-yang
Written: ca. 490–500
Published: ca. 500

[of literature] under the emperor of the Ch'in did not include medical and divinatory texts, so that afterwards all such works [from earlier times] were still extant. But when [Emperor] Hsien [181–234] of the Han dynasty had to move his residence, and later, when Emperor Huai [283–313] of the Chin dynasty had to escape in great haste, all the [old] writings fell victim to the flames; of a thousand works, not one was left. These four chapters [of the *Pen-ching*] are all that remain today [of the materia medica of Shen-nung]. It is assumed that these notes were written by Chung-ching [i.e., Chang Chi, 142–220?] or Yüan-hua [i.e., Hua T'o, 110–207], because the places of origin [of the drugs] in the *Pen-ching* are listed according to the regulations of the later Han dynasty. In addition there is also [a work on drugs entitled] *T'ung-chün ts'ai-yao lu* ["Mr. T'ung's Notes on the Collection of Drugs"], in which are described the blossoms, leaves, appearance, and colors [of the drugs]. In the four chapters of [another work entitled] *Yao-tui* ["Comparison of Drugs"], the mutual effects of the drugs [when used simultaneously] are described. Later, during the time of Wei and Chin, Wu P'u and Li Tang-chih further abridged and also supplemented these works; some editions [of the *Shen-nung pen-ts'ao*] therefore describe 595 kinds of drugs, others 431, or even 319. Sometimes the three classes of drugs remained undifferentiated, or the cold and hot [thermo-influences of the drugs] were mistakenly confused. Herbal and mineral drugs were not discussed separately, neither were drugs made from worms and quadrupeds. Furthermore, the main indications [of the drugs] and their proportions [in prescriptions] were not presented in any order to the medical people. As a result, the knowledge of them is sometimes shallow and sometimes deep. I have now taken upon me the task to collect all these scriptures, to eliminate the unnecessary and to fill up deficiencies. As primary [material] I have taken over the three drug classes of the *Shen-nung pen-ching*, with a total of 365 drugs; as secondary [material] another 365 drugs of renowned medical men. All in all, I have recorded 730 kinds of drugs. I have included detailed, as well as briefly outlined, descriptions, in order to avoid further omissions. I have divided [the material into] sections and I have distinguished different groups of substances. I have also commented on names, times [to collect substances], usable [parts], and the places of origin. Finally, I have included relevant material from the scriptures of the immortals and from the techniques of the Taoists. Together with this preface, [my work] consists of three chapters. It cannot stand in line with the excellent [*pen-ts'ao* works] of the past, but then it is my own private compilation. After I have left this world, it may be given to all those who are knowledgeable about prescriptions.

Pen-ts'ao scripture, upper chapter: a listing of the foundations of the nature of drugs; discussion of appearance and interpretation of illnesses and their names; table of all substances recorded for a detailed survey.

Pen-ts'ao scripture, middle chapter: precious stones, minerals, herbs, trees [differentiated according to] the three classes. A total of 356 kinds [of drugs].

Pen-ts'ao scripture, lower chapter: worms, quadrupeds, fruits, vegetables, grains, foodstuff [differentiated according to] the three classes. A total of 195 kinds [of drugs. Furthermore,] three sections of [drugs] known by name but obsolete, with a total of 179 kinds [of drugs]. Altogether 374 kinds [of drugs].

Of these three chapters, the middle and the lower chapter combine a total of 730 kinds [of drugs]. Each has its own separate table of contents. Also, I have differentiated in writing by means of red and black [colors the text of the original *Pen-ts'ao ching* from] writings by various other authors and my own commentaries. I have now divided this large work into seven chapters.[42]

In the bibliography of the *Sui-shu* (compiled in the seventh century), a work entitled *Ming-i pieh-lu* ("Additional Notes of Renowned Medical Men") corresponded to the additional 365 "drugs of renowned medical men" mentioned in the preface. Later, this work was often ascribed to T'ao Hung-ching. It is likely, however, that T'ao Hung-ching compiled the second half of his material from different medical-pharmaceutical writings available during his time, and that an anonymous author, encouraged by the remark in T'ao Hung-ching's preface, published shortly thereafter a work with the above-mentioned title. In the bibliography of the *Sui-shu*, the name of T'ao Hung-ching is given in its full length in connection with the *Pen-ts'ao ching chi-chu;* by contrast, only a "Mr. T'ao" is recorded as the author of the *Ming-i pieh-lu*. T'ao Hung-ching's remark, in his preface, that he "differentiated in writing by means of red and black (colors)" has been interpreted by subsequent pen-ts'ao authors to mean that he set off the parts of the *Pen-ching* from the "additional notes of renowned medical men" by different ink colors. Accordingly, he is supposed to have marked all information that he took from the *Pen-ching* with red ink, the rest with black ink.

The first chapter of T'ao Hung-ching's materia medica contains the author's preface, followed by general discussions which also include the ten general sections from the first chapter of the *Pen-ching*. T'ao Hung-ching's own knowledge of pharmaceutics and his opinions on the drug practices of the time are reflected in his commentaries on the *Pen-ching* and in his lengthy original contributions. For this reason, several excerpts and a detailed description of the structure of the first chapter are given below.

The numbers assigned here to the individual commentaries make possible a comparison with the corresponding sections in the *Pen-ching* (see C, I, 1.1.1). In several cases it is only through such a comparison that the sense of T'ao Hung-ching's explanations becomes clear.

[1] The nature of the drugs in the upper class is quite capable of expelling illnesses. But the strength and function [of these substances] is gentle; they do not produce hasty results. If [these drugs] are consumed over years and months, though, a very beneficial effect is inevitable. All illnesses will be overcome and one's existence will be extended. The way of Heaven is [characterized by] humaneness and creation. Therefore, it is said [that the effect of these drugs] corresponds to Heaven. [The] 120 drugs [of this class] should be referred to as representing the months *yin, mao, ch'en,* and *ssu.* They correspond to the time when all things come to life and flourish.

The nature of the drugs in the middle class is more closely connected with the curing of illnesses; one mentions them less frequently in connection with the liberation of the body from its material weight. If one takes these [drugs] to eliminate actual suffering, he should [use them] quickly; if they are supposed to increase one's life span, they should be taken gradually. Mankind harbors feelings and desires. Therefore, it is said that [the effects of] these drugs correspond to Man. [The] 120 drugs [in this class] should be referred to as representing the months *wu, wei, shen,* and *yu.* They correspond to the time of completion and maturity of all things.

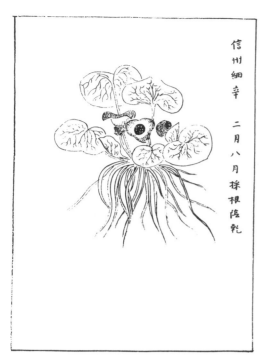

信
州
細
辛

二
月
八
月
採
根
陰
乾

haselwort root *(hsi-hsin)*—*Shao-hsing pen-ts'ao*

老
軍

國
將

The nature of the drugs of the lower class is especially suited for attack. The influences of these drugs with their markedly medicinal effectiveness upset the harmony [of the organism]. They are not to be consumed over an extended period of time. Once an illness is cured, the intake [of such drugs] must be stopped immediately. The principle of the Earth is to detain and kill. Therefore, it is said [that the drugs of the lower class] correspond to the Earth. The 125 drugs (in this class) should be referred to as representing the months *hsü, hai, tzu,* and *ch'ou.* Added to this should also be the additional dates of intercalations. [The drugs of this class] correspond to the decay and [final] concealment of all things. According to the principles of combining [drugs to prescriptions, the drugs of this class] must not be employed one-sidedly. They should be blended in accordance with a patient's suffering and then act collectively. In matching ruler and ministers, one should comply with what is said afterwards. There will be no discussion, though, on the intake of single [substances].

[2] [The use of drugs] is similar to the governing process. When there are many rulers but only a few ministers, or many ministers and only a few assistants, their power does not influence all areas. But if one examines the prescriptions in the scriptures of the immortals and also those in popular usage, [their structure] does not necessarily correspond to this [rule]. In general, those medications that are meant to nourish one's existence are composed to a great extent of rulers. Medications meant to nurture one's nature are composed largely of ministers. Many assistants are found in medications for the treatment of illnesses. In other words, when combining [drugs for prescriptions one must take into account] the properties of [the drugs on the basis of their individual] characteristics. Continual deliberation [is appropriate]. Careful usage will certainly lead to beneficial results. Furthermore, I suspect that within the class of rulers there are differences between noble and inferior [substances] since [in earlier times] the feudal lords of all individual states were termed rulers, yet they regularly had to return to and appear at the court of Chou. Among ministers and assistants, similar [distinctions] should be made. Therefore, *men-tung* and *yüan-chih* can be used both as rulers and as ministers. And [the references to] *kan-ts'ao* as *kuo-lao* ["a retired high-ranking official"], and to *ta-huang* as *chiang-chün* ["active general"] make it clear that the qualities of these drugs cannot always be ranked in accordance with the position [of these substances] in the hierarchy. Who would dare to comment on what is correct and appropriate, and [who would dare to] calculate light and heavy in order to distinguish [the proper amount of] dosages, except for followers of [Shen-]nung and Ch'i [Po]?[43]

[3] [Drugs may] be identical with respect to the [illnesses] they are able to cure. Yet, because the principles of their [curative] nature do not harmonize with each other, they may [if used together in one prescription] even cause suffering! If we look at some prescriptions, [we realize] that they are based on drugs that are said [if used together] to influence one another negatively, or whose effects [with the same indications] stand in direct opposition. Yet treatment with such drugs does not always lead to negative results, since these prescriptions also contain [ingredients] that limit [the unpleasant reactions]. This is similar to the aid that K'ou [Hsün, died A.D. 36] and Chia [Fu, died A.D. 55] together gave to the Han Empire, and that Ch'eng [P'u, ca. A.D. 200] and Chou [Yü, 175–210] gave to the Wu state. Where major issues are at stake, personal feelings are not allowed to cause any harm. Nevertheless, it might perhaps be better not to use [these kinds of drugs] together. In the prescriptions of the immortals, *fang-chi* and *hsi-hsin* are used together in the [pills named] *kan-ts'ao-wan.* In vulgar prescriptions, both *kua-lou* and *kan-chiang* are found [together] in the

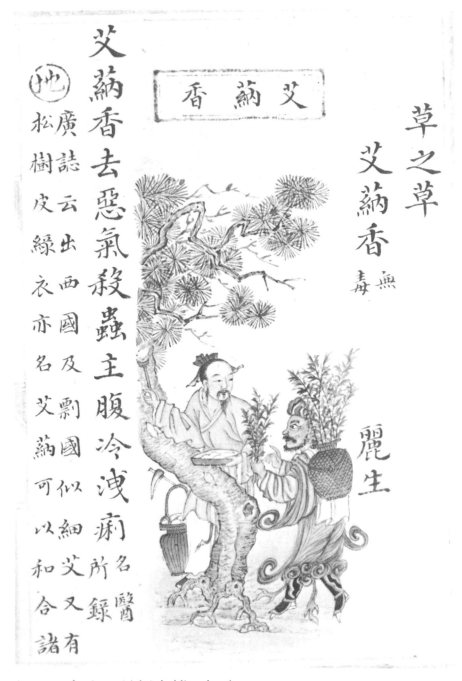

草之草

艾蒳香 毒無

麗生

艾蒳香去惡氣殺蟲主腹冷洩痢所錄名醫

松樹皮綠衣亦名艾蒳可以和合諸廣誌云出西國及㴉國似細艾又有地

A western foreigner (right), holding the plants
necessary for the production of *ai* camphor (*ai-
na-hsiang*), in conversation with a Chinese who
is scraping off the *ai-na* moss from a pine—
Pen-ts'ao p'in-hui ching-yao

34

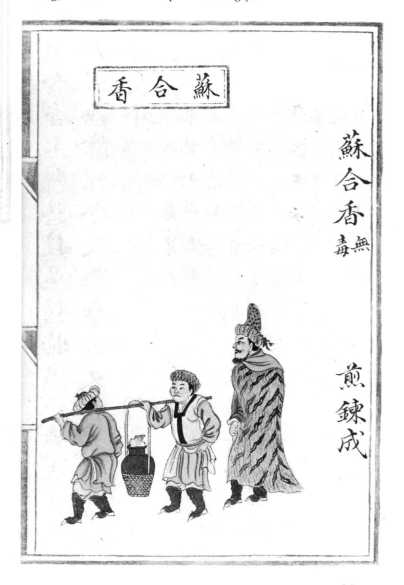

名醫
所錄

底野迦

底野迦主百病中惡客忤邪氣心腹積聚

A western foreigner presents theriaca (*ti-yeh-chia*) to a Chinese—*Pen-ts'ao p'in-hui ching-yao*

Western foreigners carrying storax (*su-ho-hsiang*) to China—*Pen-ts'ao p'in-hui ching-yao*

蘇合香

蘇合香 無毒

煎鍊成

[powder named] *yü-shih-san.* Here the principle [just mentioned] is adhered to. There are many more such instances; I have commented on them in subsequent sections. *Pan-hsia,* for example, possesses distinct medicinal effectiveness. In prescribing this drug one must always add *sheng-chiang,* thereby taking advantage of the weakening effect of combined use. [In this case] one must not use (drugs of) the kind which mutually depend on or reinforce each other! This is similar to the preparation of mild soups and balanced meals from fish, meat, vegetables, and salty items. There exist [for all ingredients of a dish other ingredients that alone are] suitable, when used together, for developing [their respective taste].

[4] In addition, one must constantly discern the weight and amount of [drug] dosage. If, in the application [of drugs], one has made use of suitable [substances], corresponding to the illness, recovery must begin as soon as [the medication] has entered one's mouth! The body will be rested, and life expectancy will have been extended. However, if one confuses the cold and hot [nature of drugs], is not able to classify genuine and false [ingredients], does not follow the necessary proportions, and disregards the proper form of medication, he will employ a preparation that inevitably acts contrary [to its purpose], even to the point of harming one's existence. [To practice] medicine [requires] conscientious reflection. In ancient times some were known as good physicians because they took the correct measures, based upon careful deliberation. A saying goes: "The general populace has no good physicians. Half [of all] deaths are untimely. No treatment at all is better than any care by an ignorant doctor." This is further illustrated by the following parable. If a cook were to use eels and tortoises for a *ch'un* soup, illness would immediately follow the meal. How could someone, who wanted to still his hunger, expect such a thing? Thus, Chung-ching [i.e., Chang Chi] has stated: [Patients] who die through such [mistakes] were killed by imcompetent physicians!

[5] Conversely, [one] also [differentiates among] illnesses those suitable for treatment by pills, those suitable for treatment by powder, decoctions, wine, or paste, and those for which several medications are equally effective. In order to prepare the [correct] medication, the origin of the illness must be investigated.

[6] In current times, who besides an enlightened physician can detect an illness before it is really an illness, just by listening to sounds, checking complexion, or testing the pulse? Furthermore, someone who does not yet feel ill will scarcely be prepared to seek treatment. For this reason, Prince Huan paid no attention to the small problem with his skin until it had developed into a chronic bone-marrow disease.[44] The difficulties today do not lie solely in the knowledge about and awareness of [an illness], for it is not easy for someone to believe [that he is sick] and accept [treatment] as well. Ts'ang-kung [i.e., Shun-yü I, ca. 180 B.C.][45] said: If a patient is unwilling to accept medication, this will be the first [reason for his] death. If a patient believes in shamans, yet does not trust the physician, this will be the second [reason for his] death. [If a patient] neglects his body, and is unconcerned with his existence, and takes care of neither, this will be the third [reason for his] death. The causes of illness are, of course, manifold, but they are all related to [something] evil. Evil is a designation for that which is not proper, that is to say, an abnormal condition of the human body. Wind, cold, heat, moisture, hunger, overeating, exhaustion, and idleness are all examples of evil—not solely demonic influences or epidemics. Man lives amidst influences as the fish live in water. If the water is dirty, the fish are emaciated. If the influences are muddled, people become ill. Harm caused to men by evil influences is most serious. The conduits pick up these influences, leading them to all depots and palaces. Illnesses then arise in these, depending upon the prevailing conditions of depletion, reple-

tion, cold, or heat. The illnesses, in turn, create one another; therefore, they drift, change, proceed, and spread. Originally the spirit resides in the body [using the latter] as its material base. If, however, the body is affected by evil [influences], the spirit will be confused too. Once the spirit is confused, demonic forces will invade his position. The power of the demons becomes greater and greater as the protection of the spirit diminishes. Who, under such conditions, could escape death? In ancient times, the people compared this with the planting of willows; the underlying principle seems to be the same.[46] But among the illnesses there are some that are caused by demonic spirits in the first place. Here it is appropriate to use prayers and sacrifices in order to chase them away. Now, although it is said here that they can be chased away [with such means, there are examples of demonic possession where] positive therapeutic results were achieved through pharmaceutical treatment. Li Tzu-yü with his red pills may be seen as an example for this from former times.[47] In the case of Duke Ching of Chin, where [the demons had settled between] the *kao* and *huang* [regions of his body],[48] we have an example where a pharmaceutical treatment remained without result, and where there was no [other way] to chase away [the demons]. In general, harm caused by demonic spirits may have many causes, but there is only one origin of illness. Then, of course, there may be more or less serious [illnesses]. In the *Chen-kao* it is said that if one, as a rule, does not serve with all respect those on high, he will bring himself to the sources of all possible illnesses, though blaming spirit forces for his misfortune. Yet, only an idiot would, when there is wind, lie down at a moist place and then charge others with the responsibility for [the consequences resulting from] his faulty behavior. To serve those on high with all respect means that one's entire conduct must be guided by respectful thoughts. If one in drinking and eating follows his unrestrained desires, and if he does not restrict his sexual intercourse, this will be the first source of all possible illnesses. [Such behavior] will result in depletions and internal injuries. If [under such conditions] wind and moisture penetrate [the body] from outside, they will cause harm together [with these internal conditions]. Now, what relationship could exist between such cases and the spirits? Here one should seek assistance from the therapeutic principles of pharmacy, and nowhere else.

[7] One simply cannot use at will one or two medicinally effective drugs alone—for example, *pa-tou* or *kan-sui*. Thus, it is said in the scripture: One ingredient, one medicinally effective drug, take one pill the size of small hemp seeds. Two ingredients, one medicinally effective drug, take two pills the size of large hemp seeds. Three ingredients, one medicinally effective drug, take three pills the size of small beans. Four ingredients, one medicinally effective drug, take four pills the size of large beans. Five ingredients, one medicinally effective drug, take five pills the size of hare droppings. Six ingredients, one medicinally effective drug, take six pills the size of *wu [-t'ung]* seeds. From here up to ten [ingredients, the size of pills is limited to] that of the *wu [-t'ung]* seeds. The preparation of pills is determined by the number [of the ingredients]. Of course, there are varying degrees of medicinal effectiveness. For example, how could the [drugs] *lang-tu* and *kou-wen* be equated with evil ones like *fu-tzu* and *yüan-hua*? [The use of] all these kinds [of drugs] must be determined in accordance with what is appropriate.

[8] As far as the individual properties of drugs are concerned, it is possible that a single drug can master more than ten illnesses. For this reason, the most potent quality [of a given drug] must form the basis [for its application in treatment]. Furthermore, one must take into account whether the patient has a condition of depletion that must be filled or a repletion that must be drained; other factors are whether the patient is male, female, old, or young; whether he manifests bitterness or cheerfulness; whether the patient is in splendid condition or shows

signs of distress. Also the area in which the patient lives, and his daily habits are different in every case. Ch'u Ch'eng [died 499] treated widows and nuns according to different principles than wives and concubines! In this manner he could achieve that his desires [toward therapeutic successes] were realized.

[9] Not only the manifold effective properties of drugs, but also the times they are taken, whether early or late, must be regulated according to certain principles. This is the reason a prescription specialist today prescribes "eating first" or "eating afterward." Furthermore, there are medications that must be taken with wine or another drink, either warm, cold, lukewarm, or hot. There are liquids that must slowly be brought once to the boiling point, and others that are repeatedly boiled. Some drugs are taken in their raw state; others must be cooked. Every application is based upon certain rules. One must pay close attention [to these rules].

[10] Here now, [in the *Pen-ching*,] only one illness is named with regard to the indications of a drug. But to be hit by wind (*chung-feng*) alone can appear in tens of variations. And the symptoms and history of harm caused by cold manifest themselves in more than twenty possibilities. One must always strive for the heart of the matter, searching for the common element [in the individual variations], and then find out the underlying principle of its course. The basic nature [of an illness should] be the starting point [of therapy]. Then, the symptoms are brought together in order to combine the [appropriate] drugs.[49]

Following these comments on the first ten sections in the *Pen-ching*, the first chapter of T'ao Hung-ching's *Pen-ts'ao ching chi-chu* continues with further general remarks by the author. In part, they treat matters previously introduced. But they also contain specific instructions for pharmaceutical technology, or deal with, for example, the standardization of units of measurement:

> The physicians do not know the drugs. They rely exclusively upon the seller in the marketplace. The sellers, in turn, do not understand the differentiation and evaluation [of drugs]; they commission others who specialize in collecting and delivering drugs. These collectors and suppliers pass down to one another their methods, and act in ignorance. Thus, there is no control over genuineness, quality, or harmfulness [of drug material].[50]

As to the time and month of collecting drugs, the *yin* [month] is always set as the beginning of the year. This has been recorded ever since the *t'ai-ch'u* period [104–101 B.C.] of the Han dynasty. Root-items are usually collected during the second and eighth months, for the following reason. At the beginning of spring, the sap begins to appear but has not yet reached the trees and leaves; [during this time] its powers are pure and undiluted. In the fall, the branches and leaves dry up and wither, and the sap flows back downwards. Investigations have shown that [collection of these drugs should take place] rather early in spring and very late in fall. Blossoms, fruits, stems, and leaves must be collected during their respective periods of maturity. One cannot always follow the letter of such instructions, since during the course of the year delays may occur, or events may take place early.[51]

The old units of measurement consisted solely of *chu* and *liang;* the term *fen* was not yet in use. Today, the following applies: ten *shu* are equal to one *chu;* six *chu* are equal to one *fen;* four *fen* are equal to one *liang;* sixteen *liang* are equal to one *chin.* Although there are other units of measurement, such as *tzu-ku* ["grain-seeds"] and *chü-shu* ["black

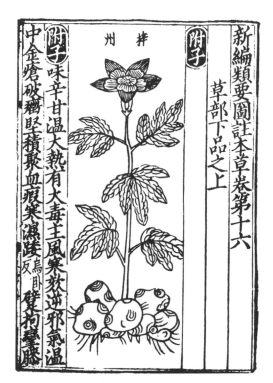

aconite tubers *(fu-tzu)—Hsin-pien lei-yao t'u-chu pen-ts'ao*

millet"], they have long since been standardized and should be used accordingly. When contemporary prescription specialists speak of "equal *fen*," this is not the *fen* of the *fen* and *liang* [units of measurements]. They [merely intend to] say that [in a given prescription] the amount of all drugs should be the same, no matter whether in *chin* or *liang*. One must first look at the size or seriousness of the illness and what it needs, then one should decide [about the amount of the ingredients in a prescription] on the basis of one's own considerations. This kind [of prescriptions with equal amounts of ingredients] is only used in pills and powders; they must be taken according to fixed standards. In decoctions and [medicinal] wines, [a provision of] "equal amounts" does not occur.[52]

All drugs used in the preparation of pills or powders must first be cut up into fine pieces. Then they are dried in the sun and pulverized. Whether a drug is to be pulverized individually or together [with the other drugs in a prescription] is determined by the prescription. For drugs containing a large amount of moisture, such as *men-tung* and *kan-ti-huang*, the following is applicable. First, they are cut, dried, and pounded individually into small pieces. Remove the fine parts repeatedly and tear [the remaining]. [Then, they are] dried again. If shady weather or rain arrives, they may also be roasted over a weak fire until they are dry. One waits a few moments until they have become cool again before they are pounded.[53]

All drugs containing moisture suffer great weight losses during the drying process. For this reason, the amounts must be carefully increased [before drying]. Weighed [again afterwards, the amounts will be] correct. This does not apply to drugs used in decoctions or [medicinal] wines.[54]

Decoctions are boiled gently over a small fire. The amount of water varies with [the volume of] the prescription. In general, one *tou* of water is used with twenty *liang* of drugs, reduced by boiling to four *sheng*. This should serve as a standard. If one wishes to prepare a laxative decoction, by means of slight processing, only a small amount of water should be used but a [relatively] large quantity [of the boiled] liquid shall be taken. If a restorative decoction is desired, which needs thorough processing, a large volume of water is used [boiled long enough so that only] a small amount of liquid [remains] to be taken [as medication].[55]

[The drugs] *lang-tu, chih-shih, chü-p'i, pan-hsia, ma-huang,* and *wu-shu-yu* must first be seasoned for a long period of time. The remaining [drugs] should be as fresh as possible.[56]

After a division of all drugs according to the eighty-three illnesses and symptoms they are able to cure, the first chapter of the *Pen-ts'ao ching chi-chu* continues with the following paragraphs:

The enumeration of forty-one possible poisonings and the suitable antidotes.

Twelve prohibitions against certain types of vegetables and meat that cannot be consumed with specific drugs.

Four general prohibitions concerning the taking of drugs.

A list of drugs not suitable for use in decoctions or medicinal wines.

A list of certain drugs according to their compatibility and incompatibility when administered together.

These tables close the first chapter of the *Pen-ts'ao ching chi-chu,* which has been devoted to more general and fundamental questions.

Following the pattern in the *Pen-ching*, T'ao Hung-ching divided the drugs in the monographs of chapters 2 through 7 into seven groups (*pu*). Only the last of these sections was totally new:

precious stones/minerals   fruits/vegetables
herbs/trees   grains/food
worms/fish   drugs known by name but
fowl/quadrupeds   no longer in use

The new commentaries added to the individual monographs treat the places or regions of origin, the appearance, the characteristics, the preparation, as well as the storage of the drugs. However, this information is not provided for every individual drug monograph according to any recognizable system.

The connection between the three sources of the text, which is composed of the old arguments in the *Pen-ching* (marked here by underlining), the "additional notes of renowned medical men" added by T'ao Hung-ching, and finally T'ao's own commentaries, can be clearly recognized in the monograph of the drug *pa-tou*:

> *Pa-tou*, taste: pungent; [thermo-influence:] warm; warm in fresh state, cold when boiled; possesses very strong medicinal effectiveness. Controls harms caused by cold, malaria fevers, fits of cold and heat; breaks up bowel obstructions of different kinds, hardenings; stagnation of drinking liquids, mucous congestions, abdominal swelling, edema, purges the five depots and six palaces; opens and breaks through obstructions; it clears the way for water and grains; removes spoiled flesh; expels poisonings caused by demons, [removes] possessions by the *ku* and [other] evil things; kills worms and fish. In women it cures stagnation of the monthly period and [induces] an overdue fetus [to leave the womb]. [It cures further] cuts and suppurations with blood, and opens passage through the sexual organs of men; it kills the poison of *pan-mao*. One can also take [this drug] after subjecting it to a process of [alchemical] refining. It has a beneficial effect on the blood vessels, gives a good coloring to humans, helps them to transform themselves, and to associate with demonic spirits. Another name [for *pa-tou*] is *pa-chiao*. It grows in river valleys in the district of Pa. In the eighth month the fruits are collected and dried in the shade. The seed coat is removed. *Yüan-hua* supports [the effects of *pa-tou*]. [*Pa-tou*] hates *jang-ts'ao*, and fears *ta-huang, huang-lien,* and *li-lu.*
> [T'ao Hung-ching's commentary:] (*Pa-tou*) comes from the district of Pa and resembles *ta-tou* ["large beans"]. It is an extremely strong laxative for humans. Fresh specimens are most suited for use. The seed coat must always be removed first, only then should [the desired amount] be weighed. (*Pa-tou*) should be roasted until yellowish-black. It should be pounded to a pulp separately [from other possible ingredients in a prescription], and, finally, it is processed into pills or powders. In Taoist prescriptions one can also find instructions for preparation of (*pa-tou*) by [alchemical] refining. It is said that one becomes an immortal after taking [the drug thus prepared]. One man took a dose of it and died immediately. A rat ate it and gained thirty pounds of weight within three years. This shows how [differently] the natures of things can tolerate each other.[57]

2.3. The fragment of Tun-huang

The next *pen-ts'ao* work in the main tradition appeared in 659 and superseded T'ao Hung-ching's herbals, which as a result were soon lost as independent editions. But the fact that later pen-ts'ao works in the main tradition took over nearly the entire contents of the *Pen-ts'ao ching chi-chu* by T'ao Hung-ching, and marked them as such, permitted in recent times an extensive reconstruction of this book. The exactness of the transmission was confirmed for the first chapter when a fragment of a copy of the *Pen-ts'ao ching chi-chu* was discovered in 1908, among the old documents found by a Japanese monk in the Tun-huang Caves in Sinkiang, West China.

The original soon disappeared in a Japanese archive; today it is in the library of the Ryukoku University in Kyoto. Until now, the basis for publications about this old text was a photostat, which the Japanese scientist Ogawa Takuji was able to make of the original decades ago. A copy came into the hands of Lo Chen-yü, who published it as a facsimile and, in an afterword, expressed the opinion that the fragment was a copy from the sixth year of the *k'ai-yüan* period of the T'ang era (718), as stated in two lines appended to the actual *pen-ts'ao* text.[58] By means of studies he was able to conduct with the original itself, however, Ogawa was able to prove later that the copy must have been completed even before the T'ang era. In the original document, one can recognize a difference in style of the writing as well as in the consistency of the ink between the last two lines and the previous text. Moreover, the taboos of the T'ang dynasty concerning certain written characters are not observed in the text of the fragment; thus, the assumption seems justified that only the appended two last lines date from the T'ang era.

With the exception of the first two lines of T'ao Hung-ching's preface, the Tun-huang fragment contains the entire first chapter of the *Pen-ts'ao ching chi-chu*. Thus, it opened up the possibility for a comparison with the work attributed to T'ao that was transmitted through the quotations in later *pen-ts'ao* works. The differences proved to be insignificant; they were confined to small deviations from the text and differences in the arrangement of the drugs.[59]

2.4. Observations on the work of T'ao Hung-ching

T'ao Hung-ching's *Pen-ts'ao ching chi-chu*, although completed before the probable beginning of T'ao's active involvement with elixir preparations in his Mao-shan retreat, contains many traces of his early interest in the transmutations of metals and minerals. Mercury played a controlling role in the preparation of drugs for a long life and often formed the basis for chemical experiments. T'ao Hung-ching recorded the following observation: "Quicksilver is able to change gold and silver into a paste."[60] Without doubt this paste refers to the amalgams; already 150 years later they were described in the *Hsin-hsiu pen-ts'ao* as suitable for filling teeth.

Pen-ts'ao ching chi-chu (also: *T'ao Hung-ching pen-ts'ao ching chi-chu*)
"Classic of Pharmaceutics, Compiled and Annotated [by T'ao Hung-ching]"
Short title: *Pen-ts'ao chi-chu*
7 chapters / 730 drug descriptions
Author: T'ao Hung-ching (452–536)
    tzu: T'ung ming
    hao: Yin-chü, Cheng-pai
    from: Mo-ling in Tan-yang
Written: ca. 500
Published: 500

typha pollen *(p'u-huang)—Ch'ung-hsiu cheng-ho pen-ts'ao*

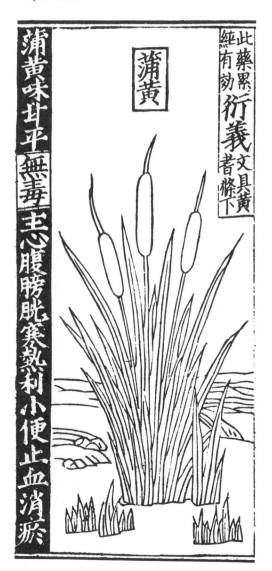

T'ao described the production of minium (Pb_3O_4; *huang-tan*), which was used in the preparation of lead plasters: "Minium is produced by treating lead with heat."[61] This reaction could be confirmed, since during the T'ang period a number of drugs were brought to Japan from China and since that time have been stored in Nara. A substance labeled *tan* was shown by analysis to be Pb_3O_4.[62]

A further example of T'ao's own observational skills—or of his familiarity with insights gained by other experimenters—can be found in his description of the two substances *mang-hsiao* ($Na_2SO_4 \cdot 10H_2O$; mirabilite) and *hsiao-shih* (KNO_3 etc.; niter). He recognized that hsiao-shih, unlike mang-hsiao, "produces a violet smoke when heated dryly."[63]

T'ao Hung-ching included in his work numerous drugs whose effects are still acknowledged in China today. He was the first to call attention to the drug *ping-lang* (the betel nut) as a remedy for tapeworms.[64] He was also the first to recommend *yin-ch'en-hao* (an *artemisia* species),[65] a drug he had taken over from the *Pen-ching*, as a remedy for jaundice. A positive effect of this drug on hepatitis is still recognized by modern scientific research.[66]

Just as significant as the numerous individual observations are the references in many of his drug descriptions to the close connection between the effectiveness of drugs, on the one hand, and the places or regions of origin and time of collection, on the other. For example, T'ao took over the assertion that the drug *ma-huang* must be collected at the beginning of fall for maximum effectiveness. Modern pharmacobiology has completely confirmed the importance of drug geography and the seasonally dependent fluctuations in potency.

One of the most important accomplishments of T'ao Hung-ching's is found in his arrangement of the drug monographs. To be sure, he did not give up the distribution of all drugs into the upper, middle, or lower class, but he was the first to subordinate this division to a classification according to the natural origin of the respective substances. As mentioned earlier, drugs in the *Pen-ching* were arranged within the three classes according to their natural origin. T'ao Hung-ching reversed this order. In the *Pen-ts'ao ching chi-chu*, drugs are distributed into six groups depending upon natural origin and then subdivided into the three classes. This new type of classification was continually refined up to the *Pen-ts'ao kang mu* of Li Shih-chen (1518–1593). During this period, the classification into three sections lost more and more of its significance and later was totally ignored in many works.

The differentiation of both sources of the *Pen-ts'ao ching chi-chu* by means of different colored ink proved itself of special value for later textual criticism. This separation was taken over by all later pen-ts'ao works in the main tradition. After the introduction of printing techniques—the first printed Chinese materia medica appeared in A.D. 973—the two sources were differentiated by white characters on a black background and vice versa.

It is noteworthy that T'ao Hung-ching introduced a tradition of plainly naming the source of newly added drug descriptions or commentaries. All pen-ts'ao works in the main tradition followed this example. Another interesting innovation by T'ao Hung-ching, however, was not able to assert itself. T'ao wrote:

> The sweet or bitter taste of a drug can be estimated, and it is easily ascertained whether or not [a substance] possesses a strong medicinal effectiveness. But whether [the thermo-influence of a drug] is cold or hot must be made clear. Here I have marked hot [thermo-influence] with a red dot, cold [thermo-influence] with a black dot, and neutral [nature] with no dot, in order to avoid a complicated commentary.[67]

T'ao's attempt to abandon the word in favor of an abstract symbol did not last long. Only the following pen-ts'ao work of the T'ang period continued this procedure. However, the first pen-ts'ao work in the succeeding Sung period, the *K'ai-pao pen-ts'ao,* contained the following passage:

> Hot, cold, and neutral [thermo-influence] were marked in the T'ang *pen(-ts'ao)* with, respectively, black, red, and no dots. This was the source of many errors. Today, we again add a written commentary to each individual monograph, as was customary in the *Pen-ching* and in the "Additional Notes [of Renowned Medical Men]."[68]

The index of drugs that T'ao Hung-ching introduced proved to be of substantial aid for the practicing physician. Drugs were listed according to the illnesses and symptoms for whose treatment they were suitable. It was this index that first made possible the use of a pen-ts'ao work as a handbook and reference work and not just a compendium of current knowledge about drugs. Thus, when a physician recognized an illness, he could consult the index listing for that illness to find the appropriate drugs for treatment. A table following this listing contained further information about the compatibility of the drug for use with other drugs. If the physician wished still further information, he had to consult the relevant section in the main part of the *Pen-ts'ao,* the drug monograph itself. As a result, T'ao Hung-ching created in China what we might call a first "Guide to Drug Usage," in which the needs of practicing physicians were already extensively taken into account.

It is in this connection that T'ao's definition of units of volume and weight and his references to the mistakes caused by undifferentiated usage of old and new units of measurement are to be seen. Certainty and clarity in units of measurement build one of the foundations not only for the successful outcome of alchemical operations but also for a successful use of drugs and for their further refinement into effective medicinal forms.

Not surprisingly, the work and personality of T'ao Hung-ching are still valued in China today, 1,500 years after this scholar published his knowledge and thoughts. There are, in fact, treatises that label T'ao Hung-ching as the Chinese Leonardo da Vinci, based upon those accomplishments that impress us today. It is only in some publications of the People's Republic of China that T'ao's achievements appear more objectively integrated into the entirety of his work (including his entanglement in the errors of his day).

millet *(liang-mi)—Shao-hsing pen-ts'ao*

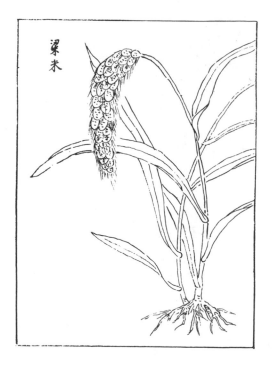

3.1. The preface of the *Hsin-hsiu pen-ts'ao*

In the fourth year of the governmental period *hsien-ch'ing* of the T'ang era (A.D. 659), the official K'ung Chih-yüeh wrote the preface for a pen-ts'ao work which he himself had helped compile, and which soon superseded the *Pen-ts'ao ching chi-chu* as an independent work. Since this preface is one of our most important sources for the development of the *Hsin-hsiu pen-ts'ao,* I present below the decisive excerpts in translation. These excerpts also show the very close connections between the newly compiled text and the preceding work by T'ao Hung-ching:

> In ancient times the Ch'in government carried out a burning [of books], with the exception of these [medical] scriptures. During the disturbances at the time of the *yung-chia* period [307–313], these teachings remained still extant. At the time of the Liang dynasty, T'ao Hung-ching took great interest in the dietetic preservation of life and studied thoroughly the art of drug [use]. He was of the opinion that the *Pen-ts'ao ching* had indeed been compiled by Shen-nung but had not yet been published as a book [by this ancient ruler]. He regretted that the time of [Shen-nung] was long past, and that, as a result, the records on wooden slabs had long since fallen to pieces. He found fault with the writings of T'ung and Lei [-kung], combined oral and written traditions, and gathered everything into his own work. Furthermore, by reshaping the classic, as well as by formulating prescriptions he provided great help for the medical world. At that time, however, one cherished alchemy, and whatever [T'ao] heard and saw had the drawback of being limited in various aspects. Thus, the general view is not expressed in his formulations; commentaries and explanations [in his work] are solely based on his personal scholarship. Therefore, he valued, for example, [the drug] *fang-chi* from Chien-p'ing, and he rejected *pan-hsia* from Huai-li. He allowed *yü-jen* to be gathered in the fall, and *yün-shih* in winter. He mistakenly confused the yellow and the white type of *liang-mi,* and he mixed up the two kinds of *ching-tzu.* He separated *fan-lou* from *chi-ch'ang* [although they are one and the same] but arranged *yu-pa* and *yüan-wei* together [although these are two different drugs]. He erroneously ascribed the same root to *fang-k'uei* and *lang-tu* and incorrectly grouped *kou-wen* and *huang-ching* into the same class. He did not differentiate lead and tin and did not separate the *ch'en*-orange from the *yu*-fruit. There are many more such examples. Since his time, the ability of combining drugs has been refined, but renowned medical men continue [T'ao's misleading] directions, passing them on to each other. Only in a few instances could corrections be made. Thus one continues to collect *tu-heng* instead of *chi-chi,* to search for *jen-tung* instead of *lo-shih. Chih-li* is still rejected and *pieh-t'eng* used instead; *fei-lien* is disregarded and *ma-chi* used in its place. As a result, doubtful things are passed on and errors are made. There has never been anyone who was truly informed about this matter. Cases of illness therefore mean great danger, and that is very sad indeed! [Finally] the [official] Su Ching took up the matter of T'ao Hung-ching's mistakes and analyzed the widespread errors. He addressed a petition to the court requesting a revision, in order to profoundly assist the intentions harbored by the emperor. Thereupon it was decreed that [the officials] [Ch'ang-sun] Wu-chi, Hsü Hsiao-ch'ung, and others, twenty-two men in all, undertook a detailed revision in cooperation with Su Ching. We took account of the fact that the appearance and the life of animals and plants show different characteristics from region to region, and also that the seasonal variations of spring and autumn affect the influences

3. The *Hsin-hsiu pen-ts'ao*

Hsin-hsiu pen-ts'ao
"Materia Medica, Newly Revised"
Short titles: *T'ang pen-ts'ao; T'ang-pen*
54 chapters / 850 drug descriptions
Authors: Su Ching (ca. 650)
        Ch'ang-sun Wu-chi (?–659); from: Lo-yang
        Li Chi (594–669); *tzu:* Mou-kung; from: Li-hu in Shan-tung and others
Written: 657–659
Published: 659

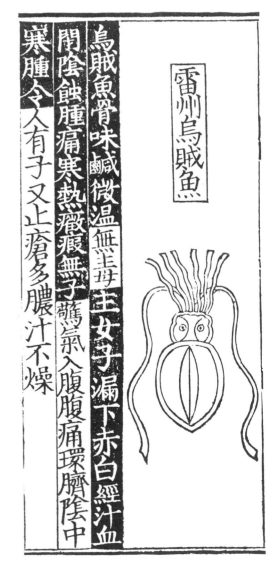

cuttlefish *(wu-tse-yü)*—*Ch'ung-hsiu cheng-ho pen-ts'ao*

[stored by herbs and animals], resulting in effects [exerted by the respective drugs] that are different from the norm. Furthermore, if [herbs and animals] leave their original grounds, the material will remain the same but their efficacy will be different. If one does not pick [herbs] in accordance with the proper rules, one will have the right thing but one may have missed the proper time. Fruits famous [for their therapeutic properties] will fail, and there will be many mistakes concerning their cold and warm [nature]. When [such faulty drugs] are used [to treat] the common people, this is bad enough, but if their application is extended to noble men, no greater act of rebellion can be perceived. For this reason, from above we took over the directions of spirits, and below we evaluated the general view. We issued a general appeal in which we requested drugs [from all regions of the empire]. Be they fowl, fur-bearing or scaly animals, or crustaceans, none should be so far away that one did not seek it. All known roots, stalks, blossoms, and fruits should be collected. Thus, in the following period, the important things were carefully examined and medical knowledge was collected on a large scale. Although the *Pen-ching* has its deficiencies, that [from its contents] which could be proven effective had to be written down. The Additional Notes did indeed still exist, but they had to be corrected without delay. Similarities and differences were examined, and a choice was made as to what should be taken over or omitted. Lead and pen were applied to determine the correctness of all words; the appearance and form of all drugs were portrayed in rich colors. The (*Hsin-hsiu*) *pen-ts'ao*, the "[drug-] illustrations" (*yao-t'u*), the "commentaries [for these]" (*yao-ching*), and a table of contents with a total of fifty-four chapters were composed, in order to enclose, as in a net, old and new, and to open ears as well as eyes. [Our work] combines all the mysteries of medicine and of the prescriptions. It will save the life of any living being. It will be handed down over tens of thousands of years without falling into obscurity, and it will be regarded highly during the reign of hundreds of kings without ever becoming useless.

Submitted in the *hsien-ch'ing* period, in the fourth year on the 17th day by the official Su Ching.[69]

藥圖
藥經

3.2. The first government-sponsored materia medica in China

Su Ching, whose name was later changed to Su Kung as a result of an imperial taboo, had already made private efforts for a revision of the *Pen-ts'ao ching chi-chu*, before he turned to the throne in 657, with a petition in which he suggested a careful and extensive new edition of the *Pen-ts'ao*. The emperor apparently reacted very quickly, for a committee of officials completed the entire work in two years, as is evident from the date of the preface.[70]

Thus began an important new phase in the development of the pen-ts'ao drug literature. Beginning already in the T'ang period, but mainly during the Sung dynasties, various aspects of medicine received the greatest and most effective attention from the state in the entire history of the Chinese Empire. It is not surprising that such attention was reflected also in the area of pharmaceutical literature. From the seventh century until the end of the Sung period, pharmaceutical books were ordered, revised, and published in China with government initiative or support, the only time before the twentieth century that this was to occur. Subsequently, herbals are reported to have been written upon order of the emperor only once during the Ming period and once during the Ch'ing period.[71] The works resulting from those later orders, however, were not intended to reach the general public and therefore cannot be considered exceptions to the thesis given above.

The committee appointed by the emperor for the compilation of an up-to-date, comprehensive materia medica consisted of twenty-two officials. The leader of the group was Su Ching, of whom we know very little. Ch'ang-sun Wu-chi became director of the editorial staff. As a former comrade-in-arms of the second T'ang emperor, he had held various high official posts after the emperor's ascension to the throne. Among other duties, he was also appointed to revise the code of laws. When, despite lucrative offers of bribes, he refused in the year 654 to participate in the seizure of power by the Empress Wu (625–705), Ch'ang-sun Wu-chi was accused of treason at her instigation five years later and, together with his family, was murdered in 659 in Szechwan. Therefore, his name no longer appears on the list of twenty-two officials, which was placed at the beginning of the completed *Hsin-hsiu pen-ts'ao.*

Replacing Ch'ang-sun Wu-chi's name is Li Chi. Originally known by the name of Hsü Shih-chi, he had risen from worker, via a period as a robber, to officer in the troops of Li Mi (582–618). In 618, he changed over to the side of the ruler of the T'ang, also changing his name to Li Shih-chi. He once again received a new name when, in 626, the second T'ang emperor, Li Shih-min (597–649) ascended to the throne, and the "Shih" portion of Li Shih-chi's name fell victim to a taboo. Li Chi, as he was now finally called, is indirectly held responsible for the rebellion of the Empress Wu, as he had persuaded the emperor to marry this woman. Thus, it is understandable that he, a favorite of the empress, was placed at the head of the pen-ts'ao editorial committee following Ch'ang-sun Wu-chi's removal.

Of the other committee members, twelve bear titles identifying them as medical or pharmaceutical officials. From among the names of the remaining members, the well-known historiographer Hsü Ching-tsung (592–672), the astrologer and soothsayer Li Ch'un-feng (602–670), and Lü Ts'ai (died 664?) stand out; the last-named was esteemed as a connoisseur of Chou-period music and had also been appointed by the emperor to revise the works of the yinyang philosophical school.[72]

As the preface makes clear, the editorial committee issued a decree requesting color illustrations of drug material from all provinces of the empire. It is unknown how effective the decree was and to what extent the desired material arrived in the capital. The fact that after only two years' work a materia medica was completed which contained only 115 more monographs than T'ao Hung-ching's work, may indicate either that, indeed, more drugs were not yet used by physicians or that the decree was not able to mobilize existing knowledge sufficiently.

In this connection, one must take into account that many of the newly added drugs were imported from India and Arabian countries during the course of the trade expansion in the T'ang period. Beside numerous aromatic drugs, which were among the new imports, we also find in the *Hsin-hsiu pen-ts'ao* a substance called *ti-yeh-chia.* This is apparently the drug combination, sometimes containing opium, whose invention is ascribed to King Mithridates of Pontus (124–62 B.C.) and which is known in Europe as *theriaca*. *Theriaca* consisted of an average of fifty to sixty ingredients and was considered the most important and most famous panacea in medieval Europe. In the *Pen-ts'ao* of the T'ang period, this exotic substance, which had probably been introduced into China from Persia, is grouped under the animal drugs with the following monograph:

> *Ti-yeh-chia,* taste: acrid, bitter; [thermo-influence:] neutral. No marked medicinal effectiveness. Masters a hundred illnesses, if one is hit by the malevolent, and evil influences, as well as abdominal obstructions. Origin: Western countries.
>> It is said: this [drug] is made from gall-bladders [of pigs]. Externally, it resembles pills that have been rotten for a long time. The color is red-black. Occasionally, [this drug] is brought here by barbarians. It is considered extremely valuable and expensive. Its effectiveness has been shown in experiments. New addition.[73]

藥典

Chinese historians have claimed repeatedly that the *Hsin-hsiu pen-ts'ao* represents the first pharmacopoeia (*yao-tien*) of China and of the world, and they have pointed out an alleged Chinese advantage of more than eight centuries over the first Western pharmacopoeia, published by the city-state of Nuremberg in 1546.[74] Such claims are unfounded, and they reveal a basic unawareness of the characteristics of the Nuremberg Code and its successors. The Nuremberg pharmacopoeia was the first such book ever to request from physicians and pharmacists strict adherence to officially defined standards of drug usage. Government supervision was initiated at the same time to enforce adherence to the code, which had legal status. Over the centuries, the drug codes have become increasingly more sophisticated and their contents have continuously adapted to new developments in chemistry and physics in general, and to new analytical techniques and insights in pharmacology, pharmaceutical technology, and other relevant sciences, in particular. Many countries have followed the Nuremberg example and it was only in 1930 that the first such Chinese drug code was published (see E, I, 2). Interestingly enough, the preface to the *Chung-hua yao-tien* of 1930 explicitly points out the Nuremberg Code as the beginning of a tradition which China joined about 500 years later. The mere fact that during the T'ang dynasty, and a few times in subsequent centuries, a government supported or initiated the compilation of pen-ts'ao works is not sufficient to term these works yao-tien, drug codes, or even pharmacopoeia. There is no evidence at all that they had any legal status similar to that held by the Nuremberg Code and its successors.

3.3. Structure and contents of the *Hsin-hsiu pen-ts'ao*

The *Hsin-hsiu pen-ts'ao* describes a total of 850 drugs, 735 of which were taken over from T'ao Hung-ching's work. The increase by five in the number of drugs over the usual number of 730 monographs given for the *Pen-ts'ao ching chi-chu* is explained by the fact that some

monographs of the *Pen-ts'ao ching chi-chu,* in which T'ao had described two different drug terms as referring to the same substance,
were divided into two separate monographs by the authors of the
Hsin-hsiu pen-ts'ao, who felt that the terms designated different drugs.

Regardless of the relatively small number of newly added drug
descriptions, the dimensions of the *T'ang pen-ts'ao* go far beyond those
of the preceding *Pen-ts'ao ching chi-chu.* Its fifty-four chapters are
divided as follows:

Hsin-hsiu pen-ts'ao (Preface, general sections, monograph section)	20 chapters
Table of contents	1 chapter
Yao-t'u ("Drug Illustrations")	25 chapters
Table of contents	1 chapter
Yao-ching ("Commentaries on the Illustrations")	7 chapters

The drug illustrations (*Yao-t'u*) and their commentaries (*Yao-ching*)
are an important innovation. Through them, the first *Pen-ts'ao* written
under governmental sponsorship also constitutes the first comprehensive illustrated Chinese materia medica known to us. The illustrations,
as well as most of their commentaries, must be considered as having
been lost since at least 1050. Consequently, they remain largely unknown. We can only conclude, from a remark in the preface of the
Hsin-hsiu pen-ts'ao, that the illustrations were colored.[75]

For the following three centuries, the *Hsin-hsiu pen-ts'ao* remained
the decisive compendium of drugs from the main pen-ts'ao tradition.
Together with a supplementary work written in the eighth century by
Ch'en Ts'ang-ch'i—the *Pen-ts'ao shih-i* from the secondary tradition
(see C, I, 3.4)—it constituted the basic pharmaceutical work of the
time, and was newly revised and brought up to date only in the tenth
century. This new version then appeared under the title *Ch'ung-kuang
ying-kung pen-ts'ao.* As a result, however, the T'ang edition became
obsolete and was lost as an independent work.

In China itself, hardly a single fragment worth mentioning of the
Hsin-hsiu pen-ts'ao has been discovered. There exist only a few min-
imal text portions which correspond to the contents of the *Hsin-hsiu
pen-ts'ao.* The contents are known today, on the one hand, from
numerous quotations in later pen-ts'ao works of the main tradition,
as well as in several other medical works and encyclopedias; on the
other hand, ten of the twenty chapters of the *Hsin-hsiu pen-ts'ao* were
rediscovered and copied in Kyoto in the years 1832 to 1842, the earliest
chapters possibly dating back to 731.[76] In 1889, a set of copies was
acquired by the Chinese military official Fu Yün-lung, who accidentally
heard about it during a trip to Kyoto; it was published later together
with the third chapter reconstructed by Kojima Hoso. Thus, by the
end of the nineteenth century, ten complete chapters of the independent
Hsin-hsiu pen-ts'ao were preserved in the original.

These fragments and the quotations mentioned above form the basis
for the reconstruction of the twenty chapters of the *Hsin-hsiu pen-
ts'ao,* which the Japanese scientist Okanishi Tameto prepared in the
1930s.[77] This reconstruction enables us to understand and evaluate

the exact structure and contents of the monograph section of the *T'ang pen-ts'ao*.

The first chapter of the *Hsin-hsiu pen-ts'ao* begins with an outline of the chapters and a list of all drugs described. The total number of drugs is mentioned for each group, and the sources are given, for example, *Shen-nung pen-ching, Ming-i pieh-lu,* or "New Addition" (*hsin-fu*). K'ung Chih-yüeh's preface, from the year 659, follows; appended to this is the list of names and ranks of the twenty-two members of the editorial committee. The first chapter concludes with T'ao Hung-ching's preface to the *Pen-ts'ao ching chi-chu* and the ten general sections of the *Pen-ching* annotated by T'ao.

新附

The second chapter of the *Hsin-hsiu pen-ts'ao* in Okanishi's reconstruction gives the additional text of the first chapter of the *Pen-ts'ao ching chi-chu*. Scattered throughout this chapter we also find brief commentaries by the T'ang editors, each clearly introduced by the two characters *chin-an* ("carefully annotated").

謹按

The third through twentieth chapters comprise the drug monographs. Their arrangement corresponds to T'ao Hung-ching's work insofar as their division into the three classes remains subordinated to the grouping according to origins. In the arrangement of the individual sections, however, the authors did not follow T'ao, but the *Pen-ching,* by again expanding their number from seven—as in the *Pen-ts'ao ching chi-chu*—to ten:

precious stones/minerals	chapters 3–5	83 drugs
herbs	chapters 6–11	256 drugs
trees	chapters 12–14	100 drugs
quadrupeds/fowl (incl. man)	chapter 15	56 drugs
worms/fish	chapter 16	72 drugs
fruits	chapter 17	25 drugs
vegetables	chapter 18	37 drugs
rice/grains	chapter 19	28 drugs
known by name but obsolete	chapter 20	193 drugs

Each individual section in the monograph part is again preceded by a list of the drugs described in it, and their source.

Within the monographs, the drugs of the *Pen-ching* and those of the "Additional Notes by Renowned Medical Men" (*pieh-lu*) were distinguished by red and black ink, according to T'ao Hung-ching's supposed example. Newly added monographs were also written in black ink but were marked by the two characters *hsin-fu* ("New Addition").

T'ao Hung-ching's monographs were again taken over complete and unchanged, as I have already mentioned, a characteristic of the main tradition. Each new commentary by the T'ang authors, marked by the two characters chin-an ("carefully annotated"), was appended only after T'ao's commentaries on the "Additional Notes by Renowned Medical Men" or on the monographs taken over from the *Pen-ching*.

The T'ang commentaries did not add any new elements to the work; they were mostly intended to complete T'ao Hung-ching's statements or to correct faulty information. This, too, is a characteristic of the main pen-ts'ao tradition: in general, the errors of previous authors were not removed and replaced by new views, but were left in to give the reader the opportunity of weighing and judging greatly diverging statements.

Therefore, Okanishi remarked correctly in the preface of his reconstruction of the *Hsin-hsiu pen-ts'ao* that it was not the intention of the T'ang authors to create a completely new book.[78] Instead, they endeavored—as did T'ao Hung-ching—to preserve the old texts, to correct their faulty commentaries and incorrect arrangement with annotations, and to enrich the work through the knowledge acquired in the meantime.

This knowledge was taken mainly from the works of the so-called secondary pen-ts'ao tradition. It was integrated during the T'ang and Sung periods into the works of the main pen-ts'ao tradition, and in the Ming period into two outstanding encyclopedic works of the sixteenth century. The works in the secondary tradition, it is true, were less extensive, but they should not be underestimated in comparison with the works of the main tradition, which are discussed here in such detail. Including the materia medicas mentioned so far, the bibliographical chapter of the T'ang dynastic history already lists at least forty-one titles that can be defined as pharmaceutical works. These books were either outlines or supplements of works in the main tradition which had already been published, or the authors had concentrated on the description of certain groups of drugs, such as the area of dietetics, or on other peculiarities. These books presented local knowledge, and we may assume that these less extensive, and thus more easily copied and cheaper editions, were often more widely distributed than the voluminous and costly works of the main tradition.

An important work from the large secondary tradition is the *Pen-ts'ao shih-i*, described in the following section, which was written as an immediate supplement to the *T'ang pen-ts'ao*. Other representatives of the secondary tradition will be discussed in the second part of the present work, which is devoted to the specialized pen-ts'ao literature.

3.4. A supplement to the *T'ang pen-ts'ao*—the *Pen-ts'ao shih-i*

Ch'en Ts'ang-ch'i had been appointed as a military official in the district of San-yüan of the prefecture of Ch'ing-ch'ao when he wrote the widely respected supplementary work *Pen-ts'ao shih-i* during the governmental period *k'ai-yüan* (713–741). Since, in Ch'en Ts'ang-ch'i's opinion, the *Shen-nung pen-ts'ao ching* had considerable deficiencies—in spite of the expansions through the works of T'ao Hung-ching and Su Ching—he himself wrote a supplement with the necessary corrections. The ten chapters of his work included one chapter with preface and introduction, six chapters on "matters that have been neglected," and three chapters on "explanations of obscure points." Numerous important commentaries and drugs described for the first time were taken over from the *Pen-ts'ao shih-i* by subsequent

Pen-ts'ao shih-i
"Additions to the Materia Medica"
10 chapters / number of drug descriptions: unknown
Author: Ch'en Ts'ang-ch'i (8th century)
　　　　from: Szu-ming
Written: ca. 713–741
Published: date unknown

pen-ts'ao works of the main tradition and handed down to modern times. The original, however, thus became superfluous and was lost as an independent work, probably during the Sung period.[79]

The following are some of the innovations from Ch'en Ts'ang-ch'i's *Pen-ts'ao shih-i.*

In a bibliographical work of the Ch'ing period, the *T'u-shu chi-ch'eng ch'üan-lu,* we find the remark that Ch'en Ts'ang-ch'i had recommended eating human flesh as a treatment for anorexia. This is said to explain the fact that, later, dutiful children frequently gave their own flesh to save their parents.[80] In subsequent pen-ts'ao works, one finds references to a total of ten drugs with human origin which are supposed to have been described for the first time by Ch'en Ts'ang-ch'i in a materia medica. Among them are the "human placenta,"[81] "human blood," and "human bile," but also "boy's pubic hair," "pillows of deceased men," and "excrement from the navels of newborn babies."

In the area of metals, Ch'en Ts'ang-ch'i was the first to mention, among other things, rock crystal (*shui-ching*)[82] and glass (*po-li*)[83] in a materia medica. Concerning glass he wrote:

> *Po-li,* taste: acrid; [thermo-influence:] cold. No marked medicinal effectiveness. Masters fear and agitation, as well as heat in the heart. It is able to pacify the heart, to clear the eyes, and to cure red eyes. If pressed [on any part of the body], it eliminates heat and swellings. This is a treasured article from Western countries. It is the "king of the water." Some say ice transforms into it in the course of a thousand years, [a process which makes] it belong to the class of precious stones. It originates from minerals in the earth, but it does not necessarily constitute ice. Among rock crystal and gems, it is the most brilliant and clear [article]. It is a gem which, if one places it into water, becomes invisible. If one presses it on the eyes, it drives out hot tears. Some call it "fire-flames-gem." If turned towards the sun it may pick up the [solar] fire.[84]

One reference in the *Pen-ts'ao shih-i* has attracted interest as possibly the earliest known remark about the location of ores and their surrounding materials. Ch'en Ts'ang-ch'i mentions a mineral called *fen-tzu-shih,* which can no longer be identified, as covering natural deposits of gold. It may be the same substance named *pan-chin shih* ("gold-accompanying stone") in the *Pen-ts'ao yen-i.*[85]

The use of the iron solvate *t'ieh-chiang* (which was later found as an antidote for lead poisoning) as a detoxicating agent was first mentioned by Ch'en Ts'ang-ch'i, who wrote:

> Take any iron, place it into a pot, and add water to cover it. After a long time, when a foam of virid color has emerged, remove [the iron]. [The liquid] is suitable for black-dying. Also, it dissolves all poisons that enter the abdomen. Its intake can also calm down one's heart. It masters fits, development of heat, mad walking by domestic animals, humans with fits of madness. If someone has been injured by snake, dog, tiger, or wolf poison, or was bitten by evil insects, and if he takes this [drug, the poison will] not enter [his body].[86]

In the area of plants, Ch'en Ts'ang-ch'i introduced, for example, certain hygienic effects of the soap-tree *kuei-tsao-chia*:[87] "From *kuei-tsao-chia* a decoction is prepared which serves as a detergent. It removes skin ailments, such as scabies. One can clean clothes and remove dirt from the hair by rubbing them with the leaves."[88]

The *mi-hsiang* tree is also mentioned by Ch'en Ts'ang-ch'i for the first time in a pen-ts'ao work. Its place of origin was Annam, and it was used in China for the production of *mi-hsiang* paper. The earliest reference to this tree in any Chinese work is found in a botanical text of the third century, the *Nan-fang ts'ao mu chuang* ("Herbs and Trees of the South").[89]

As a last example the *ku* should be mentioned, which was already found in the *Pen-ching* as an illness-causing agent but which was described for the first time in the *Pen-ts'ao shih-i* as a curative and preventive drug. Ch'en Ts'ang-ch'i recommended as an antidote, obviously on the basis of concepts of magic correspondence, the *ku* poison of those animals that, in nature, are able to subdue the animal diagnosed as the source of the *ku* poisoning being treated.

The exact number of monographs in the *Pen-ts'ao shih-i* has not come down to us. Later pen-ts'ao works of the main tradition took over a total of 488 *Pen-ts'ao shih-i* monographs of drugs described for the first time in this text. Since the *Pen-ts'ao shih-i* was recognized without reservation as a supplement to the *T'ang pen-ts'ao*, we may assume that the number of 488 monographs is a fairly complete reflection of the contents of the six chapters on "matters that have been neglected." The extent of the other three chapters, however, is completely uncertain.

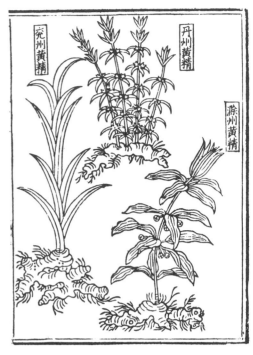

species of Solomon's seal *(huang-ching)*—*Ch'ung-hsiu cheng-ho pen-ts'ao*

During the years 934 to 965, a small state called Hou Shu existed in Szechwan. Its second emperor, Meng Ch'ang (died 992), is generally known for his unpredictable and extravagant life-style; less noted is the fact that during his reign, extensive work was done on the classics and in other areas of literature.

Meng Ch'ang apparently possessed a certain interest in Taoist activities. According to a remark in the official history of the *Wu-tai* period on the state Hou Shu, "Meng Ch'ang intended to devote himself to magical and sexual practices. For this purpose, he filled the rear sections of the palace with numerous daughters of free families."[90] Similar interests in the possibilities of a healthy life-style and the prolongation of life may have created the incentive for ordering a revision of the *T'ang pen-ts'ao*.

The *Ch'ung-kuang ying-kung pen-ts'ao* was written by Han Pao-sheng, an official of the Han-lin Academy, in cooperation with physicians and other scholars. Emperor Meng Ch'ang himself wrote the preface. As the title indicates, the work constitutes an "expansion of Ying-kung's materia medica." *Ying-kung* was an honorary title of Li Chi, the later head of the editorial committee for the *T'ang pen-ts'ao*.

Han Pao-sheng took over the *Hsin-hsiu pen-ts'ao* part of the *T'ang pen-ts'ao* and also inserted a section of the T'ang period "Commentary on the Drug Illustrations" (*T'u-ching*) into the orginal monographs. He strove for a careful revision of the work, and included some com-

4. The *Ch'ung-kuang ying-kung pen-ts'ao*

Ch'ung-kuang ying-kung pen-ts'ao
"Enlarged Materia Medica of the *Ying-kung*"
Short titles: *Shu pen-ts'ao;*
           Shu-pen
20 chapters / number of drugs: unknown
Author: Han Pao-sheng
Written: ca. 934–965
Published: date unknown

mentaries of his own, which were quoted in later pen-ts'ao works as "Commentaries of the Shu Edition" (*Shu-pen chu*).

The *Shu pen-ts'ao* did not contain any illustrations. Li Shih-chen, however, wrote that the *Shu pen-ts'ao* had contained a *T'u-ching*, from which one might also conclude that there had been pictures. Li Shih-chen's error here originates from the unclear method of quotation in a subsequent *Pen-ts'ao* of the main tradition, the *Chia-yu pen-ts'ao* by Chang Yü-hsi (992–1068). In this work one often finds the following remarks at the beginning of quotations: "*Shu-pen t'u-ching:* . . . ." Correctly interpreted, these four characters have the meaning, "The Shu edition [quotes the] *T'u-ching* [of the *T'ang pen-ts'ao* with the following words]: . . . ." Several passages transmitted in the even later *Ta-kuan pen-ts'ao* support this view—for example, the twenty-first chapter:

> The official [Chang] Yü-hsi and his colleagues carefully quote the Shu edition [which says]: "In the *T'u-ching*, [the *tse-shan* cicada] is considered the singing cicada. It is collected, steamed, and dried in the sixth and seventh month." T'ao Hung-ching wrote: "[The *tse-shan* cicada] is the silent cicada. The female cicadas cannot sing." There is a contradiction between these two statements. We will follow the *Yü-p'ien*.[91]

A similar statement can be found in the twenty-seventh chapter of the *Ta-kuan pen-ts'ao*:

> The official [Chang] Yü-hsi had his colleagues quote carefully from the Shu edition, whose commentary reads: Su [Ching] said: "[The white melon seeds] are the sweet melon seeds." The *T'u-ching* reports: "In addition, there are also *hu*-melons with a yellow-red color and no taste." Neither of these statements seems reliable today.[92]

When, and in what form, the *Shu pen-ts'ao* was published is uncertain. It was probably already lost as an independent work during the early Sung period. Only several of the commentaries have come down to us in the form of quotations in the *Chia-yu pen-ts'ao* and *Ta-kuan pen-ts'ao*.

5. The Works in the Main Pen-ts'ao Tradition of the Sung Period

5.1. The intellectual situation during the time of the Northern Sung and its influence on the development of medicine

The Sung period is one of the most important epochs of Chinese intellectual history, and consequently, of Chinese science. The close association of these segments of Chinese culture is clearly evident in the similar influence which the multifaceted changes in Chinese society during the Sung period exerted, for example, at the same time upon philosophy and medical thought.

The characteristics of the intellectual currents, which have often earned the Sung period the designation as a turning point in Chinese history, did not originate by pure chance. The elevation of Confucianism, directed toward secularity and the social order of life, to the state ideology during the Han period had changed Taoism, many adherents of which appear to have turned away from the aspiration of influencing the legal power, into a popular religion which promised the individual the possible fulfillment of his desires even beyond the perceptible world and outside the sphere of earthly temporality. Shortly thereafter, in the first century, Buddhist ideas penetrated into China, soon gaining domination. Above and beyond the beginnings of transcendence of earthly entanglements in Taoism, Buddhism offered a genuine metaphysics with subtle concepts of the redemption of beings in the hereafter. The post-Han period disturbances brought many simple and educated people into close contact with the contents of Buddhism and Taoism. This situation was by no means always a result of religious conviction. Economic necessity or mere opportunism often determined whether one, for example, joined a Buddhist, tax-free monastery, or traveled as a mendicant friar through the countryside.

The strong influence of Buddhism during the T'ang period was paralleled by an opening of the Chinese Empire to the outside world. Traveling monks and extensive trade brought numerous contacts with foreign countries and ideas, which led to a diversity in Chinese intellectual life. To some extent in the T'ang period, but mostly in the Sung period, some scholars strove to reestablish the attraction that Confucianism had visibly lost, by means of a syncretism of the actual socioethical elements of Confucianism, and the Taoist knowledge of nature. In addition, ideas were developed to compete with Buddhist metaphysics. These efforts are given expression in scores of writings in the form of a nationalistic striving for unity that was supposed to supplant the T'ang period's pluralism of world views.[93] The result was the so-called Sung-Neoconfucianism which, first of all, made it theoretically possible to win over to the expanded Confucian ideological system those people who had earlier favored Buddhism or Taoism. Moreover, the interest of Confucians was now expanded to areas previously closed to the Confucian world view. Unlike in the T'ang era, when a cultural blossoming had been carried to China from the outside, Chinese intellectual life during the Sung period developed to a peak from within.

The influence that this movement had on Chinese medicine is complex and occurred in two phases. The first phase rests on the opening and expansion of the Confucian horizon, connected with the inclusion of Taoist and Buddhist elements in the official state philosophy. The syncretic tendency of the Sung-Neoconfucianism influenced medical thinking and pharmaceutical literature only in a second phase at the beginning of the twelfth century, resulting in the so-called Chin-Yüan medicine (to which I have devoted chapter C. sec. II of this book).

During the Sung period, an exceptional governmental interest in medical practice can be observed, an interest which a "pure" Confucianism probably would not have supported. The increased influence of Taoism and the Buddhist therapeutic ethic may be perceptible here.

In this connection, it is important to note that, owing to climatic changes in northern China, large segments of the population began to migrate to the south in the eighth century. Until the middle of the eighth century, only 40 to 45 percent of the Chinese population lived

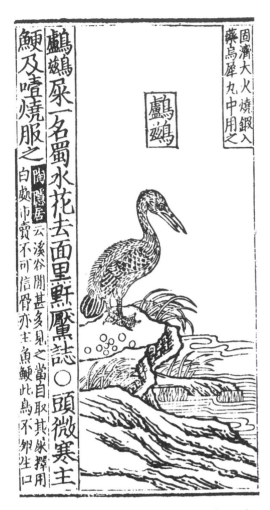

cormorant *(lu-tz'u)—Ch'ung-hsiu cheng-ho pen-ts'ao*

in the Yang-tzu Valley and farther south. Near the end of the thirteenth century, this figure had reached 85 to 90 percent. Many peasants from the plains in the north could find no arable land in the hilly and mountainous countryside of the south, however. Urbanization thus assumed unsuspected proportions.[94] Possibly the government recognized the need for effective medical care for residents of these densely populated areas, where cities with over a million inhabitants were no longer exceptions. The old antipathies against experts practicing medicine could no longer be sustained here. The conditions forced the government into a first welfare system, which brought with it the establishment of a number of apothecary shops under official supervision, on the one hand, and public physicians' clinics, with civil servants or at least physicians in governmental service, on the other.

Other external circumstances, such as the spread of printing, also contributed to the development. The classic writings of Chinese medicine were no longer restricted to the libraries of the emperors and the privileged few. Until the Sung period the medical classics, such as the *Huang-ti nei-ching* and the *Nan-ching,* as well as the *Shang-han lun,* a work on prescriptions, had existed only in a few handwritten copies. These editions were frequently incomplete and riddled with mistakes, in addition to being too expensive for the mass of general practitioners. Consequently, during the pre-Sung centuries the practitioner was restricted to the oral transmission of theories and prescriptions gained through personal experience.

During the Northern Sung period, a department for the editing of medical works was established in the imperial publishing house. The officials Kao Pao-heng, Lin I (ca. 1070), and Sun Ch'i were commissioned to revise the medical works, which were then published. Private publishing houses were founded and followed their example. In this manner broader segments of the population gained access to medical literature, and the formation of educated societies was encouraged. This activity encompassed not only theoretical writings but also those works meant specifically for medical practice, that is, books on prescriptions and the pharmaceutical literature.

5.2. The *K'ai-pao hsin hsiang-ting pen-ts'ao*

K'ai-pao hsin hsiang-ting pen-ts'ao
"Materia Medica, Newly Examined and Determined during the *K'ai-pao* Period"
Short title: *K'ai-pao pen-ts'ao*
21 chapters / 983 drug descriptions
Authors: Liu Han (ca. 975); from: Lin-chin in
    Ts'ang-chou
    Ma Chih (ca. 975)
    Lu To-hsün (?–986); from: Ho-nei in
    Ho-nan
    and others
Written: 973
Published: 973

In the fourteenth year of his rule (973), Emperor T'ai-tsu (927–976), the first sovereign of the Sung dynasty, issued an order to revise the materia medica. For the completion of this task he appointed a board of authors, headed by the high pharmacy official Liu Han and the Taoist Ma Chih. The association of these two personalities symbolizes, on the one hand, a certain polarity, and, on the other hand, the urge for joint action based upon otherwise diverging concepts.

At the side of the practicing Taoist Ma Chih, who had made a name for himself with amazingly effective prescriptions and numerous successful cures, was placed Liu Han, a Confucian scholar-physician, whose family was known for generations for having transmitted medical abilities. In addition, the editorial board included seven officials

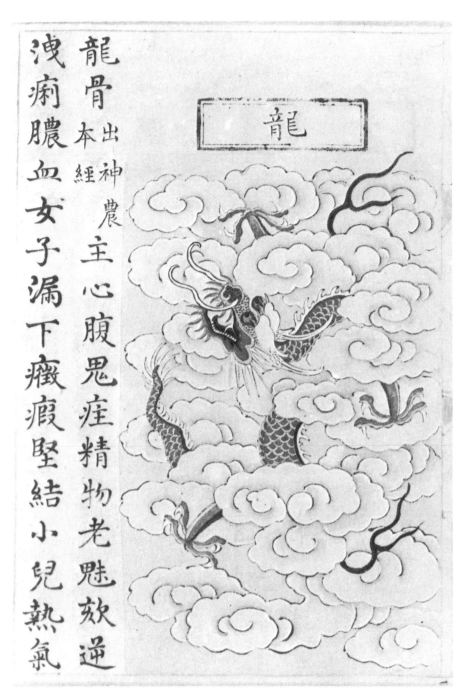

龍骨本經 出神農 主心腹鬼疰精物老魅欬逆洩痢膿血女子漏下癥瘕堅結小兒熱氣

龍

dragon *(lung)—Pen-ts'ao p'in-hui ching-yao*

益氣長肌肉肥健生子○眼平主驚癇腹
白馬莖 本經 出神農 主傷中脉絕陰不起強志

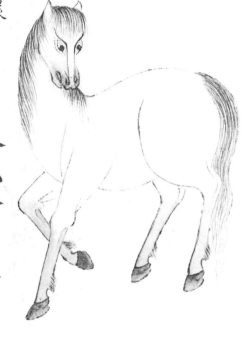

white horse *(pai-ma)—Pen-ts'ao p'in-hui ching-yao*

musk deer *(she)—Pen-ts'ao p'in-hui ching-yao*

毒癰瘡去三蟲頭服除邪不夢寤厭寐 上以
麝香 本經 出神農 主辟惡氣殺鬼精物溫瘧蠱

麝

57

of the Han-lin Academy, among whom the Imperial Physicians Wu
Fu-kuei, Wang Kuang-yu, and Ch'en Chao-yü were especially prominent. Ch'en Chao-yü had attracted the attention of his contemporaries
through his extensive knowledge in the area of pharmaceutics and
medicine. Above all, his precise diagnoses had contributed to his reputation. Like Liu Han, he too came from a family with an obvious
medical tradition. We encounter his name and that of Wu Fu-kuei
again a little later in history, since the second ruler of the Sung dynasty,
Emperor T'ai-tsung (939–997), also appointed them to the editorial
committee of a medical work.

Even as a prince, T'ai-tsung is said to have been very open-minded
towards medical problems and to have established a collection of 1,000
effective prescriptions. After his ascension to the throne, he ordered
all effective secret prescriptions to be published. In the course of this
action, over 10,000 formulas were gathered. Under the direction of
Ch'en Chao-yü, Wu Fu-kuei, and Wang Huai-yin, a former Taoist
monk and later medical official in the directorate of the Han-lin Academy, the results were combined in the extensive prescription collection,
T'ai-p'ing sheng-hui fang.[95]

After Liu Han, Ma Chih, and their colleagues had completed the
manuscript of the revised *Pen-ts'ao,* Lu To-hsün was charged with the
final revision of the work. In contrast with the committee, whose
members (as far as we know) were all considered specialists in the
medical-pharmaceutical field, Lu To-hsün was regarded primarily as
an expert on the Confucian classics and historical works. In 955 he
had passed the central exams, in 979 he rose to president of the War
Ministry. Lu To-hsün is usually named as the author of this first Sung
period materia medica in the main pen-ts'ao tradition. The work,
which comprised twenty chapters of text and an additional chapter
with table of contents, was printed by the government publishing
house.[96]

5.3. The *K'ai-pao ch'ung-ting pen-ts'ao*

Emperor T'ai-tsu does not appear to have been content for very long
with the revision of the materia medica by the authors of the *K'ai-
pao hsin hsiang-ting pen-ts'ao,* for after only one short year, in the
seventh year of the governmental period *k'ai-pao* (974), he issued a
new order to revise the *Pen-ts'ao.*

Again, Liu Han and Ma Chih were charged with the preliminary
work, but this time the final version was prepared by Wang Yu, Hu
Meng (915–986), and Li Fang. Hu Meng was a historian and had
contributed substantially to the preparation of the dynastic history of
the *Wu-tai* period. Both he and Li Fang were also among the authors
of the encyclopedia *T'ai-p'ing yü-lan.* The second official materia medica of the *k'ai-pao* period was published in the same year the order
was issued. Li Fang is commonly given as the author.[97]

The *K'ai-pao hsin hsiang-ting pen-ts'ao* and the *K'ai-pao ch'ung-
ting pen-ts'ao* were jointly designated and quoted as the *K'ai-pao pen-*

K'ai-pao ch'ung-ting pen-ts'ao
"Materia Medica, Newly Determined during
the *K'ai-pao* Period"
Short title: *K'ai-pao pen-ts'ao*
21 chapters / 983 drug descriptions
Authors: Liu Han (ca. 975); from: Lin-chin in
　　Ts'ang-chou
　　Ma Chih (ca. 975)
　　Li Fang (924–995); *tzu:* Ming-yüan;
　　from: Jao-yang in Chih-li
　　and others
Written: 974
Published: 974

ts'ao in later literature. Differences between the contents of the two works can no longer be determined, since both editions were lost as independent works. Most of the commentaries and drug descriptions that had been newly added to previous knowledge in these texts have been preserved in the quotations of subsequent pen-ts'ao works in the main tradition, along with, of course, the preface, which is again able to give us some insight into the problems and working methods of the authors, as well as their self-awareness within the pen-ts'ao tradition.

Of the three great works of antiquity, Shen-nung wrote one. After he had differentiated hundreds of drugs, he recorded his notes in the *Pen-ts'ao*. The three chapters of the old classic were handed down from generation to generation. [In addition,] another work was compiled from the "Additional Notes of Renowned Medical Men." Then, in the Liang period, Cheng-pai T'ao [Hung-] ching combined these "Additional Notes" with the "Original Classic," [but still] distinguished [the two sources] through red and black script. This was considered very clear. Furthermore, [T'ao Hung-ching] examined the applicability [of the drugs] and added appropriate commentaries. Thus, he wrote a total of seven chapters, which were then circulated in the Southern Empire. In the Tang period, another expansion and revision [of the *Pen-ts'ao*] took place; the number of drugs was increased to over 800, with new commentaries raising the total to twenty-one chapters. Whatever was missing in the *Pen-ching* was supplied; T'ao Hung-ching's mistakes were made clear. But after another four centuries, there no longer existed any editions which agreed with respect to the red and black script. Old commentaries were lost in some, extant in others, and vice versa.

If the Cycle of Great Harmony were not subordinated to the [current] emperor's majesty, and if, as a result, our good fortune did not last forever and beyond all boundaries, then how would it be possible to revise and correct [this work]? Therefore, we were ordered to examine thoroughly the errors handed down from the past, and to edit a final work.

If a drug monograph was not arranged correctly, we have changed that. Thus, for example, [the drug] "brush-tip ash" is from rabbit's hair, but it was classified among herbs. We have now arranged [this drug] following [the drug] "hare's skull bones." *Pan-t'ien-ho* and *ti-chiang* are both waters. They, too, were grouped among the herbs. We have now placed them in the group of soils and minerals. We have regrouped [the drug] "old drumskin" with the animal skins, *hu-t'ung-lü* with the tree drugs. *Tzu-k'uang* is also a tree [drug]; we removed it from the section of precious stones and minerals. Bats belong in the group of [flying] animals; we have placed them there from the group of worms and fish. *Chü* and *yu* are now classified as fruits. We have arranged table salt with *kuang-yen;* fresh and dried ginger were combined into one monograph. We have grouped *chi-ch'ang* with *fan-lou,* and *lu-ying* with *shuo-tiao,* because they are of similar type.

Moreover, we consulted the [*Pen-ts'ao*] *shih-i* of Ch'en Ts'ang-ch'i and the [*Pen-ts'ao*] *yin-i* by Li Han-kuang. We have traced some material in works [outside of the *pen-ts'ao* tradition]; the benefits of other material were handed down by physicians. We have examined all this information and separated the useful from the useless. Thus, for example, according to the old interpretation [the drug] *t'u-ch'ü-pai* was classified among ashes. Today, we group it under the tree roots. [The drug] *t'ien-ma-ken* was [until now] considered identical with *ch'ih-chien;* now we know that these two drugs are completely different. Thus we have discarded incorrect [information] and have adopted the facts,

[in this case] establishing a new monograph. The other corrections we
have made are impossible to enumerate here. We have taken into consideration all the opinions of the people and recorded them for printing.
[The share of] Shen-nung was set in white characters, the ["Notes of]
Renowned Medical Men" in black. Additions from the T'ang period
and from modern time have been clearly indicated by commentaries.
The explanations are detailed, appearances and properties (of the drugs)
have been examined. We have marked [our own] clarification of mistakes and the differentiation of unclear points with the words "modern
commentary" (*chin-chu*). Whenever we ourselves have checked literary
records and written down the results [of these examinations], it is indicated by the words "newly examined" (*chin-an*).

今註

今按

In this manner, we have determined meaning and clarified principles.
Old and new drugs now total 983; together with the table of contents,
they have been recorded in twenty-one chapters. May they be widely
circulated in the entire empire.[98]

The two pen-ts'ao works of the k'ai-pao period are the first known
printed Chinese materia medicas. Their structure, as that of the following works in the main tradition, does not show any significant
innovations. They all continued the characteristics of the main tradition and differed mainly in the increasingly comprehensive sources
and in the constantly growing number of drugs and commentaries.

5.4. The *Chia-yu pu-chu Shen-nung pen-ts'ao*

In the second year of the governmental period *chia-yu* (1057), an
imperial decree ordered the officials Chang Yü-hsi, Lin I, Su Sung,
Chang Tung, Ch'in Tsung-ku, and Chu Yu-chang to revise the *K'ai-
pao pen-ts'ao*. Of these six men, only the last two are known as
specialists in the medical-pharmaceutical field. Chang Yü-hsi wrote
geographical treatises; Chang Tung acquired the emperor's good will
on the basis of his knowledge of the Confucian classics.

Chia-yu pu-chu Shen-nung pen-ts'ao
"Shen-nung's Materia Medica, Expanded and
Annotated during the *Chia-yu* Period"
Short titles: *Chia-yu pen-ts'ao;*
 Pu-chu pen-ts'ao
21 chapters / 1084 drug descriptions
Authors: Chang Yü-hsi (992–1068); *tzu:* T'ang-
 ch'ing; from: Yen-ch'eng in Hsü-chou
 Lin I (ca. 1060)
 Su Sung (1020–1101); *tzu:* Tzu-jung;
 from: Nan-an in Ch'üan-chou
 Chang Tung (1019–1067); *tzu:*
 Chung-t'ung; from: K'ai-feng
 and others
Written: 1057–1060
Published: 1061

In 1060, after exactly three years' work, the authors submitted the
completed manuscript to the emperor; after another inspection, it was
published in the year 1061.[99]

The extensive preface, which I give here in its entirety, shows, even
more clearly than those quoted so far, the procedure of the authors
and the sections of the work that they deemed particularly worthy of
emphasis. For the first time, the authors reported difficulties of in-
corporating newly added drugs into the old three-class division. This
classification had apparently already lost any remaining vitality. They
managed the problem by grouping similar items together, and thus
introduced, within the already common arrangement of sections (*pu*),
the subdivision according to relation of types (*lei*); this was carried
out with reference to a similar procedure in the *T'ang pen-ts'ao* which,
however, was not specifically expressed in that work.

部

類

As we shall see, more and more space is devoted to the history of
the development of pen-ts'ao drug literature:

According to old tradition, the *Pen-ts'ao ching* is said to have been
written by Shen-nung. That, however, is not indicated in the classical

本草石之寒溫
原疾病之深淺

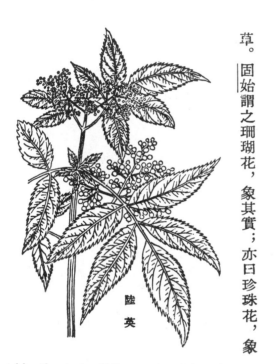

草。

固始謂之珊瑚花，象其實；亦曰珍珠花，象

陸
英

elder *(lu-ying)*—*Chih-wu ming-shih-t'u k'ao*

部
門 類

records. There is no such entry in the section *I-wen chih* of the *Han-shu*. In the annals (of the governmental period) of the Emperor P'ing-ti [8 B.C.–A.D. 6] it is written: "In the fifth year of the governmental period *yüan-shih* [A.D. 5], all scholars of prescription techniques and *pen-ts'ao* from the whole empire were summoned [to the court]. They were sent to the capital by horse drawn carriages." The following sentence is to be found in Lou Hu's biography: "Already at an early age [Lou] Hu had mastered the medical classics, the *pen-ts'ao*, and the art of prescriptions; a total of several 100,000 words." Accordingly, [the term] *pen-ts'ao* appears [for the first time] in these quotations. Li Shih-chi, [whose honorary title was] *ying-kung*, and others cited Pan Ku's annotations for the *Huang-ti nei wai ching* in their commentaries, where it says *pen ts'ao shih chih han wen, yüan chi ping chih shen ch'ien* ["the cold and warm (nature) of herbal and mineral drugs and the different types of illnesses were investigated"]. But this is only a discussion of regulations in the [*Huang-ti nei wai ching*], the term *pen-ts'ao* is not contained in it. Only in the Liang period work *Ch'i-lu* is there a *Shen-nung pen-ts'ao* work with three chapters listed, and [some people are of] the opinion that this is the first [record of this name]. That, however, is a gross mistake. Others have speculated that the names of places of growth and origin of drugs listed [in the *Shen-nung pen-ts'ao*] are terms from the later Han period, and have arrived at the conviction that Chang Chung-ching and Hua T'o should be considered the authors. But that, too, is not true. In the *Huai-nan tzu* it is written: "Shen-nung has tested the tastes of the herbs; in one day he discovered 70 with medicinal effectiveness. This is the beginning of medicine and of prescriptions." There were no written characters in antiquity; the tradition had always been passed from teacher to pupil, and it was called *pen-ts'ao*. During the two Han dynasties, the number of renowned medical practitioners increased greatly. Chang Chi and Hua T'o followed, above all, the old teachings, expanded them through new views, and recorded [this knowledge] in written works. From this time on, the *Pen-ts'ao* appears in the bibliographies of the classics. The oldest edition of the *Pen-ts'ao ching* contained no more than 365 drugs in three chapters. During the Liang period, T'ao Yin-chü contributed the additional notes of renowned medical men, also containing 365 drugs. In addition, he provided [his own] commentaries and divided the entire work into seven chapters. During the T'ang era, at the time of the governmental period *hsien-ch'ing*, the chancellery head of the palace guard, Su Kung, took up the matter of deficiencies and errors [in previous editions] and addressed a petition to the emperor, requesting a definitive new edition. Thereupon, the director for public works, Li Shih-chi *yin-kung*, and others, together with [Su] Kung, were ordered to examine the work for its advantages and disadvantages. Once again, 114 drugs were added and arranged according to a subdivision into natural groups (*men*), sections (*pu*), and related types (*lei*). The whole work was expanded to twenty chapters. It is generally known (under the title) *T'ang pen-ts'ao*. During the present dynasty, at the time of the *k'ai-pao* period [968–975], the emperor ordered the medical practitioner Liu Han and the Taoist Ma Chih to compile a collection [on drugs]. They included another 133 types of drugs which have often been used successfully by medical men, adding them to the existing drug repertory. Subsequently, the emperor ordered Lu To-hsün, Li Fang, Wang Yu, and Hu Meng, scholars at the Han-lin Academy, to write a new definitive edition [of the *Pen-ts'ao*]; this resulted in two publications—the *Hsiang-ting* and *Ch'ung-ting*. Both were published and distributed. From that time on, the medical practitioners were familiar with the suitable [criteria] for the application of drugs. Earlier, Emperor Meng Ch'ang of the unrecognized Shu dynasty had ordered his scholar Han Pao-sheng and others to combine the T'ang edition and the *T'u-ching* into a somewhat expanded compendium. The result was the so-called *Shu-pen-ts'ao*, a work still in circulation today.

Thus, this [*pen-ts'ao*] work has now existed from the Han period to the present, almost exactly 1,000 years. Within this time span it was expanded through constant collection, and one may indeed speak of a great accomplishment.

Medical practitioners, however, are of the opinion that since the [*Pen-ts'ao*] has already been handed down for such a long time and, in later centuries, attempts were always made to add numerous new items, a comparison with the material used today shows that much in the *Pen-ts'ao* is missing or presented too superficially. Therefore, a work should be written now that is completely suited to strengthening life and preventing illnesses.

In the eighth month of the second year of the governmental period *chia-yu* [1057], an imperial order was issued to the officials [Chang] Yü-hsi, [Lin] I, [Su] Sung, and [Chang] Tung to undertake a new revision and correction [of the *Pen-ts'ao*]. Under this order, we have subsequently carried out very thorough examinations and have arrived at the following opinion. The medical practitioners of previous times used drugs according to their diagnoses. If the effect was positive, they wrote it down. Gradually this material increased; an examination of the works today shows that they are extremely varied and can hardly be understood completely. Although new items were added or superfluous ones omitted [for every edition], the selection was different each time. Some things are already recorded in the *Pen-ching*, but in vague and overly simplistic statements. Other things, however, have been used by people for a long time but remained unknown to imperial physicians. Thus, until now no exact description [of pharmaceutics] has existed which was closely oriented on the available facts; for this reason, much [information] has remained unnoticed or scattered. Therefore, our aim was to fill in the gaps and explain the contradictions. So we have selected and combined the uses of all drugs, as they were recorded in the medical works and drug treatises of all kinds of authors. We rejected only those descriptions that seemed too vague to us or absurd. In addition, some rather incidental references to drug effects are also to be found in numerous classics and historical works, although they are not specifically pharmaceutical or dietetic texts. If this information on drug effects was comparatively reliable, we have adopted it as well. We endeavored to create a comprehensive and consistent work, in order to comply with the intent of the imperial order.

Different works are concealed under the title *Pen-ts'ao*. We have consulted the *k'ai-pao ch'ung-ting* edition as a standard work. It is divided into chapters and related types [of drugs], and the original statements of the [*Pen-*]*ching* are interspersed with [later] commentaries. [These two parts of the text, i.e., quotations and commentary] have been differentiated by means of red and black characters. We have followed the old example and there shall be no further reform. When we corrected deficiencies or wrote commentaries, we followed the reference works. If their views were similar to those found in older works, we have made cuts or eliminated such passages entirely, in order to avoid repetition. If some views were recorded incompletely in the old works and then continued in later works, we have given both quotations side by side, in order to create a detailed and easily understandable work.

We have written the beginning characters of each monograph in red as follows: "We officials have carefully examined what the work *x* says about the matter *y*." Whenever we had to write a new, separate monograph, we have added the note "see work *xy*" at the end. n all quotations from books, the *T'ang pen-ts'ao* and the *Shu pen-ts'ao* have been listed first, the remaining works in the chronological order of their composition. In all quotations from works that had earlier [already]

crabs (*hsiu-mou:* right; *yung-chien:* left)—*Hsin-pien lei-yao t'u-chu pen-ts'ao*

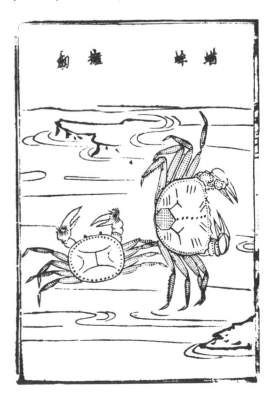

carried the title *Pen-ts'ao,* we have given only the author's name, with the exception of the T'ang and Shu editions, which we cite as "The T'ang edition states" and "The Shu edition states." The division through red and black script is done in such a manner that all parts from the *Shen-nung pen-ching* are written in red characters; on the other hand, all supplements that were added to Shen-nung's old explanations as additional notes of renowned medical men have been marked in black characters to distinguish them from the red ones. All other later additions have been listed in separate sections and in black characters. Everything inserted by T'ao Yin-chü bears the designation *Ming-i pieh-lu,* which is always appended to the section in question. We have marked material added during the *hsien-ch'ing* period by a commentary "first presented in the T'ang edition" (*T'ang-pen hsien-fu*) at the end of each quotation. All material newly added during the *k'ai-pao* period has been marked by the commentary "modern addition" (*chin-fu*). Finally, everything at the end of the quotation that we ourselves have added or supplemented, and which did not yet exist in the old works, is clearly marked with the words "newly supplemented" (*hsin-pu*).

唐本先附

今附

新補

類

All drugs were originally arranged according to an upper, a middle, and a lower class. It is very difficult to arrange the recently added drugs carefully into this pattern. Therefore, we have arranged them according to related types (*lei*) and have, for example, placed [the drug] *lü-fan* after *fan-shih,* *shan-chiang-hua* after *tou-k'ou,* and *fu-i* after *shui-yang.*

續註

If a certain drug and its use were not yet listed in the *Pen-ching* but old commentaries for it existed which are in agreement with modern views [about other drugs], we did not write a separate monograph for it; instead, we added the designation "continued commentary" (*hsü-chu*) as an explanation at the end of the description. Therefore, we have discussed [the drug] *ti-i* following *yüan-i,* *yen-fu* after *t'ung-ts'ao,* and *ma-tsao* after *hai-tsao.*

陶隱居元

唐本註

今註

今詳　今按
　　　　又按

All old commentaries that originate with T'ao have been marked with [the words] "T'ao Yin-chü said" (*T'ao Yin-chü yün*). The commentaries that originate in the *hsien-ch'ing* period bear the note "commentaries of the T'ang edition" (*T'ang-pen chu*), and those from the *k'ai-pao* period are marked as "modern commentary" (*chin-chu*). If, in addition, the origin of the quotations included in [the *Pen-ts'ao*] of the *k'ai-pao* period has been examined and stated, this is made clear by the designations "examined now" (*chin-an*), "now presented in detail" (*chin-hsiang*), or "reexamined" (*yu-an*). These remarks have always been set off from the monograph itself by red characters.

Some drugs are already listed by name in the *Pen-ching,* but their use was not yet described in detail. If such information has been added only now, this [new description] is also to be found at the end of the original commentary.

新定

Some drugs are in general use today but have not yet been listed in any book, so that there is no possibility of identifying and explaining them. Here we must mention, for example, [the drugs] *hu-lu-pa* and *hai-tai.* In such cases, we have asked the imperial medical officials to meet for a joint discussion; we have then recorded the result [of these efforts] in a separate monograph, designating it with the words "newly determined" (*hsin-ting*). The previous number of drugs was 983; 82 drug [monographs] were added by us, not including the additional commentaries. Seventeen drugs were newly determined. The total of new and old monographs is now 1,082. All drugs have been roughly sketched according to their relation of type: there are 15 different groups in all. The meaning of all revisions and explanations is thus made clear. The three prefaces from the older works of the *k'ai-pao* period, the *ying-kung,* and of Mr. T'ao are all of such great significance that we did not want to omit them and have again placed them at the beginning of the work.

Total number of new and old drugs: 1,082. From the *Shen-nung pen-ching:* 360 [drugs]; from the *Ming-i pieh-lu:* 182 [drugs]; first included in the T'ang edition: 114 [drugs]; modern additions: 133 [drugs]; known by name but obsolete: 194 [drugs]; newly supplemented: 82 [drugs]; newly determined: 17 [drugs].[100]

Together with the manuscript, the authors of the *Chia-yu pen-ts'ao* submitted an accompanying letter, in which they also gave a description of the development of their work. This description, in part, corresponds exactly to the one given in the preface. In this report the enumeration of the sources is of particular interest to us. Of the sixteen pen-ts'ao works mentioned among the total of fifty sources, four belong to the main tradition and twelve to the secondary tradition. As through a wide funnel, the most important pharmaceutical information up to that time flowed again into the "official" collection:[101]

Sources from the main pen-ts'ao tradition: *K'ai-pao hsin hsiang-ting pen-ts'ao, K'ai-pao ch'ung-ting pen-ts'ao, T'ang Hsin-hsiu pen-ts'ao,* and *Shu Ch'ung-kuang ying-kung pen-ts'ao.*

Sources from the secondary pen-ts'ao tradition: *Wu-shih pen-ts'ao, Yao-tsung-chüeh, Yao-hsing lun, Yao-tui, Shih-liao pen-ts'ao, Pen-ts'ao shih-i, Ssu-sheng pen-ts'ao, Shan-fan pen-ts'ao, Pen-ts'ao hsing shih lei, Nan-hai yao-p'u, Shih-hsing pen-ts'ao,* and *Jih-hua tzu chu-chia pen-ts'ao.*

5.5. The *T'u-ching pen-ts'ao*

Following the example of the *T'ang pen-ts'ao,* which consisted of a monograph section (the *Hsin-hsiu pen-ts'ao*), drug illustrations (the *Yao-t'u*), and several chapters of commentaries on these illustrations (*Yao-ching*), nearly the same group of authors who compiled the *Chia-yu pen-ts'ao* was charged with the task of writing an annotated volume of illustrations for it at the same time.

They explained their work in the preface:

In antiquity, Shen-nung tried the tastes of all herbs, in order to provide relief for the sufferings and illnesses of humanity. Posterity [therefore honors] him as teacher and ancestor. From this origin, the *pen-ts'ao* learning developed. During the Han and Wei dynasties, famous medical practitioners continuously passed down respective books; there were the drug registers by Wu P'u and Li Tang-chih, and the commentaries by T'ao Yin-chü and Su Kung. At the beginning of the present dynasty, court officials were twice ordered by the emperor to compile, with the help of outstanding medical practitioners, the statements of all authors [in this field]. The result was the *K'ai-pao ch'ung-ting pen-ts'ao.* The information it contained concerning harmless and medicinally effective [drugs], cold and warm nature, and sweet or bitter taste [of drugs] can be called detailed and complete. But the products from all five cardinal points require different [handling] because of [the respective] climatic conditions and influences (prevailing at their places of origin), and there are many names and species. Mistakes are difficult to distinguish. Thus [the drug] *hui-ch'uang* is presented as [being similar to the drug] *mi-wu, chi-ni* is incorrectly passed off as *jen-shen.* Even the people in

T'u-ching pen-ts'ao (also: *Pen-ts'ao t'u-ching*)
"Materia Medica with Illustrations"
21 chapters / 634 drug descriptions
Authors: Su Sung (1020–1101); *tzu:* Tzu-jung; from: Nan-an in Ch'üan-chou
Chang Yü-hsi (992–1068); *tzu:* T'ang-ch'ing; from: Yen-ch'eng in Hsü-chou
and others
Written: 1058–1062
Published: 1062

antiquity already suffered from these errors, but all the more so do modern medical practitioners, for the drugs they use come from the markets, and the markets obtain the drugs from the people who gather them in the wilderness. These people gather as they please, at any time, and the origin of the drugs is never checked later. If one uses these products for the treatment and cure of illnesses, must not the achievement of this goal lie far in the distance? Earlier [in the T'ang era] during the *yung-hui* period [650–655], there were also "[drug] illustrations" and "commentaries" on these, in addition to the revised *Pen-ts'ao*. They supplemented each other and were widely circulated. The illustrations noted the appearance and color [of drugs]; the commentaries pointed out differences and similarities. [Both parts were] compiled at the emperor's order. Furthermore, there was the *T'ien-pao tan-fang yao-t'u* ["Illustrations of Drugs Employed in One-Ingredient Prescriptions, from the *t'ien-pao* period"]. The discussions [in these works] of all matters were so true-to-life and detailed that one easily perceived a correct treatment. Suitable criteria existed for the combination of prescriptions. Both of these works have been lost already for a long time; hardly anything of them is extant. Even in the closed libraries of the capital, there is not a single copy. Only one chapter still exists from the prescription book of the *t'ien-pao* period [742–755], from which one can roughly see the division and explore the structure of the entire work. Apparently [it is a book] for which a wise ruler and an intelligent minister devoted their entire attention to the collection and arrangement [of the material]. At the beginning [of the present period], Confucian officials were ordered by the emperor to revise anew the *Shen-nung pen-ts'ao* and seven other works. The archivist [Chang] Yü-hsi, [whose honorary title is] *kuang-lu ch'ing*, [Lin] I, the secretary for sacrifices in the ministerial council and archive editor, [Su] Sung, professor in the office of imperial sacrifices and editor in the imperial library, Chien, the executive secretary in the palace chancellery, and [Kao] Pao-heng, executive secretary in the office of imperial banquets, were chosen for this task. In addition, the order was also issued to the two medical officials Ch'in Tsung-ku and Chu Yu-chang. The annotations and editing extended over several years, but finally the *Pu-chu pen-ts'ao* was completed and presented to the emperor. The emperor then issued another order that, in all *chün* and *hsien* administrative districts, samples of all herbs growing in these areas be recorded in illustrations and sent to the court. Originally, on the basis of the old example of [the compilation of the *T'u-ching* during] the *yung-hui* period, a new order for a compilation [of commentaries on the requested illustrations from all over the country] was issued. However, the official [Chang] Yü-hsi remarked that all works should be examined and corrected, taking into account all possible views; in this manner, good results could be achieved. If, however, the individual treatises came from different hands, the work as a whole would not be a uniform product. The thousands of different [drug] specimens that have now been drawn in illustrations in the empire and presented to the court represent, in their commentaries and arrangements, only those which the respective medical practitioners have heard and seen. Thus, there are detailed and superficial explanations, and the mode of expression is often based on overly simplified language. If one specific [expert] were not charged with the task of going through and comparing the entire material and correcting the explanations in a suitable language, it would not be possible to bring order into this work, and it would be difficult to use this book and the information that is sought. Therefore, [Chang Yü-hsi] pointed out that the official [Su] Sung had, for a long time, shown profound interest in this work, and that he should be placed in charge of the preparation of the edition. The official [Su] Sung received the order and collected all records. He arranged [the drugs] according to related groups, prepared annotations,

光 祿 卿

chianghuo rhizomes *(ch'iang-huo)—Ch'ung-hsiu cheng-ho pen-ts'ao*

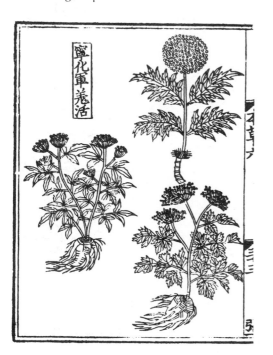

and established sequences, and made rough divisions into monographic sections; these were further divided according to the names of precious stones, minerals, metals, and soils, and, further, according to the distinctions between herbs, trees, worms, and fish. If different geographical regions had been given as the place of origin for one and the same item, and if completely different drugs were concealed behind the same name and appearance, he consulted old and new statements and adopted them all [in spite of their contrary nature], for reciprocal explanation. If, for example, the old information concerning the strength of roots and stalks or the degree of maturity of blossoms and fruits completely contradicted [more recent statements], he nevertheless adopted both. If a summary was incomplete, he included some old commentaries in order to complete the meaning of the argument. If the commentaries were insufficient, he also used explanations from outside sources, from classics or historical works, from other medical works and novels, in order to trace and comprehend the beginning and origin [of the point in question]. For example, [the drug] *lu-ying* was incorrectly claimed to be *shuo-tiao-hua*. Here the explanations of the *Erh-ya* were used to discuss [this particular drug]. All aromatic drugs are basically the same. Here, the *Ling-piao lu-i* was used for proof. The *Pen-ching* served as the first source for the places of drug origin. The suitable places of origin for the present were added as secondary. [The drug] *t'u-szu*, for example, originally comes from Korea; today, however, it comes from Yüan-chü. [The drug] *hsi-tu* previously came from Shao-shih; today one receives it from San-shu. If there were different opinions concerning the [best] times [for collection of an item, and concerning] collectible [parts], the author included them all together. For example, the *Pen-ching* states that only the root of [the drug] *ch'ih-chien* should be gathered. Today, however, the stalks and shoots are also taken. In the matter of [drugs] that originate abroad, [Su Sung] has followed oral reports and written records. For example, it is said today only that [the two drugs] *yü-hsieh* and *yü-ch'üan* are both jade and come from Yü-nieh. But one does not investigate the background—how they are obtained. In this case the *P'ing-chü hui hsing-ch'eng chi* was used as a source. [Su Sung] arranged the drugs, which are divided into the upper, middle, and lower class, according to the *Pen-ching*. [Those drugs] that strongly resemble one another with respect to properties but are not really well known, and [those drugs] that come from distant regions and cannot be described correctly, were appended to a preceding monograph. [The drug] *sou-su*, for example, was discussed following *kou-ch'i*, [the drug] *hou-p'o* following *fu-ling*. Furthermore, in ancient prescription works, the people of former times, restricting themselves to simple [language] and essential [points], had already recorded the obvious effects [of certain drugs] that are in frequent use up to this very day. [These] as well as those drugs that have proven their effectiveness in the practice of physicians from all possible regions for a long time already, were also all recorded with their prescription formulas. The work from the *t'ien-pao* period served as a model. We have not dared to record further material not yet handed down in the literature, and which also cannot be explained by modern medical practitioners, because the [resulting] text would have consisted of forced interpretations based on personal opinions and superficial views. In addition, there are those drugs that are used by modern medical men but are not listed in the old texts. These were included at the end of the [appropriate] chapters, according to their relationships [with the other drugs described already]. They were designated by the term "[Drug] types [listed] outside of the original scriptures" (*pen-ching wai-lei*). However, those [drugs] from this group whose use has proven to be particularly effective, and whose names resemble [drugs] long recorded [in the *Pen-ts'ao*], have been inserted immediately following the respective monographs [of those items they

"stone snakes," fossils *(shih-she)—Ch'ung-hsiu cheng-ho pen-ts'ao*

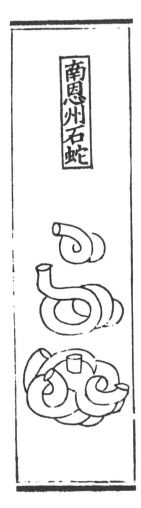

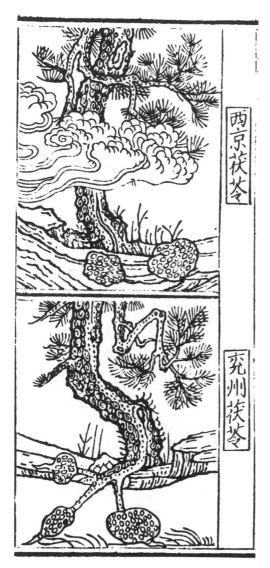

fungus sclerotium *(fu-ling)—Ch'ung-hsiu cheng-ho pen-ts'ao*

resemble]. [The drug] *t'ung-t'o*, for example, appears after *mu-t'ung*, [the drug] *shih-she* follows *shih-hsieh*. The whole work has twenty chapters and an additional chapter with the table of contents.[102]

The imperial decree for the procurement of illustrative material from all areas of the empire, mentioned at the beginning of the preface, was published in 1058 as the result of a petition by the authors. The decree stated, among other things:

> Shape, color, and size of roots, stalks, shoots, leaves, blossoms, and fruits, as well as worms, fish, birds, quadrupeds, precious stones, and minerals, if suitable for pharmaceutical use, should be drawn in illustrations one by one, accompanied by an explanatory comment, describing, for every single object, the time of blooming, of ripening of the fruit, and of gathering, as well as the use and effect [of the drugs in question]. Concerning [those] drugs that come from other countries, inquiries must be made at custom posts, in all boroughs and marketplaces, on ocean ships and with merchants and visitors. [The foreign drugs] are to be included on the basis of these [inquiries]. The evidence [gathered in this manner is] to serve as a basis for the creation of *pen-ts'ao* illustrations. In addition, commentaries are to be written for the illustrations. [Illustrations and commentaries are then] to be distributed with the *Pen-ts'ao* [compiled in the] present [governmental period], so that in the future, the appropriate criteria for the use of drugs will be known to the people.[103]

The number of drugs described in the *T'u-ching pen-ts'ao*—634— was 250 fewer than the number of monographs in the *Chia-yu pen-ts'ao*. It is likely that most of the drugs not listed were imported from foreign countries and therefore were not available in the original form— plant, animal, and mineral—necessary for the drawings. Other drugs described in the *Chia-yu pen-ts'ao* were perhaps known only through hearsay and thus could not be obtained. Furthermore, there were numerous drugs whose illustrations would scarcely have been useful— for example, those of drugs derived from humans; after all, it was rarely the item used as medication that was to appear in the illustrations but rather the original herb, animal, or mineral from which a drug was produced. Finally, we do not know the effect of the above-mentioned decree.

Some drug commentaries in the *T'u-ching pen-ts'ao* contained several illustrations of different variations of one and the same item, resulting in a total of 917 illustrations.

Like the *Chia-yu pen-ts'ao*, the *T'u-ching pen-ts'ao* has been lost as an independent work, and only fragments of its text can be reconstructed from quotations in later works. The type of illustrations is completely unknown to us, unless we justly assume that the illustrations in the *Ta-kuan pen-ts'ao* of 1108, the first pen-ts'ao work of the main tradition that has been completely preserved, were taken over from the *T'u-ching pen-ts'ao*. In the subsequent illustrated pen-ts'ao works of the Sung period, there seems to have been no urge to prepare new illustrations of the plants, animals, and minerals for each new edition of the materia medica—unless they were listed for the first time. The revised editions adapted not only the old texts but also the

old illustrations from preceding works. Therefore, it is possible that
the illustrations that are still available today from the above-mentioned
pen-ts'ao edition of 1108 originate with sketches from the *T'u-ching
pen-ts'ao*. Li Shih-chen appears to have seen the *T'u-ching pen-ts'ao*
in the sixteenth century. He wrote:

> During the Sung period, Emperor Jen-tsung [1010–1063] ordered
> Chang Yü-hsi and others to write a *pen-ts'ao* [work]. It was completed
> after several years. In addition, he issued an order that illustrations of
> the drugs should be sent to the court from all districts in the whole
> empire. [A similar decree from] the *yung-hui* period during the T'ang
> era served as a model. The professor in the Imperial Office of Sacrifices,
> Su Sung, was specifically charged with the completion of this work. It
> contains a total of twenty-one chapters. Its statements are detailed and
> clear. It attained a wide circulation. However, illustrations and texts do
> not correspond. Some illustrations remained without explanations; in
> other cases the drug is described, but the illustration is missing! In
> addition, the wrong picture was occasionally added to the commentary.[104]

5.6. The *Ch'ung-kuang pu-chu Shen-nung pen-ts'ao ping t'u-ching*

The first pen-ts'ao work of the main tradition compiled on private
initiative during the Sung period was written by Ch'en Ch'eng, a
physician from Liang-chung. As we learn from the following preface,
as a medical practitioner he was disturbed by the fact that the monographs of the *Chia-yu pen-ts'ao* and the only very briefly annotated
illustrations of the *T'u-ching pen-ts'ao* were contained in two separate
works. He saw the most important goal of his own contribution in
combining, for the first time, the drug monographs with the appropriate illustrations, thereby substantially facilitating the use of the pen-
ts'ao literature for the practitioner.

We also encounter in this preface the first harsh criticism of what
is apparently a large number of medical practitioners. Such criticism
certainly cannot be understood only as politeness on the part of the
author of the preface, Lin Hsi, towards the author of the work, so as
to set him off against his colleagues in this manner. We must probably
view these critical remarks, which will occur frequently from this time
until the Ch'ing period, as the beginning of a conflict with those groups
of physicians to whom the main pen-ts'ao tradition no longer seemed
the *non plus ultra* of pharmaceutical literature and drug knowledge,
and whose opinions were reflected in the works of the so-called Chin/
Yüan tendency, the second phase of Neoconfucian influence on medical
thought:

> Just as a good physician is unable to cure any illnesses without med-
> ications, a talented general cannot conquer any enemies without sol-
> diers. The soldiers can easily be recognized as such by their appearance;
> he who makes masterly use [of them] is able to preserve men's lives by
> means of their abilities to kill. In comparison, the qualities of drugs are
> difficult to comprehend; he who does not use them to perfection will
> kill people with their powers of preserving life! This is frightening,
> indeed!

Ch'ung-kuang pu-chu Shen-nung pen-ts'ao ping t'u-ching
"Shen-nung's Materia Medica, Enlarged, Re-
vised, and Annotated, and Combined with the
Volume of Illustrations"
Short title: *Ch'ung-kuang pen-ts'ao t'u-ching*
23 chapters / number of drug descriptions:
unknown
Author: Ch'en Ch'eng
        from: Liang-chung in Szu-chuan
Published: 1092

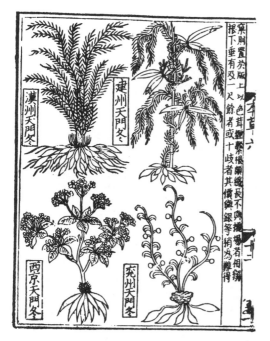

asparagus root (t'ien-men-tung), Ch'ung-hsiu
cheng-ho pen-ts'ao

[There are drugs with] cold, hot, cool, and warm [nature, with] acrid or sweet [taste, and drugs which are] able to act slowly or quickly, each in all variations imaginable. So who would be capable of distinguishing all this except for [Shen-nung who discovered] seventy medicinally effective [drugs] in one single day? Countless prescriptions have been handed down from ancient times by the *Yü-han* [*fang*], the *Chin-kuei* [*yao-lüeh*], the *Chou-hou* [*pei-chi fang*], the *Nang-chung*, and the *Ch'ien-chin* [*fang*], or were secretly stored in the Outer Tower (*Wai-t'ai pi-yao*). Taking these [books] as a starting point, one may say that the difficulties [of using drugs] are not only in taking the pulse [of the patient] and then administering the [appropriate] prescription but mainly in distinguishing the drugs. The treasures among the metals and minerals, the marvelous in the area of herbs and trees, and the great number of animals or plants that fly in the air or hide in waters are exceedingly abundant. Moreover, the winds and the climatic influences differ [regionally and seasonally]; north and south are not the same. Some articles do not exist in China, others are unattainable with human power alone. Whoever wants to master the distinction of right and wrong is offered the possibility by the *Pen-ts'ao* and the *T'u-ching* of not being uncertain for even one moment. . . . [Now follows the usual description, omitted here, of the development of the *pen-ts'ao* literature from Shen-nung to Su Sung's *T'u-ching*.] But the medical practitioners of our time practice what is old and preserve what is common. Their false ideas border on absurdity. They acquire a number of guidelines for the preparation of decoctions, and if they are lucky they may have frequent success. They themselves call this sufficient to be able to cure all illnesses. But if their talk is more closely examined, their carelessness and ignorance [become apparent]. They consider the *Pen-ts'ao* and the *T'u-ching* to be almost senseless writings. Even if there were someone in remote provinces and unimportant places who would be willing to take [these works] into consideration, who would sell them to him? Already in his youth, Ch'eng, of the Ch'en family from Liang-chung, showed pleasure in studying. He was especially enthusiastic about medicine. It is said that he understood the teachings of all authors. He regretted that the circulation of the two works mentioned above [the *Pen-ts'ao* and the *T'u-ching*] was limited, and that those who endeavored to study them did not have access to both of them. For this reason, he combined them into one work, further expanding them by statements from earlier and more recent times, as well as by knowledge he had acquired through his own ears and eyes. He arranged the work in twenty-three chapters and entitled it *Ch'ung-kuang pu-chu Shen-nung pen-ts'ao ping t'u-ching*. It contains both the written explanations [of the drugs] and the illustrations which show the appearance [of the drugs]. Thus one needs to open only one book cover to have both parts. It has become unnecessary to travel to foreign places and remote areas, to mountain tops and river banks: The ten-thousandfold multiplicity lies immediately before the eyes [of each reader]. When one looks at maps and statistics in a discussion of geographic problems, or when one goes into the armory to inspect war weapons, the situations are similar.

For generations, Ch'eng's ancestors were generals and ministers. This is what master Ou-yang means when he says, "In four generations six lords." Ch'eng was their great-grandson and had already lost his father while still a youth. He then devoted himself to his mother, living in the area between the Yang-tzu and the river Wei. He locked his door [to visitors] and fed her a vegetarian diet. Noble men called him a person who exercises true filial piety. At that time, a strange illness appeared. Numerous physicians failed with their knowledge and knew no way out. Ch'eng carried out conscientious pulse-diagnoses and then explained that taking a specific medication in a specific preparation would provide the cure. This proved to be true in all cases without exception. This demonstrates that while Ch'eng's learning may have been based on illustrations and books, his intellectual wisdom was beyond comparison. How could anyone define the borders of both? Kuei Yü-ch'ü and Ch'i Po are [persons] of a distant past now; I have no way of becoming acquainted with them. But if one looks at how Ch'in Yüeh-jen, Shun-yü I, Ts'ang-kung and Hua T'o acted [in treating illness], this is what the educated should be able to familiarize himself with! Preface by [the official] Lin Hsi, written during the new moon, in the ninth month of the seventh year of the *yüan-yu* period [1092].[105]

This work, too, was soon outdated and was eventually lost. Some of Ch'en Ch'eng's own commentaries have been preserved in the *Cheng-lei pen-ts'ao* by T'ang Shen-wei (ca. 1082). In his own work, he had introduced them with the words "further statements" (*pieh-shuo*); in the *Cheng-lei pen-ts'ao* they are quoted as "further statements say . . ." (*pieh-shuo yün*).[106]

別說

別說云

5.7. The *Ching-shih cheng-lei pei-chi pen-ts'ao*

The last phase and, at the same time, the climax in the development of the pen-ts'ao works of the main tradition was initiated by a physician named T'ang Shen-wei. Like Ch'en Ch'eng, he came from Szechwan, the Chinese province richest in drugs, and he wrote his materia medica with similar intentions. He, too, combined, on private initiative, the *Chia-yu pen-ts'ao* with the *T'u-ching pen-ts'ao* into a single work more suitable for the practitioner. T'ang Shen-wei, however, did not stop with this combination, but inserted 662 additional monographs of drugs which had not yet been described in the *Pen-ts'ao*, and whose names he marked with a black border; moreover, he expanded the work by approximately 2,900 instructions for the application of individual drugs (*tan-fang*), which greatly increased the practical benefits of the work.

Ching-shih cheng-lei pei-chi pen-ts'ao
"Materia Medica, Annotated, Arranged by Types, Organized for Speedy Use, and Based upon the Classics and Historical Works"
Short title: *Cheng-lei pen-ts'ao*
31 chapters / 1744 drug descriptions
Author: T'ang Shen-wei
        tzu: Shen-yüan
        from: Chin-yüan in Szu-chuan
Written: between 1080 and 1107
Published: see *Ta-kuan pen-ts'ao*

單方

Unlike Ch'en Ch'eng, who expressed his own opinions in the commentaries he wrote, T'ang Shen-wei preferred to quote the views of other authors and did not present his own.[107]

With respect to the sources T'ang Shen-wei consulted for his work, it is important to remark that the later annotators of the *Cheng-lei pen-ts'ao* pointed out that T'ang took into consideration the Confucian classics and historical works, the Taoist canon, and, thirdly, the literature of Buddhism. This may reflect the tendencies of Sung Neoconfucianism.

T'ang Shen-wei referred to a total of approximately 250 sources. Nine of these belonged to the *Pen-ts'ao* category, 89 titles came from other medical literature, and of the remaining works, 35 were Taoist, and 1 was Buddhist.[108]

While in his youth, Yü-wen Hsü-chung (1079–1146), a scholar from Hua-yang in Szechwan, had met T'ang Shen-wei. In the afterword of a later, revised edition of T'ang's work, he wrote:

T'ang Shen-wei—his *tzu*-name was Shen-yüan—came from Hua-yang in Ch'eng-tu. His manners were very simple, his language natural and reserved. He was, however, extremely intelligent; he was able to cure every illness he treated. He usually said only little about the symptoms and the further progress of the illness. If one asked him again, he became quite angry and answered nothing. He did not differentiate people according to rich and poor. When he was called [to a patient], he complied without fail. Neither cold nor heat, neither rain nor snow could detain him. When he gave medical treatment to scholars, he did not take any money, but he asked these people for famous prescriptions and secret records. He was, therefore, extremely well liked by scholars. Whenever they came upon the name of a drug or found the discussion of a prescription in the classics or historical works, they copied it and gave it to [T'ang Shen-wei]. He collected [all of this] and then wrote the present work. The executive secretary to the Ministry Council of the Left, Mr. P'u Ch'uan-cheng, wanted T'ang Shen-wei to accept the position of an official entitled to petition on the basis of political merits. But [T'ang Shen-wei] excused himself and did not accept the offer. His two sons [aged] fifty-one and fifty-four—unfortunately, their names have been forgotten—and son-in-law, Chang Tsung-shuo—whose *tzu* was Yen-lao—carried on all the abilities [of T'ang Shen-wei]: they were well-known medical practitioners in Ch'eng-tu. At the time of the *yüan-yu* governmental period [1086–1093], when I was still a child, my late grandfather suffered from being affected by wind poison. Shen-yüan cured him as if he were a spirit. In addition, he sealed a written directive and determined in advance on which day of which year and month it should be reopened. At this time, the old illness reappeared and one looked at the contents of the opened note. It contained three prescriptions. The first one concerned the treatment of a recurrence of the wind poison, the second one dealt with the treatment of wind poison slowly attacking the upper [parts of the body] with the result that one feels an urge to pant and cough. [My grandfather] followed the instructions of T'ang Shen-wei in taking [the prescribed medications] and was completely cured after half a month. From this can be seen the miraculous skills of that [medical practitioner]. Written during the full moon in the ninth month of the third year of the *huang-t'ung* governmental period [1143] by Yü-wen Hsü-chung from Ch'eng-tu.[109]

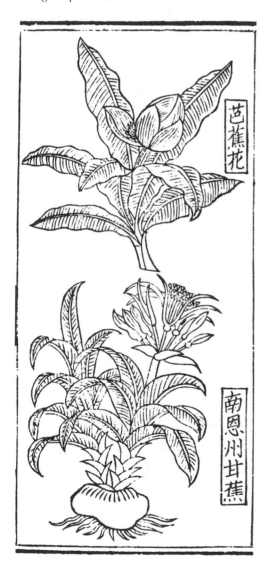

banana blossoms (*pa-chiao-hua:* above) and bananas (*kan-chiao:* below)—*Ch'ung-hsiu cheng-ho pen-ts'ao*

A precise dating of T'ang Shen-wei's life has not yet been possible. Various studies suggest that he was occupied with the revision and expansion of the *Pen-ts'ao* since at least the year 1080. Watanabe Kōzo assumed that, in the years 1082–1083, when P'u Ch'uan-cheng held the post of an official responsible for the transmission of petitions in Ch'eng-tu, the capital of Szechwan, he offered a position to T'ang Shen-wei, expressing recognition of his merits in the revision of the *Pen-ts'ao*.[110] The completion of the manuscript apparently took place after 1097, since the latest work quoted by T'ang Shen-wei bears a date from this year.[111]

The manuscript remained unpublished for the time being. It is nevertheless the first work of the main pen-ts'ao tradition to have been preserved, since it was published some time after its completion by someone other than the author and also under a different title, and since, unlike the preceding works in the main tradition, it was not subsequently superceded by any actual revision.

5.8. The *Ching-shih cheng-lei ta-kuan pen-ts'ao*

Only a few years after its completion, the as yet unpublished manuscript of T'ang Shen-wei's *Cheng-lei pen-ts'ao* came into the hands of two literati, the officials Sun Ti and Ai Ch'eng. Under the patronage of Sun Ti, Ai Ch'eng added forty-four commentaries from the only recently published work of Ch'en Ch'eng and Lin Hsi's preface, as well as his own introduction to the manuscript. Owing to an imperial taboo on the character Shen, T'ang's personal name is given here as Chin-wei:

> In ancient times it was said: Among all things that exist between Heaven and Earth, there is nothing that does not also find use between Heaven and Earth. This is truly so! Just look at what is listed in the *Pen-ts'ao*. Everything from precious stones, minerals, herbs, trees, worms, fish, fruits, and vegetables to dirty clothes, bruised furs, airborne dust, and collected filth is useful in curing illness.
>
> The old classic of Shen-nung consisted of only three chapters. The number of drugs was limited to a few hundred. During the Liang period, T'ao Yin-chü took over this work and doubled [its size]. During the T'ang period, the work was adopted by Su Kung and Li Chi and their colleagues and expanded again. In this manner, the work achieved a thorough degree of completion. Already during the governmental periods *k'ai-pao* [968–975] and *chia-yu* [1056–1063] of the present dynasty, several Confucian officials were ordered to discuss and compile [this work anew]. They were to prepare again an extensive collection. Everything that had previously been disregarded, that had been known by name but not used, and was in use but not recorded, was supposed to be taken into account and included in these editions. Since numerous drugs were added, [the total number of all monographs] rose to more than 1,000. Almost nothing was left out.
>
> Medical men, prescription specialists, and even peasants and old village women achieve, from time to time, speedy and inexplicable successes with prescriptions from individual drugs or strange ingredients. Much of this was not recorded in earlier works and remained unknown to larger circles. In response to this situation [T'ang] chin-wei, on the basis of what he saw and heard, acquired an extensive collection and carefully recorded everything. In addition to those drugs already contained in the *Pen-ts'ao* and *T'u-ching*, he became acquainted with several hundred more articles. In addition, he took from the prescription works, from the classics and from specialized literature, from biographical reports, from Buddhist writings, and from the Taoist canon, whatever was recorded on the effects of items and which should be made known, placing it beside the [descriptions] of the original drugs. In this manner, he composed a text containing more than 600,000 characters, with thirty-one chapters, and an additional chapter devoted to the table of contents. The title of this work is *Ching-shih cheng-lei pei-chi pen-ts'ao*. One can see the strength and care that T'ang chin-wei devoted to it. However, the work was not distributed and was only rarely mentioned. [The manuscript] finally came into the possession of the literary official Sun [Ti], who valued it highly. In his spare time, outside of his duties for the state, he commissioned an official to revise and correct [the work again], and then had it cut into printing plates. He thus intended to promote the circulation of the work. This shows the humanity in his character.
>
> Illnesses do not necessarily have to kill people, but it often happens that medicines do! Medical men today seldom make the effort to as-

Ching-shih cheng-lei ta-kuan pen-ts'ao
"Materia Medica of the *Ta-kuan* Period, Annotated and Arranged by Types, Based upon the Classics and Historical Works"
Short title: *Ta-kuan pen-ts'ao*
31 chapters / 1744 drug descriptions
Authors: T'ang Shen-wei (end of the 11th century); from: Chin-yüan in Szu-chuan
Ai Ch'eng (ca. 1100); *tzu:* Tzu-hsien; from: Chen-chou
Written: see *Cheng-lei pen-ts'ao*
Published: 1108

certain whether the nature of a root is warm or cool, or whether its effect occurs slowly or violently. On the basis of false opinions they increase or decrease [the number of drugs in prescriptions]. When they use [such medications] for the treatment of illnesses, it happens often enough that luck is not with them and that the lives [of patients] are endangered. How is this different from grabbing a spear and stabbing somebody to death in bed? If someone thinks [about these problems] and goes so far as to conduct investigations, he will consult literature in order to explore the theories under consideration. He will check illustrations to be certain about the appearance of things and study prescriptions, so as to recognize their effectiveness. As a consequence, he does not have to wait until [he has discovered] seventy medicinally effective [herbs] in order to know the drugs, and until he has healed a triple fracture of the upper arm until he knows medicine. If there [are now people who act in] such [a responsible manner], the dissemination of the present work will be of enormous benefit to all!

Chin-wei's family name was T'ang. Who he was is not known to me. Those who handed down his work omitted a description of his birth-place and family. I can contribute nothing on this subject.

In the tenth month of the second year of the *ta-kuan* period [1108]. Preface by Ai Ch'eng, police president of the administrative district Jen-ho in the prefecture Hang-chou, with the rank of a *t'ung-shih lang* and jurisdiction over educational matters.[112]

通仕郎

The official whom Sun Ti commissioned was probably Ai Ch'eng himself. In the same year in which Ai Ch'eng's preface is dated, 1108, Sun Ti arranged the printing and publication of the work. The so-called *ta-kuan* edition of the *Cheng-lei pen-ts'ao* has been handed down continuously to the present day. The oldest existing editions in China were printed in 1211 and 1302.

After the first edition in 1108, the work was reprinted numerous times during the Sung period and in the following centuries. Despite later editions, with only negligible revisions, the original did not fall into oblivion. The second edition appeared in 1185; in 1195, only ten years later, another printing was necessary. After the above-mentioned version of 1211, there are editions known from the Chin period (1214), and Yüan period (1302), and later.[113]

5.8.1. The structure and contents of the *Ta-kuan pen-ts'ao*

It was unavoidable that the continuous combination of old and new material in the pen-ts'ao works of the main tradition resulted in poorly arranged encyclopedias, filled with repetitions and contradictions. The reader was offered a bundle of differing opinions from various authors in widely separated time periods, from which he could choose the suitable answers for his particular questions. This conservatism of form, which I mentioned at the beginning of the characterization of the main pen-ts'ao tradition, finally led into a dead-end and, along with the other factors, caused the demise of the tradition itself.

The hesitation of authors to make decisions whose consequences would not only have been the rejection of antiquated opinions but the exclusion of them in the first place, inflated the pen-ts'ao works more

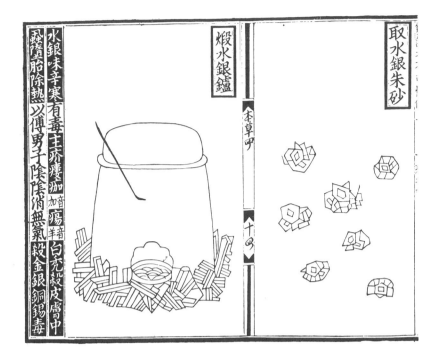

cinnabar (*tan-sha:* right) and oven for the production of quicksilver *(shui-yin)*—*Ta-kuan pen-ts'ao*

and more, prevented sufficient recognition of the real innovations, and, probably most important, continually diminished the practical benefits of these texts. Practitioners confronted with pressing questions of curative treatment needed concrete answers, not a history of the development of each individual opinion—even though it certainly was of literary interest!

As the prefaces have demonstrated sufficiently, the authors of the pen-ts'ao compendia were quite aware of the need for continuously corrected information. Perhaps the unfortunate form they adopted was necessary—in a Confucian society, whose essential pillars included fundamentalism—in order to express, under this cover, many new opinions and discoveries which stood in blatant contradiction to the original ones.

Another kind of development, the presentation of only new and correct information, might have led inevitably to splinter movements; representatives of a "traditional direction" might have accused proponents of modernization of a lack of understanding for time-honored traditions. As it happened, however, everything was collected under one roof, though at the price of practical use. The *Cheng-lei pen-ts'ao,* along with the subsequent, only negligibly revised editions, marked the saturation point and, thus, the necessary conclusion of this development. Its structure, given in detail below for purposes of comparison with the earlier works in the main pen-ts'ao tradition, beginning with the *Pen-ching,* reflects strikingly what has been said:

Chapter 1
Ai Ch'eng's Preface
Complete table of contents of all drugs, arranged according to chapters and drug sections, and in each case with an introduction to the

respective section—for example, in the following manner: "precious stones/minerals, upper class, a total of 73 kinds.

18 kinds from the *Shen-nung pen-ching,* white characters

3 kinds from the *Ming-i pieh-lu,* black characters

唐附   1 kind listed for the first time in the T'ang edition, marked 'T'ang addition' (*T'ang-fu*)

今附   3 kinds were added for the first time in this edition; these are effective drugs, frequently used by medical practitioners. They are designated 'added now' (*chin-fu*).

5 kinds newly added to the drug repertory

5 kinds received their own monographs

3 kinds, in addition, come from the *Hai-yao (p'u)*

35 kinds, in addition, come from Ch'en Ts'ang-ch'i

All drugs whose names are framed in black have been recently included in the *Cheng-lei (pen-ts'ao).*"

Preface of the *Chia-yu pen-ts'ao*

Preface of the *T'u-ching pen-ts'ao*

Preface of the *K'ai-pao pen-ts'ao*

Preface of the *T'ang pen-ts'ao*

Preface by T'ao Hung-ching

The general sections from the *Pen-ching,* and T'ao Hung-ching's commentaries on these sections

A general introduction by Chang Yü-hsi—a careful commentary on Hsü Chih-ts'ai's *Yao-tui,* Sun Szu-mo's *Ch'ien-chin fang,* and Ch'en Ts'ang-ch'i's *Pen-ts'ao shih-i*

Preface of the *Ch'ung-kuang pu-chu Shen-nung pen-ts'ao ping t'u-ching*

Preface of the *Lei-kung p'ao-chih lun*

Chapter 2

A list of 82 illnesses and symptoms, including the drugs suitable for treatment

A list of 39 possibilities for poisoning and the appropriate antidotes

A list of remedies for indisposition caused by an overdose of drugs

Instructions for diet during the period of taking medications

A list of drugs and their compatibility for simultaneous administration with other drugs

A five-line quotation from the *Yao-tui*

Chapters 3–31

Monograph section. The arrangement of the individual sections of the monographs corresponds to the *Hsin-hsiu pen-ts'ao,* with the exception that vegetable drugs follow, rather than precede, rice/grains:

precious stones/minerals	upper class	chapter 3	73 drugs
	middle class	chapter 4	84 drugs
	lower class	chapter 5	93 drugs

herbs	upper class	chapter 6	87 drugs
	upper class	chapter 7	53 drugs
	middle class	chapter 8	62 drugs
	middle class	chapter 9	78 drugs
	lower class	chapter 10	62 drugs
	lower class	chapter 11	105 drugs
trees	upper class	chapter 12	72 drugs
	middle class	chapter 13	91 drugs
	lower class	chapter 14	99 drugs
man		chapter 15	26 drugs
quadrupeds	upper class	chapter 16	20 drugs
	middle class	chapter 17	17 drugs
	lower class	chapter 18	21 drugs
fowl		chapter 19	56 drugs
worms/fish	upper class	chapter 20	50 drugs
	middle class	chapter 21	56 drugs
	lower class	chapter 22	81 drugs
fruits		chapter 23	53 drugs
rice/grains	upper class	chapter 24	7 drugs
	middle class	chapter 25	23 drugs
	lower class	chapter 26	18 drugs
vegetables	upper class	chapter 27	30 drugs
	middle class	chapter 28	13 drugs
	lower class	chapter 29	22 drugs
known by name but not in use		chapter 30	194 drugs
herbs/trees not included in *pen-ts'ao* works		chapter 31	98 drugs

The individual monographs in the *Cheng-lei pen-ts'ao* and, consequently, in the *Ta-kuan pen-ts'ao* had grown to unwieldy proportions. The above-mentioned disadvantages for the practitioner apply not so much to the first and second chapters as to the unclear monographs.

The description of the drug *pa-tou* can once again serve as an example. A complete translation here, however, no longer makes any sense; it would stretch over too many pages, without adding anything essentially new. For this reason, a survey of its arrangement will suffice.

An illustration of the trunk of the tree with branches, leaves, and blossoms is reproduced at the beginning of the monograph; it combines the name of the drug with its preferred place of origin. The text begins with the portions of the *Pen-ching* and *Ming-i pieh-lu;* the commentary of T'ao Hung-ching and the commentary from the T'ang edition follow. After the respective introductory notations come the explanations of this drug by Ch'en Ts'ang-ch'i, Chang Yü-hsi, and Jih-hua tzu, as well as from the *T'u-ching pen-ts'ao* and *Lei-kung p'ao-chih lun.* A list of fourteen prescriptions containing *pa-tou* is appended; in each case, the source works (here there are nine) are cited.

The complexity of this type of monograph form derives from the fact that the nine commentators cited above each treated all, or at least several, aspects of the characteristics of the drugs, so that a practitioner seeking information about the appearance or effectiveness of a drug against a specific illness was forced to study the entire lengthy text. Since the statements of the most diverging authors of the previous centuries were grouped together, the reader ran into varying literary styles and levels of difficulty, occasionally making a comprehensive education highly recommendable for an understanding of the texts. Nevertheless, only in the most exceptional cases did the reader find a definitive answer. Contradictory opinions were frequently arranged together; thus, the solution to the problem in question was usually left to the reader.

It was not until five centuries later, as we shall see, that a new form of organization appropriate for such an enormous compendium and more suited to the needs of the practitioner was found. Only then could the *Cheng-lei pen-ts'ao* be effectively supplanted as a comprehensive materia medica. Since the requirements of practitioners remained the same, the times had to change in order to make possible a new form. Such a change did not occur during the Sung period.

5.9. The *Cheng-ho hsin-hsiu ching-shih cheng-lei pei-yung pen-ts'ao*

Cheng-ho hsin-hsiu ching-shih cheng-lei pei-yung pen-ts'ao
"Materia Medica, Based on the Classics and Historical Works, Annotated, Arranged by Types, and Organized for Practical Use, Newly Revised during the *Cheng-ho* Period"
Short title: *Cheng-ho pen-ts'ao*
30 chapters / 1748 drug descriptions
Authors: T'ang Shen-wei (end of the 11th century); *tzu:* Shen-yüan; from: Chin-yüan in Szechuan
Ts'ao Hsiao-chung (ca. 1116)
Written: see *Cheng-lei pen-ts'ao*
Published: 1116

It was Emperor Hui-tsung (1082–1135), a ruler of the late Northern Sung dynasty much inclined towards Taoism, who gave the order to the medical official Ts'ao Hsiao-chung, as chairman of an editorial board of eight officials, to revise the *Ta-kuan pen-ts'ao*. Ts'ao completed this task by 1116, only eight years after the appearance of the first edition of the *Ta-kuan pen-ts'ao*.

The *Cheng-ho pen-ts'ao* recorded only five new drugs and eliminated one old monograph (on human saliva), so that a total of 1,748 drugs were described. Since the authors combined the last two chapters of the *Ta-kuan pen-ts'ao* on known but obsolete drugs, and drugs that did not come from pen-ts'ao works, the number of chapters was reduced to thirty.

As already mentioned, in 1143 Yü-wen Hsü-chung, a scholar at the Han-lin Academy, wrote an afterword to the *Cheng-ho pen-ts'ao* (see pp. 70–71).

All original editions of this work have been lost. Only a further revised and expanded version, the *Ch'ung-hsiu cheng-ho pen-ts'ao*, has been preserved.[114]

5.10. The *Shao-hsing chiao-ting ching-shih cheng-lei pei-chi pen-ts'ao*

Wang Chi-hsien, a medical practitioner from K'ai-feng, was highly honored by the emperor Kao-tsung (1107–1187), a son of Emperor Hui-tsung, for his successful treatment of the emperor's mother. Although he appears to have possessed some notable medical abilities—for he was called "teacher of medicine Wang"—his biography did not end on a very positive note in the Sung history. Characterized as cunning and sycophantic, continually striving for higher positions, his star began to fade after the death of the emperor's mother. He was finally banished to Fu-chou, where he died.[115]

Wang Chi-hsien is credited with having compiled the *Shao-hsing pen-ts'ao*, which is listed in some subsequent bibliographies as having thirty-two chapters; others record twenty-two chapters. Although none exist in China today, various fragments have been preserved in Japan.

Okanishi Tameto assumes that Wang Chi-hsien first revised the *Ta-kuan pen-ts'ao*, expanding it by one chapter to a total of thirty-two and then submitting it to the throne in 1157. In Okanishi's opinion, this revision was then improved stylistically by the court chancellery and published by the School of Princes. This edition has not been preserved.

Subsequently, Wang Chi-hsien carried out an imperial order, probably directed to him personally, for a further comprehensive revision and annotation of the *Pen-ts'ao* which was to include new drugs. Wang Chi-hsien delegated this task to three subordinates—Kao Shao-kung, Ch'ai Yüan, and Chang Hsiao-chih—who completed it in 1159. Wang himself contributed the following preface:[116]

> We have heard that the *Pen-ts'ao* was the work of Shen-nung. In later times it was honored and served as a guideline. It was considered a magnificent compendium. There is no more beneficial source of aid for someone who deplores early death and the illnesses of life, and who seeks help in drugs made from plants and minerals. In the past and future, over thousands and hundreds of years, no one will dare disregard [the *Pen-ts'ao*]! During the Ch'in period, when the literature of earlier centuries was burned, this classic was grouped with medical and prophetic works, and its circulation was in no way diminished. Only during the centuries of the Han and Chin dynasties can [these] texts have been lost. Nothing but three chapters of Shen-nung's old classic were preserved, with no more than 365 drugs [being recorded]. As a result, succeeding generations could no longer consult the complete work of that exemplary man. How regrettable!
>
> T'ao Yin-chü [who lived during the] Liang period was endowed with superior abilities. He combined Shen-nung's old classic with the additional notes of renowned medical men and differentiated both [sources] by means of red and black characters. He introduced classificatory sections and added his own commentaries. However, he had based everything only upon his own personal knowledge and on his own ideas; [his perspective] was biased and [he developed] few insights. Thus, the advantages in his work are offset by the disadvantages.
>
> After the beginning of the T'ang dynasty, Su Kung submitted a petition requesting a revision and correction [of the *Pen-ts'ao*]. The result was a significant expansion [of this work], but the annotations are occasionally muddled—harmful and positive [effects of drugs] cannot be distinguished, and cold and hot [nature] are not [sufficiently] differentiated.
>
> Then came the establishment of the great Sung dynasty. Perfected men brought peace; their good deeds affected the entire world, and their humanity resembled that of heaven! During the *k'ai-pao* period, these men commissioned Lu To-hsün and others to correct again [the *Pen-ts'ao*]. Later, during the *chia-yu* period, they ordered [Chang] Yü-hsi and others to undertake an expanded commentary. In addition, Ch'en Ch'eng contributed his own statements [as a private citizen] and

Shao-hsing chiao-ting ching-shih cheng-lei pei-chi pen-ts'ao
"Materia Medica, Revised during the *Shao-hsing* Period, Based upon the Classics and Historical Works, Annotated, Arranged by Types, and Organized for Speedy Use"
Short title: *Shao-hsing pen-ts'ao*
32 chapters; later 22 chapters / number of drug descriptions: unknown
Authors: Wang Chi-hsien (?–1181);
       from: K'ai-feng and others
Finished: 1159
32-chapter version remained unpublished
Date of publication of 22-chapter version: unknown

cherry species (*ying-t'ao*)—*Shao-hsing pen-ts'ao*

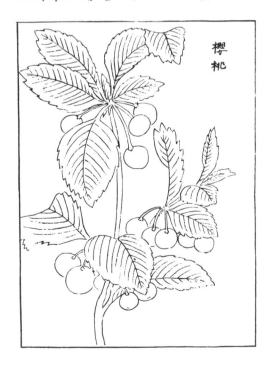

during the *ta-kuan* period, T'ang Shen-wei compiled the [*pen-ts'ao*] collection *Cheng-lei*.

Careful, detailed examination of the old and new commentaries in which the views of all authors are expressed shows that confusion and contradictions were abundant. Although the comments of the T'ang period corrected errors and contradictions [in the work of] T'ao, they themselves were marked by omissions and flaws. Commentators of the present [dynasty] have pointed out, in turn, the mistakes of the T'ang period and are, on occasion incomplete themselves. One [statement] is true, another [statement] is wrong, and both stand in contradiction to each other. If the *Pu-chu* [*pen-ts'ao*] of [Chang] Yü-hsi and the *Cheng-lei* [*pen-ts'ao*] of [T'ang] Shen-wei are examined, one finds the diverging views of all authors recorded in an overly complete manner, so that it is impossible to decide the validity [of any information]. [In these works] items with cold nature are sometimes [mistakenly] listed as a cure for cold, while other drugs with hot nature are [mistakenly] listed as a cure for heat. Some drugs, which [in reality] replenish [conditions of deficiency], are recorded as suitable for relieving conditions of surplus; [conversely], drugs that relieve [conditions of surplus] are termed beneficial in the treatment of [deficiencies]. The principles and the facts of the differentiation of the hot, cold, replenishing, or relieving properties of drugs have been turned on their heads! In addition, some medicinally effective items are said to exert no curative effects; [conversely], items that exert no curative effects are said to be medicinally effective. Thus, the true differentiation of drugs according to their medicinal effectiveness has also been completely distorted! Even the results achieved by the frequent use of certain drugs in prescriptions are not to be found anywhere in the commentaries on the classic. Also, the suitability of individual drugs for external or internal use, which must determine their application, has not been clearly recorded. Because it has such a long history already, the distinction between red and black characters has fallen into disarray. One can no longer count the [deficiencies] individually. If the [above-mentioned works] were consulted in the application [of drugs], grave mistakes would result! Wherever later generations departed from what was right, we have corrected it. In days worth thousands of gold each, a praiseworthy exemplary period of rule has raised the virtue of the appreciation of life. Fighting has been stopped and punishment is carried out in an orderly way. [The conditions are] quite sufficient to bring the people closer towards the Golden Age of Longevity, and, as a result, there is no more suffering from an unexpected early death! Thus, the illustrious imperial mind harbored sorrowful considerations leading to the statement that there are discrepancies and contradictions in the original text and the commentaries of the *pen-ts'ao* book and that there are faulty advices for treatment. Therefore, taking [the activities of] his ancestors during the *k'ai-pao* and *chia-yu* periods as an example, the emperor issued a decree to us, his civil servants, to the effect that additional revisions should be made and controversies be settled, so that [the materia medica] could be respected as an achievement of utmost sage-like humanitarianism and virtue. We now [present the result of our work and we] dare [to say that we may] not have fully explored all the great thoughts [of previous men]. We have collected prescription techniques on a wide scale, and we have compared all authors. We have analyzed where they agree and where they differ, and in cases where, for instance, the principles of the nature of a substance, such as cold or hot [thermo-influence], filling or draining [capacities], or its therapeutic strength, were turned upside down, so that [a particular statement] contradicted a correct interpretation, we have differentiated the original meaning, and we have considered it to be our duty to follow only what is appropriate. As to the shape and appearance [of the items discussed], we have based [our own presen-

male magpie (*hsiung-ch'iao*)—*Shao-hsing pen-ts'ao*

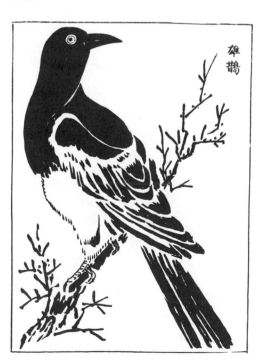

tation] on old illustrations. Although we have gathered knowledge as
with a large net, we have not dared to give as evidence what was, in
reality, only unfounded talk. We have investigated more than 500 famous prescription formulas, and we have proven more than 8,000
characters to be wrong. Because those who utilize this work will not
be misled, and because any application of this [book] will result in
success without fail, one will be able to advance towards longevity and
to reach the full extent [of one's lifetime]. Above, we thus support, if
only in a minor aspect, the rule of the Exemplary, and below we wish
[this work] to be handed on to the future. How could anybody say this
was only a small amendment [of the existing *Pen-ts'ao*]? We officials
are of sincere awe and sincere apprehension. We bow our heads and
our words are full of respect. Submitted to the Throne in the 29th year
of the period *shao-hsing* (1159) by the . . . Imperial Physicians and
temporary Professors of the Imperial Medical Office Kao Shao-kung,
Ch'ai Yüan, Chang Hsiao-chih, and Wang Chi-hsien.[117]

There is no proof whether this work was indeed presented to the
emperor; it was probably never published, a fact that may be connected
with the death of the emperor's mother six months later. This event
also signaled the end of imperial favor for Wang Chi-hsien.

The preface does not mention the number of chapters. Okanishi
conjectures, however, that the number was the same as in the *Ta-kuan
pen-ts'ao*, which Wang Chi-hsien had expanded earlier. According to
Okanishi, a shortened version of twenty-two chapters was then constructed from this first *Shao-hsing pen-ts'ao* with its thirty-two chapters, and contained only Wang Chi-hsien's new commentaries, additions,
and drug illustrations. According to an entry in the *Shu-lu chieh-t'i*,
the work was published by the Court Department of Construction.[118]

The twenty-two-chapter version was apparently still extant during
the Ming period: it is listed in two bibliographies of that epoch. But
already during the Ch'ing period, it is no longer mentioned.

In Japan, however, a number of incomplete handwritten copies have
been preserved. All these fragments, in turn, can be traced to a nineteen-chapter and a five-chapter copy. In any case, the arrangement of
drugs in these copies is identical to that in the *Ta-kuan pen-ts'ao*, with
only the subdivision into chapters being different. All of these fragments lack the section "Drugs from Humans" and the conclusion
following "Vegetables, middle class," so that they are probably based
upon one and the same original. The main difference between the
nineteen-chapter line of manuscripts and the five-chapter line is that
the former has more text to the illustrations than the latter. Apparently,
a Japanese person prepared a copy of the twenty-two-chapter version
of the *Shao-hsing* edition and brought it to Japan, where various copies
of the original, which itself was perhaps no longer complete, were
produced.

In 1933, the Shunyōdō Press in Tokyo published a manuscript in
five chapters and five volumes; the editor was Nakao Manzō. In 1971,
the same publisher produced a photo-reprint edition of a handwritten
copy in twenty-eight chapters and six volumes which belongs to the
nineteen-chapter line. The editor was Okanishi Tameto, who also
contributed a detailed introduction. This edition is distinguished in

紹興校定

particular by the beautiful, true-to-life drug illustrations and a text that is, in every case, significantly shorter than that in the *Ta-kuan pen-ts'ao*. In many monographs the text corresponds word for word (although incompletely in some cases) to the *Pen-ching* expanded by the *Ming-i pieh-lu*. Only in a few instances has a commentary by the authors themselves been added, introduced with the words "revised and determined during the *shao-hsing* period" (*shao-hsing chiao-ting*). Many of the drug illustrations lack a description of any kind.

Li Shih-chen criticized the *Shao-hsing pen-ts'ao* as insignificant. If the text of the Japanese manuscript does indeed reflect the original, one can, in agreement with Li Shih-chen, describe the work of Wang Chi-hsien as inadequate. The work was apparently intended to serve the author's prestige more than medical-pharmaceutical interests.

5.11. The *Ch'ung-hsiu cheng-ho ching-shih cheng-lei pei-yung pen-ts'ao*

Ch'ung-hsiu cheng-ho ching-shih cheng-lei pei-yung pen-ts'ao
"Newly revised Materia Medica of the *Cheng-ho* Period, Annotated, Arranged by Types, Organized for Practical Use, and Based upon the Classics and Historical Works"
Short title: *Ch'ung-hsiu cheng-ho pen-ts'ao*
30 chapters / 1746 drug descriptions
Authors: T'ang Shen-wei (end of the eleventh century);
　　　tzu: Shen-yüan;
　　　from: Chin-yüan in Szechuan
　　　Chang Ts'un-hui (thirteenth century);
　　　tzu: Wei-ch'ing;
　　　from: P'ing-yang
Published: 1249

Like the *Cheng-ho pen-ts'ao*, the *Ch'ung-hsiu cheng-ho pen-ts'ao* represents a work whose structure and contents correspond closely to the *Ta-kuan pen-ts'ao*. Nevertheless, this edition may, with some justification, be included here as an independent work.

The first difference from preceding editions can be seen in the first chapter, which includes the prefaces. It coincides word for word with that of the *Ta-kuan pen-ts'ao* but contains two additional entries. The first, less important addition, appended to the "General Introduction of Chang Yü-hsi," is a "List of Cited Works" taken over from the *Chia-yu pen-ts'ao*. A total of sixteen pen-ts'ao works are listed, with title, author, and a brief description of content, which the authors of the *Chia-yu pen-ts'ao* had consulted. The second, significant addition is the adoption of the first three chapters of the *Pen-ts'ao yen-i*, in which the author, K'ou Tsung-shih (fl. 1116), explains the theoretical background of his comments, as well as some practical instructions (see pp. 86–100). The particular quality of the *Pen-ts'ao yen-i* can only be suggested here; a detailed analysis of this work will be undertaken in the next chapter.

The *Pen-ts'ao yen-i* can be seen as a forerunner to the drug works of the Chin-Yüan epoch: certain elements already indicate the combination of the classical medical theory of the *Huang-ti nei-ching*, that is, the yinyang and Five Phases paradigms of systematic correspondence—with the practice of actual drug usage. Such a tendency stood in contrast to the preceding contents of pen-ts'ao works in the main tradition; these works were oriented totally for pragmatic use, without any explicit theoretical trimmings. The knowledge expressed in them rested on purely primary experiences or observations and on simple speculations based on the paradigm of magic correspondence.

During the thirteenth and fourteenth centuries, various editions of the *Ta-kuan pen-ts'ao* carried the complete text of the *Pen-ts'ao yen-i* as a final appendix. The author of the *Ch'ung-hsiu cheng-ho pen-ts'ao*, though, went one step further. He divided the text of the

Pen-ts'ao yen-i and added the sections individually to the corresponding monographs in the *Cheng-ho pen-ts'ao*.

As we shall see, the pen-ts'ao authors of the Chin-Yüan period distanced themselves from the main tradition. Although the *Ta-kuan pen-ts'ao* and the *cheng-ho* editions were subsequently often reprinted, with some editions also undergoing insignificant revisions, they were never expanded in accordance with the contents of the contemporary secondary tradition, that is, of the Chin-Yüan period pen-ts'ao works. The contrasting conceptions about drugs and the use of remedies were too strong to allow their integration. It was only in the sixteenth century that an author, Li Shih-chen, was able to bridge this gap. He replaced the former confrontation of the two diverging approaches with a rather pragmatic eclecticism.

5.12. The *Hsin-pien lei-yao t'u-chu pen-ts'ao*

Like the *Ch'ung-hsiu cheng-ho pen-ts'ao*, the *Hsin-pien lei-yao t'u-chu pen-ts'ao* represents an attempt to combine the *Ta-kuan pen-ts'ao* with the *Pen-ts'ao yen-i*. The structure is similar to that of the *Ch'ung-hsiu cheng-ho pen-ts'ao* and, therefore, still follows the form of the main tradition.

The authorship is uncertain. The table of contents is preceded by the lines "Revised and corrected by Liu Hsin-fu from T'ao-chi." Before the main text, however, the following comment is recorded: "Written by K'ou Tsung-shih; revised and corrected by Hsü Hung, Assistant Teaching Official and Official for the Differentiation of Drug Material in the Office of the Composition of Medicinal Drugs!" Because K'ou Tsung-shih can be eliminated with certainty as the author of the complete work, the conjecture follows that the entire remark before the main text is a forgery.

The work was not successful; two editions from the Sung period and one from the Yüan period are known.[119] Only a fragmentary copy of the Yüan edition has been preserved, located in Tokyo in the Library of the Imperial Household, where I received the kind permission to examine it.

The illustrations of the Yüan edition are very similar to those in the *Ta-kuan pen-ts'ao* and the *Ch'ung-hsiu cheng-ho pen-ts'ao*. A striking difference from these earlier works, however, is the elimination of black-white and white-black printing of respective characters as a means of separating the sections taken over from the *Pen-ching* and the *Ming-i pieh-lu*.

During the Yüan period, Hui Ch'ang completed a work on drugs entitled *Lei-pien t'u-ching chi-chu yen-i pen-ts'ao*. This work is basically a new edition of the *Hsin-pien lei-yao t'u-chu pen-ts'ao*. Hui Ch'ang's work is also known in only three editions: one from the Yüan period, a *Tao-tsang* edition, and an unidentifiable edition. The first is located in the Library of the Imperial Household in Tokyo; the edition in the Taoist canon is entitled *T'u-ching chi-chu yen-i pen-ts'ao*.[120]

Hsin-pien lei-yao t'u-chu pen-ts'ao
"Illustrated and Annotated Materia Medica, Newly Compiled and Containing the Most Important Information, Arranged According to Types"
Also: *Hsin-pien cheng-lei t'u-chu pen-ts'ao*
"Illustrated and Annotated Materia Medica, Newly Edited and Arranged by Types"
42 chapters
Author: Liu-Hsin-fu (ca. 1200)
        from: T'ao-chi
Written: beginning of the thirteenth century
Published: date unknown

6. Conclusions

6. Concluding Remarks on the Main Pen-ts'ao Tradition

The main pen-ts'ao tradition spanned approximately 1,300 years before coming to a halt. Later reprintings of the *Ta-kuan pen-ts'ao* or the cheng-ho editions could not change the situation.

The structure of the main tradition, as I have pointed out repeatedly, brought about its own end. The most important causes for this development may be summarized as follows.

The *Pen-ts'ao,* originally a compendium of pharmaceutics with an emphasis on prolongation of life rather than on actual therapy, had been transformed in the course of the main tradition into a genuine materia medica, satisfying the demands of medical and pharmaceutical practice. Like a parabola, the tradition approached the requirements of curative therapy and then withdrew again with increasing obscurity and complexity of form and content. The last editions were unsuited, as the reasons presented above indicate, for use in daily therapeutic practice.

The form of the pen-ts'ao works in the main tradition was exceedingly conservative, possibly as a concession to Confucian ideology. It appears that only this form of near-complete citation of all earlier opinions could give the authors the opportunity to express, within an officially sanctioned framework, new conceptions which frequently contradicted the old beliefs. This same form, however, also caused the increasing chaos of these works. In the end, it could not be improved in accordance with the needs of medical practitioners.

The main tradition was easily able to absorb the first phase of the effect of Sung-Neoconfucianism: Confucian, Taoist, and Buddhist sources served T'ang Shen-wei as a foundation. The second phase of the impact of Sung teachings on medical thought could no longer be reconciled with the main pen-ts'ao tradition: knowledge based upon experience and simple speculations stood in opposition to new deductions based upon a sophisticated theory. The pluralism of opinions expressed in the works of the main tradition was not compatible with Neoconfucian attempts at integration. Three additional centuries had to pass before a new perspective was able to eliminate this contrast. Nevertheless, a progressive reasoning, beyond all external stagnation, was concealed in the main tradition beneath a conservative form. The continuous correction of errors of earlier authors, the steady expansion by means of recent knowledge, and the compulsion of medicine, perhaps underlying all such efforts, always to try new drugs and prescriptions on strange, new, or even previously incurable illnesses, brought forth a long series of pharmaceutical works which need not be ashamed of any comparison with similar contemporary writings in the West.

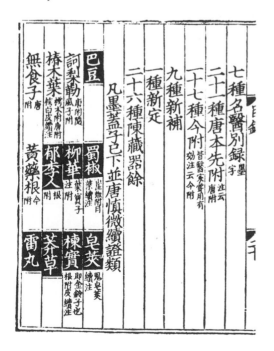

A portion of the table of contents of the *Ch'ung-hsiu cheng-ho pen-ts'ao* showing white on black and black on white print, and containing information on the sources of the drug descriptions.

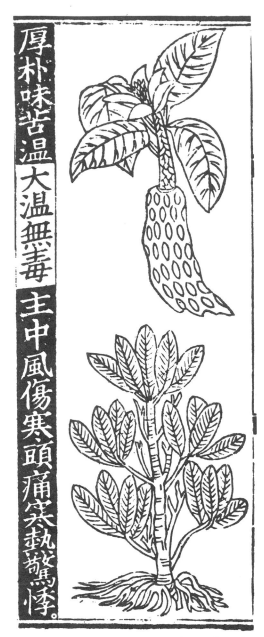

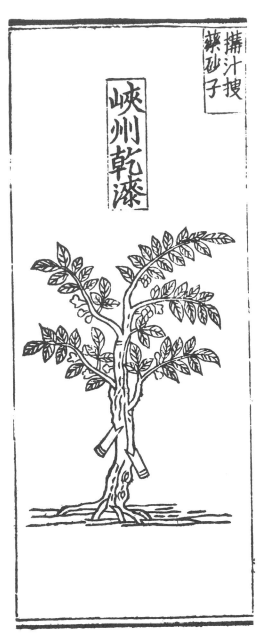

magnolias (hou-p'o)—Ch'ung-hsiu cheng-ho pen-ts'ao

dried varnish (kan-ch'i)—Ch'ung-hsiu cheng-ho pen-ts'ao

1. Toward a Pharmacology of Systematic Correspondence

1.1. Symbolic syncretism

The second important tradition in the development of Chinese pharmaceutical literature was the so-called Chin-Yüan pen-ts'ao works. To appreciate the accomplishments of this tradition as well as to elucidate its position in the entire course of Chinese medical history, the effects of Sung-Neoconfucianism upon medical thought must be examined. These effects, as I have indicated above, found expression in two phases.

The efforts to unify previously diverging world views and tendencies—which had been a leading motive for the creators of Neoconfucianism and which were supposed to create a central, that is, Chinese, doctrine—affected medicine only in the second phase of Neoconfucian influence. If the intellectual expansion that took place during the first phase produced an interest in sources that, at least officially, were not exactly closely associated with Confucians, Chinese medical writers in the second half of the eleventh century began to produce works that conscientiously combined—at the beginning in an almost symbolic manner—Taoist and Buddhist, as well as Confucian, elements. This process represented the first period in the transfer of Neoconfucian syncretism to the field of medicine.

The *Pen-ts'ao yen-i* can be seen as a characteristic example of this first period in the second phase of Sung doctrine influence on medical thought. It has been frequently recognized by Chinese and Japanese authors as a forerunner to the drug literature in the Chin-Yüan epoch—without, however, any reference being made to its relationship with contemporary intellectual currents.

1.2. The *Pen-ts'ao yen-i*

Pen-ts'ao yen-i
"Elucidation of the Meaning of Pharmaceutics"
20 chapters / 466 drug descriptions
Author: K'ou Tsung-shih (ca. 1116)
Completed: 1116
Published: 1119

The otherwise unknown official K'ou Tsung-shih wrote the *Pen-ts'ao yen-i* in 1116; his nephew, K'ou Yüeh, published it in 1119.[121] In terms of form, this work is written as an explanatory supplement to the *Chia-yu pen-ts'ao* and the *T'u-ching pen-ts'ao*. It contains no illustrations. An examination of its contents, carried out at the emperor's behest by medical authorities, brought K'ou Tsung-shih high praise and the title of an expert for the purchase of drugs.

As can be seen from various remarks in monographs of the *Pen-ts'ao yen-i,* K'ou Tsung-shih traveled extensively as a civil servant perhaps attaining his pharmaceutical knowledge in this manner. He obviously possessed a sufficiently critical attitude not to believe every statement in the older pharmaceutical literature and to examine personally what appeared doubtful to him. Most of all, though, his work illustrates quite clearly the urge for ideological unity, that is, the tendency to integrate the hitherto rather pragmatic use of drugs into the theories of systematic correspondence.

K'ou's work soon gained a good reputation. In 1195, it was added for the first time to an edition of the *Ta-kuan pen-ts'ao*. Since the contents of the *Pen-ts'ao yen-i* mark an important point in the development of Chinese medical-pharmaceutical thought, I shall treat this work in some detail in the pages that follow.

1.2.1. The first three chapters of the *Pen-ts'ao yen-i*

In a total of twenty-nine sections in chapters one and two of his work, K'ou Tsung-shih presents his views on medical theory and its application in actual health care. The third chapter, in eight sections, enumerates actual cases of illness and their therapies, with numerous references to the Han physician and author of various early prescription collections, Chang Chi (142–220?). The chapter concludes with a purely theoretical discussion.

K'ou's thoughts and, consequently, the position he takes in his work are clearly expressed in the following translations of a major portion of the first chapter and one section from the second. K'ou Tsung-shih did not write an actual preface. However, he expressed his intentions in the first section of the general treatises.

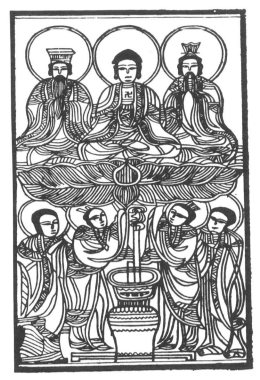

Buddha, Lao-tzu, and Confucius united on a lotus blossom

Heaven and earth have creation and perfection as their virtues. Their most important creation is the human body. The body has peace and joy as its foundation. Peace and joy may be obtained if one takes protection and maintenance [of life] as its foundation. All men must base [their existence] on this foundation, and, as a result, the foundation [of their body] will be firm. If the foundation [of the body] is firm, how can illness arise? How could early death or unexpected suffering occur? This is the principle of the preservation of life; nothing can equal it.

Trees and herbs are without knowledge. Nevertheless, they base their existence upon watering. Man stands above all things. Why should he not have the means to protect and maintain [his existence]? Theoretically, the meaning of protection and maintenance allows for ten thousand strategies, but, in short, there are [only] three actual methods. The first consists of the nourishment of the spirit. The second requires careful treatment of the influences [in one's body] and, finally, the third concerns the avoidance of illness.

When one forgets the emotions and is not concerned with wisdom, when one finds [the condition of] tranquility and achieves liberation from any preoccupation, when one is able to leave behind [superficial] matters and be completely absorbed in the truth, and when one is able to avoid internal and external distraction, the spirit cannot cause destruction from within, and the environment will not be able to cause deception from outside. [One achieves] true unity without confusion, and the spirit can obtain peace from within itself. This is the nourishment of the spirit.

When one continually holds fast to the foundations of his origins and firmly supports the return of the true influences that constitute one's finest matter, then the triple burner will be fixed in its positions and the six robbers will lose their form. As a consequence, one's inner world of knowledge will be empty, and great harmony will be achieved. Finally, [the economy] of one's influences will regulate itself. This describes the careful treatment of the influences.

When a person consumes drink and food at a suitable time and adjusts the body's temperature [by means of appropriate clothing] to external conditions, when one does not violate the eight evils either while traveling or at home, and does not force sleep or waking, the body will automatically achieve a state of peace. This is what is meant by the prevention of illness.

These three types of behavior are easily followed, and if people maintain that it is difficult, it is only because they do not have the will for it. Thus, a method for the prolongation of life exists, but men only seldom deem it important, and therefore they proceed toward death.

The exemplary men [of times past] regretted that continuous suffering and sudden illness followed each other and that the natural harmony [of the body] was often lost. For this reason, they acquainted [the rest of mankind] with the techniques to protect and preserve [life]. In addition they made known the medications that eliminate illnesses, so that experts and laymen could achieve together the goal of longevity. With similar intentions, the state compiled the [prescription collection *T'ai-p'ing*] *sheng-hui* [*fang*], revised and corrected the *Su-wen*, corrected the *Pen-ts'ao* again, and, furthermore, prepared the *T'u-ching*. Works such as Chang Chung-ching's *Shang-han lun*, the *Ch'ien-chin* [*fang*], the *Chin-kuei* [*yao-lüeh*], and the *Wai-t'ai* [*pi-yao*] are excellent and are preserved in archives.

Today, physicians in the empire are selected by repeated examinations. Title and office are bestowed upon them, and they become civil servants. In this manner, attempts are made everywhere to eliminate illness and the sufferings of mankind. This is due to the fact that the noble rulers, who possess consummate wisdom and the greatest virtue, matching the utmost humaneness of heaven and earth, assist in improving the life [of the populace], and reward the empire fully. Thus, there are no drugs in the wild that have been neglected and no illness that has remained unknown. There are, however, sections in both *pen-ts'ao* works [mentioned, i.e., the *Chia-yu pen-ts'ao* and the *T'u-ching pen-ts'ao*] in which the respective authors express their personal opinions, disregarding discussions and comparisons [with other authors and works]. As a result, students consulting them will inevitably be misled.

I have now examined the statements of all authors and compared them with the facts. I have expanded incomplete or erroneous [drug descriptions] in order to show their true nature.

This applies to [the description of] *tung-pi t'u, tao-liu shui,* and *tung-hui.*

I have explained unclear and ambiguous [descriptions] in order to make evident the characteristics [of the drugs in question].

This applies to [erroneous statements], such as that "aromatic water" originates from water that springs up beneath chrysanthemums, and that rats engender their young through the dropping of seminal fluid on the ground.

I have indicated when I found mistakes or omissions in the text, in order to clarify the meanings.

This applies to *yü-ch'üan* and *shih-mi.*

If the name [of some drug] had been changed as the result of a taboo, I traced it back to the original, so as to preserve the old designation.

Thus, *shan-yao* falls under a taboo of the present dynasty; during the T'ang period, [the name of the emperor] Tai-tsung was banned.

Therefore, as a result of my endeavors, that which is correct and that which is false have been traced back to a single [truth]; curative treatment rests on a solid foundation, and clarity, not doubt, controls the selection and use [of drugs]. For more than ten years I have conducted

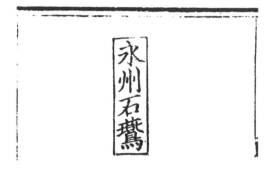

"stone swallows," fossils *(shih-yen)*—Ch'ung-hsiu cheng-ho pen-ts'ao

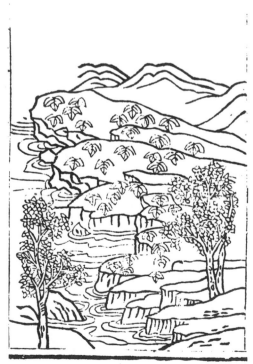

investigations and inquiries and have gathered everything that is valuable, in order to eliminate suffering and cure illnesses. The effects of
harmonization and of accumulation should be felt everywhere.

Illnesses are, of course, matters with which the exemplary men [of
times past] were diligently concerned, and [as Confucius once pointed
out], without consistency one cannot act as a physician. How could
anybody claim that this is an easy matter? K'ou Tsung-shih has repeatedly stated that in case of an illness one may depend on the physicians. The physicians depend on prescriptions, and the prescriptions
depend on drugs. Now, even if someone is able to differentiate whether
a given illness results from a depletion or repletion [in influences] and
knows whether a prescription [in a certain case] is applicable or not,
how should it be possible for him to eliminate the long endured *ku*
poisoning of the Taoist

> During the T'ang period, Chen Li-yen held the position of executive
> secretary in the Office of Imperial Sacrifices. He was well versed in
> the practice of medicine. A Taoist who had already been suffering
> from pressing sensations in his heart and abdomen for two years
> [once came to him]. After the examination [Chen] said: "There is a
> *ku* in your body because you have eaten human hair inadvertently!"
> He gave the patient a dose of *hsiung-huang* and only a short time
> later, the Taoist spit out a finger-thick, eyeless snake. The snake was
> then burned and developed the odor of hair. Thereupon, the Taoist
> was cured.

or to stimulate the crowded, clean teeth of Chang Kuo into growth,

> During the T'ang period, when Chang Kuo had obeyed the emperor's
> summons to the court, [the emperor] Hsüan-tsung once said to Kao
> Li-shih: "I have heard that it takes a remarkable scholar to drink
> unharmed a [decoction of] aconite!" It was a cold day and [Chang]
> Kuo was called in for a drink. After he had taken [the decoction
> offered to him] three times, he leaned back exhausted and remarked:
> "That was not a good wine!" He then rested for a while, and a short
> time later it could be seen that his teeth were burning and drawing
> together. Thereupon he glanced to the right and to the left, grasped
> an iron scepter, and smashed [his teeth] out. He kept them in a belt
> and took out a medicament which he proceeded to rub on his gums.
> After a while, the teeth had grown in again—lustrous, straight, and
> clean. The emperor praised him, believing his abilities to be
> supernatural.

if he does not know whether a drug is harmless or medicinally effective,
if he is not able to differentiate whether it is still early enough, or already
too late, for the use of a certain prescription, if he confuses counterfeit
for genuine drugs, or, finally, is unable to distinguish fresh from aged
drugs?

The meaning of the present work has been directed towards the
attainment of all the above-mentioned abilities. Compilation, arrangement, and completion of this book follow carefully the example of the
two scriptures [mentioned above]. I have divided it into sections and
monographs and have expanded the prefaces and general treatises to
three chapters. I have not included those [items] known only by name
but no longer in use or those drugs whose significance has already been
treated exhaustively. In addition, I have not continued the labeling [of
monographs] with such annotations as *"Shen-nung pen-ching,"*
"Ming-i pieh-lu," "first listed in the T'ang edition," "modern addition,"
"new listing," and "newly determined," because this [information] is
already recorded in the [*Chia-yu pen-ts'ao* and *T'u-*] *ching*, which I

took as my starting points. Following the old example, the work has twenty chapters, with an additional chapter for the table of contents. I have chosen the title *Pen-ts'ao yen-i.*

If there are among learned men, dedicated to the preservation of life, those who in their endeavors are in accordance with my intentions, they will be able to elucidate and expand my work, taking up the virtue of loving life, [so characteristic] of our present exemplary dynasty.[122]

A quotation from Confucius and elements of Confucian thought, such as the superiority of man above all things, are combined in this section with concepts that might be better classified in the Taoist and Buddhist sphere—for example, the postulate of forgetting all emotions, of not being concerned with knowledge, and of being free of desires.

A section on the origins of the pen-ts'ao literature then follows, similar to those we have already seen in the prefaces of the main tradition. The derivation here, however, is only very briefly sketched and is concerned solely with the appearance of the term *pen-ts'ao* and the authorship of Shen-nung. The section then proceeds immediately to a critique of what was, for the author, the last work in the main tradition and the work that needed revision—the *Chia-yu pen-ts'ao.*

The next section leads the reader from the pragmatic aspects of the old pharmaceutics to the theorization of drug knowledge. For the first time in a pen-ts'ao work, the drugs themselves are not mentioned as direct opponents of illnesses, but rather the characteristics of the drugs stand for principles of effect that apparently could be standardized. These comments are the earliest known attempts in the pen-ts'ao literature to systematically assign principles of effect to drugs, in accordance with the drug qualities, and therefore to create a theoretical basis for their successful use. K'ou Tsung-shih recognized here the physiological effects of the five influences (ch'i) of the environment and the corresponding therapeutic effects of the five tastes (wei) as exerted, for instance, by drugs. K'ou Tsung-shih's "influences" included cold, heat, wind, dryness, and the so-called ch'ung-influence, a difficult-to-define influence originating from the earth and penetrating the entire body. K'ou's influences only partly correspond to the five thermo-influences hot, cold, warm, cool, and neutral, defined as primary drug qualities by later authors of the Chin-Yüan era. In contrast, the five tastes listed by K'ou Tsung-shih coincide with later usage. Before I quote K'ou Tsung-shih's own words, a graphic summary might clarify his argument:

TABLE 3

Influences	Effects	Corresponding tastes	Effects
cold	hardens	salty	draws together
heat	draws together	bitter	hardens
wind	disperses	sour	gathers
dryness	gathers	acrid	disperses
ch'ung-ch'i	harmonizes	sweet	soothes

When heaven and earth had already been separated, the creation of all things was due solely to the five influences. After the five influences had been determined, the five tastes arose. Following the genesis of the five tastes, the thousand transformations and the ten thousand changes continued without end. Thus, it is said that the influences bring forth things, and the tastes complete them. That which was created individually becomes a pair when complete; that which was created as a pair becomes an individual entity when complete. Cold hardens; thus, the corresponding taste can be used to draw things together. Hot influence draws things together; thus, the corresponding taste can be used to harden [things]. The influence of wind disperses; thus, the corresponding taste can be used to gather. The influence of dryness gathers; thus, the corresponding taste can be used to disperse. The *ch'ung*-influences originate in the soil. They are able to harmonize everything; thus, the corresponding taste can be used to soothe. If the influences are firm, strength results. For this reason, the influences [circulating in the body] can be nourished with bitter [things]. If the vessels are drawn together, they are in harmony. Thus, the vessels can be nourished with salty [things]. If the bones are gathered together, they are strong. Therefore, the bones can be nourished with sour [things]. If the muscles are dispersed, they are not cramped. Thus, the muscles can be nourished with acrid [things]. If the flesh is soothed, it is not blocked. Therefore, flesh can be nourished with sweet [things]. If a soothing effect is wished for, then something sweet should be used; if soothing is not wanted [something sweet] should not be used. No applications may be exaggerated; excessive amounts can also cause illness. Anyone in ancient times who wanted to nourish life and cure suffering first had to understand what has been said here. Only very rarely is suffering relieved without such understanding.[123]

In the next paragraph, K'ou Tsung-shih stresses a healthy life-style as the best preventive measure against the formation of illness. The origin of illness is brought into connection with the yearly course and the influences of items belonging either to the yin or yang category of all phenomena; a quotation from the *Su-wen* indicates the origin of this concept:

The way of peace and joy will be reached by those who are able to protect and preserve [life]. Unfortunately, one must observe that, in general, harmonizing drugs are used rarely, while aggressive drugs find frequent use. This [practice and the fact that, nevertheless, numerous men become sick and die prematurely] leads to the recognition that human life depends upon protection and preservation, and that in order to maintain life, one cannot violate the healthy balance of influences. If one wants to preserve what has already been lost, then illnesses will certainly arise. If [a ruler] bases his reign on unsuitable methods, his fall will soon be observed. The prevention of sorrow must occur in a time free from cares. Thus, it is said: "Do not forget danger in peacetime; in life, do not forget death!" This is a warning issued by the sages.

The principles, by means of which one nourishes and maintains [life], are best realized in the preservation of a mean. If moderation is maintained, no harm can result from too much or too little. The classic states: "If, in the four seasons of spring, autumn, winter, and summer, *yin* or *yang* [influences] cause illnesses, this is due to an excessive adoption [of either of them]." Therefore, if one, not in accordance with his nature, forces himself to pursue [certain goals], illnesses will arise where this force has been applied. The five depots receive the influences [from outside], and there is a normal share [which they must maintain]. If

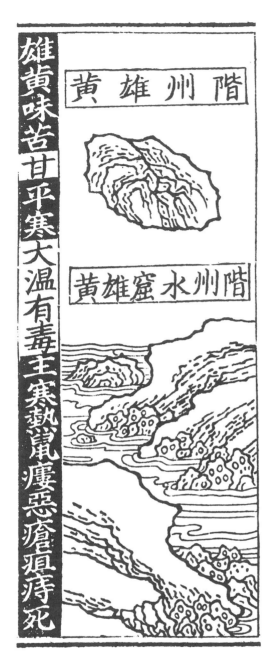

realgar (*hsiung-huang*)—*Ch'ung-hsiu cheng-ho pen-ts'ao*

they are burdened excessively [too many influences are drawn away from them], and illness will occur. Those people who understand well the process of maintaining their life will not make the mistake of overstepping the limits of exhaustion, and they are able to preserve their true origins. How could they suffer from being hit by external evil? For this reason it is better to understand the protection and preservation [of life] than the administration of medications. If, however, the protection and preservation [of life] is not understood, it is certainly advisable to be well versed in the area of medications. There are also people who know nothing about the protection and preservation [of life] or about medications. When such people suddenly fall ill, they put the responsibility on the spirits or the heavens. Yes, this matter does not receive enough consideration—how can one be insufficiently cautious in this respect?

Those who have not yet heard of *tao* allow their mind free reign and act contrary to the generation of joy. The mind should be brought into harmony with knowledge; sorrow and fear with gain and loss. Exhaustion and suffering should be harmonized with rites and regulations; one's style of life should follow one's material means. Where these four agreements do not occur, the heart will fall ill.

When someone overtaxes his strength and exhausts his appearance, when someone is noisy and violent and lets his influences stream contrary [to what is becoming], when someone delivers himself to the extravagant and succumbs to wine and prefers acrid and salty foods, the liver will fall ill. If raw food and cold liquids are consumed, if the limits of warmth and coolness are overstepped, if one sits or sleeps too long, if one eats or hungers too much, illness of the spleen will result. If one roars too much, engages in debates or argument, violates [the requirements of] cold and warmth, and if too many salty and bitter things are consumed, the lung will fall ill. If a person sits too long on moist places, enters the water violently, indulges the passions to the point of exhaustion, and if the three [cinnabar] fields run over from excess, illness in the kidneys occurs. In this manner, the five illnesses arise. They result in exhaustion before old age, and [if one behaves as indicated] there is illness before exhaustion. If the illness breaks out, it is serious; when it is serious, death must occur. Woe, all this is the result of the lack of careful thought—man himself is the cause of it. Learned men concerned with the preservation of life who study carefully these five [etiological categories] are able to complete their lives without suffering. In the classic it is written: "They treated those not yet ill, and not those already sick." This is exactly the meaning of this paragraph.[124]

A quotation from the work of the Taoist Chuang-tzu (fourth to third century B.C.) supplements the explanations in the following paragraph:

Those who understand how to nourish life, nourish the interior. Those who do not understand, nourish the exterior. He who nourishes the exterior brings about an external excess, filling himself with joy and enriching his well-being. Wishes and desires become obligatory. That abundance in the exterior is the cause of a void in the interior is unknown to such people. Those who understand the nourishment of the interior bring about an internal abundance. The depots and the palaces achieve a condition of harmony, the triple burner maintains its positions, and food and drink correspond to the requirements. For this reason, Chuang Chou says: "Where the greatest dangers threaten men—at night in bed, at drinking and eating fests—they do not know how to warn one another. That is a mistake!" If one lives carefully along these lines, how

can illnesses arise? Why should life not be long-lasting? Exemplary men
nourish the body and understand it; ignorant men stand unknowingly
before illnesses. This is truly appalling![125]

The next section, in contrast, refers to Buddhist concepts:

> It is difficult to tie anything together on the basis of softness and
> sentiment, or to cut anything apart. Decisions can only be made on the
> basis of knowledge and intelligence. This demands the renunciation of
> human pleasures. Such words are easily stated, but it is difficult to carry
> out their consequences. For the knowledge and intelligence of man are
> shallow and stand on weak legs; they are unable [to induce one] to
> overcome his desires. Thus, the following statement can be found in
> Buddhist literature: "Desire is the cause of all suffering. What, then,
> ceases when desires are eliminated?" Consequently, it is known that the
> end of suffering is impossible without the end of desires. Thus, the end
> of desires will also bring with it the end of suffering. The exemplary
> men [of the past] discussed that which was close at hand but called
> attention to that which was distant. This should be considered and
> carefully taken into account. Those who know how to nourish life will
> not exhaust their spirits and will allow no harm to come to their body.
> If body and spirits are in peace, wherefrom could misfortune and suf-
> fering arise?[126]

In the following treatise, K'ou Tsung-shih gives a concrete example
of a total illness of the organism, affecting, in succession, all five depots
of the body. The five depots were here, according to the theories
expressed in the *Su-wen*, brought into connection with the Five Phases
(*wu-hsing*). Just as these could be arranged in various series of mutual   五行
relationships, the five depots also have the corresponding series of
mutual relationships. In the example given below, in which the suc-
cessive spread of an illness from one depot to the other four is portrayed, we will find the mother-child relationship of the depots. The
depots are arranged in accordance with the "mutual production order"
of the Five Phases. A summary of the basic elements of the example
is as follows:

1. The Heart corresponds to Fire; Fire brings forth Earth
2. The Spleen corresponds to Earth; Earth brings forth Metals
3. The Lung corresponds to Metal; Metal brings forth Water
4. The Kidneys correspond to Water; Water brings forth Wood
5. The Liver corresponds to Wood; Wood brings forth Fire

The five phenomena—fire, earth, metal, water, and wood—are not
to be viewed as static elements but as symbols of change in a continuous cycle; they represent only the individual phases in the ceaseless
process of change. In a similar manner, the relationship of the five
depots of the body to one another must also not be construed as static
but in continuous interchange. It is on this theoretical foundation that
the following insights are based: that illnesses in one depot cannot be
viewed as detached from the other depots, and, as a consequence, that
when illness arises in one depot, immediate consideration should be
given to the possible consequences in other depots and to the subsequent spread of the illness.

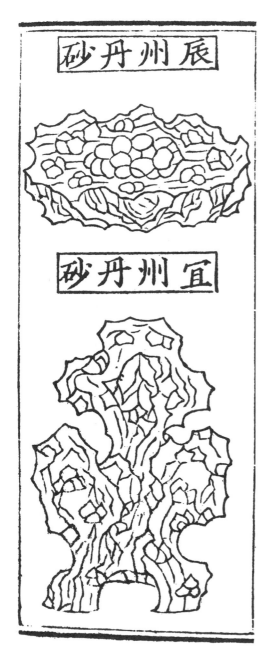

砂丹州辰

砂丹州宜

cinnabar *(tan-sha)—Ch'ung-hsiu cheng-ho pen-ts'ao*

The foundations of human life are the finest influences and the blood. All human illnesses begin with injury to the influences or to the blood. It has always been the case that young men and unmarried girls harbor thoughts in their hearts. When these thoughts overstep what is appropriate, exhaustion and damage result. For young men it means the premature dissemination of their spirit and [healthy] complexion; for young women it means the premature drying up of the monthly period. How does such a thing happen? Well, sadness and pondering injure the heart. If the heart has been damaged, the blood will flow contrary to its proper direction and will soon be exhausted. When the blood flows contrary to its proper direction and becomes exhausted, the result is premature dissipation of one's spirit and complexion and the premature drying up of the monthly period. If, thus, an illness arises in the [depot corresponding to] fire, and if one is unable to strengthen its child [depot], one will feel no need to eat. Consequently, a condition of depletion arises in the spleen, which in turn leads to a loss of influences in the [depot corresponding to] metal. A cough is the result. A cough ties up the influences in the [depot corresponding to] water, leading to a drying up of the four limbs. If the influences in the [depot corresponding to] wood are then present in insufficient quantities, frequent anger will result. Hair on the top of the head and on the temples withers; muscles are paralyzed. Finally, all five depots have been affected. Thus, one will not die of a sudden death, but then does succumb. Of all types of exhaustion, this is the type most difficult to cure. Once illness has afflicted all five depots, there is no expectation for a cure; all the strength of drugs will be insufficient. If [the patient] himself is capable of changing his mind from within, and if, in addition, support is provided by drugs, then it is possible to save a life in one case out of ten. This should serve as an example. All other types of exhaustion can be treated according to pulse and symptoms.[127]

In the course of the following discussion of the "eight important points for the treatment of illnesses," further theoretical concepts are introduced. The list of "six errors" that make the cure of illnesses impossible, also found in the next section, reflects important perceptions of possible mistakes by physician and patient.

There are eight important points in the treatment of illnesses. If these eight important points are disregarded, illnesses cannot be overcome. That does not mean, however, that illnesses cannot be overcome, but rather that the capabilities for a [possible] elimination are lacking. Thus, a careful consideration of the eight important points is indispensable, for mistakes and violations against them must be avoided at all costs.

The first is *depletion*. This signifies the five [symptoms of] depletion. A fine [movement in the] vessels, cold skin, shortness of breath, polyuria, and diarrhea, inability to ingest food and drink; these are the five [symptoms of] depletion.

The second is *repletion*. This signifies the five [symptoms of] repletion. A full [movement in the] vessels, hot skin, bloated abdomen, urinary retention, and constipation, depression; these are the five [symptoms of] repletion.

The third is *cold*. This signifies concentrations of cold in the body's depots and palaces.

The fourth is *heat*. This signifies concentrations of heat in the body's depots and palaces.

The fifth is *evil*. This signifies illnesses that do not originate proper among the [influences] in the body's depots and palaces.

The sixth is *proper*. This signifies that one was not hit by an external evil.

The seventh is called *internal*. This signifies that the illness is not in the external [sections of the organism].

The eighth is called *external*. This signifies that the illness is not in the internal [sections of the organism].

[In the treatment of illnesses] careful consideration should first be given to these eight important points. The six [locations where movement in the] vessel [can be felt] should be examined to discover the origin [of the illnesses]. If observations [of the patient's complexion, etc.] have been made, smells and voice have been perceived, questions have been asked, and the [movement in the] vessels has been felt, how could there be an incurable illness? If, however, [an illness] cannot be cured, this is due to the six errors. [These are] the errors to undertake diagnosis carelessly, to have no faith, to overstep a time limit, not to call a physician, not to recognize the illness, and, finally, to lack knowledge of medications. If even one of these errors is made, it will be difficult to cure the [illness]. As can be seen, it is not only the mistakes of medical practitioners that play a role but also the erroneous conduct of the patients. If a physician is not guided by feelings of sympathy and humanity, if a patient harbors doubts and lacks respect for the [physician], and if both of these attitudes come together, this is certainly not helpful [in the struggle] against illness. Thus, a physician must be guided without fail by sympathy and humaneness. Otherwise, he causes misfortune. Under no circumstances may a patient doubt or lack respect for the physician. Otherwise, he, too, causes misfortune. Only exemplary men are able to recognize the essence of things. They are able to attain peace and joy in every field. This is also true for the treatment of illnesses.[128]

The only concrete statements concerning an earlier, deficient treatment or use of drugs are found in two further sections of the first chapter, one of which is reproduced below. Such statements form a significant portion of the prefaces and introductions in pen-ts'ao works of the main tradition. In K'ou Tsung-shih's work, they seem to receive more a symbolic meaning than intentional informational value, especially when referring to works of the distant past:

In the *Ho-yao fen-chi liao-li fa tse* ("Quantitative Regulations for the Preparation of Medications from Individual Drugs") it is said: "The following is valid for all prescriptions: A *ch'ih*-long piece of the cinnamon drug should be used. The rind should be completely peeled and discarded. The correct weight is one-half *liang*." This is a very vague and by no means detailed description. Why should exactly one-half *liang* be the correct weight? In addition, cinnamon is, of course, a rind drug. When one reads in this work that the rind should be completely peeled and thrown away, that which remains is anything but a cinnamon drug! I would like to offer the following definition: The drug should be one *ch'ih* long and one *ts'un* wide. The rough, hollow, and tasteless [bark] sections should be removed from the rind. One-half *liang* then remains. However, I still cannot understand why it was a *ch'ih*-long piece of cinnamon that was required as a daily dose. This is, undoubtedly, a mistake of the people in earlier times.[129]

K'ou Tsung-shih also took up a problem of terminology. There were numerous such problems, and he chose as an example the term *ch'i* which, like few other terms in Chinese medicine, was connected 氣 with innumerable meanings and associations. As we have seen above,

K'ou Tsung-shih had already employed the term ch'i to designate five specific external influences. This brought him into terminological conflict with the usage of the term ch'i in the *Su-wen* and also in the general sections of the *Pen-ching,* where it was employed to designate a primary quality of edible substances and drugs, that is, the thermo-influence. K'ou attempted to solve this confusion as follows, but, as one may note today, not all subsequent authors followed his suggestions. The term ch'i remained as multifaceted as ever.

氣

性

> In the introductory section [of the *Pen-ching*] it is written: "Drugs possess the five tastes, sour, salty, sweet, bitter, and acrid, and, in addition, the four [thermo-]influences (*ch'i*) cold, hot, warm, and cool." I would like to examine this statement further. Always, when the term *ch'i* is used, an odor is meant. Cold, hot, warm, and cool are, however, the nature (*hsing*) of drugs. Thus, as the monograph on the common goose reads: "The fat of the white goose possesses cold *hsing*." "Cold *ch'i*" would be impossible here, for it is, of course, the nature (*hsing*) of drugs that is being discussed! When the four *ch'i* are mentioned, what is meant is aromatic-fragrant, putrid, penetrating, and strong-smelling. There is no connection [to the terms and concepts of] cold, hot, warm, and cool. If we take garlic, asafetida, dried fish, or sweaty socks, as examples, their odor can be described as putrid. The odor of the flesh of chickens, fish, duck, and snake can be termed penetrating. The odor of kidneys, foxes, of white horse penis, of underwear attached to the genitals, as well as of urinary sediments can be described as strong. Finally, the odors of *ch'en(-hsiang)*, sandalwood, camphor, and musk can be characterized as aromatic. In such cases the use of the term *ch'i* is appropriate. I fear that the character *ch'i* was mistakenly placed in the introductory sections [of the *Pen-ching*] later. It should be changed to *hsing,* which would correspond exactly [to the statement in question].[130]

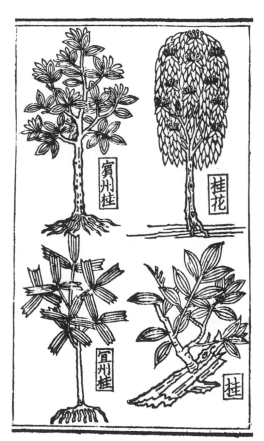

cinnamon tree *(kuei)—Ch'ung-hsiu cheng-ho pen-ts'ao*

The final section of the first chapter of the *Pen-ts'ao yen-i* contains a veiled, indirect critique of the principle of treating illnesses with only one effective drug. We recall that T'ang Shen-wei, at nearly the same time, included approximately 2,000 prescriptions in his *Cheng-lei pen-ts'ao* for the use of individual drugs. Although K'ou Tsung-shih did not treat this subject further or present alternatives, this paragraph can still be seen as an endorsement of the preparation of prescriptions from drugs of various degrees of effectiveness and functions, better taking into account the respective factors of the patients, which vary from case to case. Such a method of differentiating treatment belongs to the most essential maxims in the explanations of the *Huang-ti nei-ching* and was also postulated accordingly in the following period by the adherents of the newly emerging Chin-Yüan tradition.

> It is true that one can find in all directions on quantity such remarks as "one ingredient, one effective component" and "take one pill the size of a fine hemp seed," but these statements require further explanation. Because there are men whose finest influences are depleted and others whose finest influences are replete; because there are old and young people; because some illnesses have just arisen, while some have continued for a long time; because there are drugs with more or less medicinal effectiveness; and because it is necessary to think about a

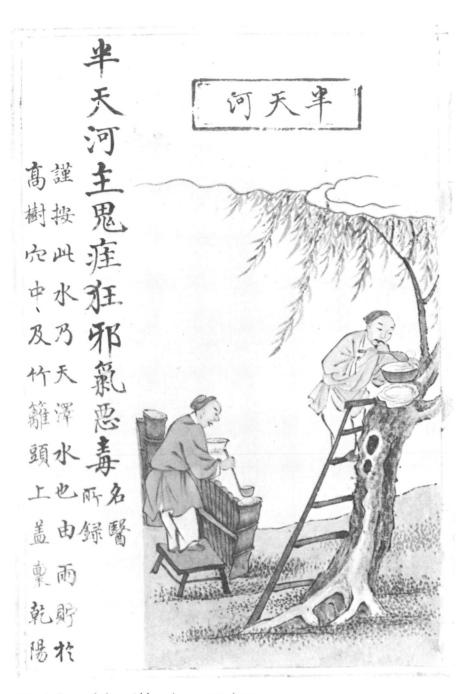

半天河

半天河主鬼疰狂邪氣惡毒名醫所錄

謹按此水乃天澤水也由兩貯於
高樹穴中及竹籬頭上蓋棄棗乾陽

The ladling of the midday river water *(pan-
t'ien ho)—Pen-ts'ao p'in-hui ching-yao*

96

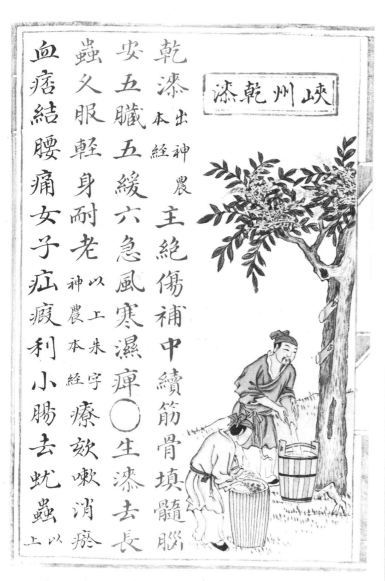

血痞結腰痛女子疝瘕利小腸去蚘蟲蟲久眼輕身耐老 神農本經 療欬嗽消瘀 安五臟五緩六急風寒濕痺〇生漆去長 乾漆 本經 出神農 主絶傷補中續筋骨填髓腦 以工朱字 神農本經 以上

the production of dried varnish *(kan-ch'i)*—
Pen-ts'ao p'in-hui ching-yao

fennel fruit *(hui-hsiang tzu)*—*Pen-ts'ao p'in-hui ching-yao*

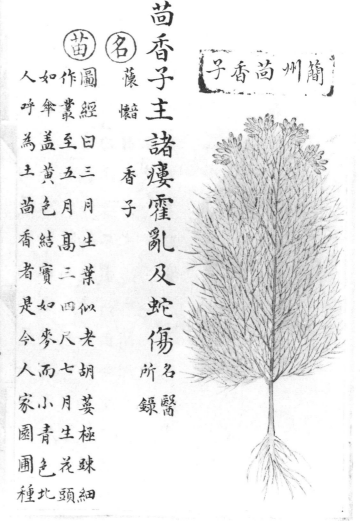

茴香子主諸瘻霍亂及蛇傷所錄 名醫

名 蘹懤 香子

圖經曰三月生葉似老胡荽極踈細作叢至五月高三四尺七月生花頭如傘蓋黃色結實如麥而小青色北人呼為土茴香者是今人家園圃種

97

correct dosage in each individual case, the example above cannot be followed in every instance. For always, in earlier times, when an example was established, it concerned a specific hypothetical situation. How could it be considered a firm rule?[131]

Other paragraphs of the first chapter are devoted to such subjects as the technology of medicinal forms and the preparation of drugs. However, there is by no means a more or less complete list of possible medicinal forms or methods of preparation.

In the second chapter of the *Pen-ts'ao yen-i*, K'ou Tsung-shih introduces further concepts of the theory of systematic correspondence as outlined in the *Huang-ti nei-ching*. For the first time in a pharmaceutical work, yin and yang are placed in relation to human existence.

The life of men is truly founded on a concentration of *yin* and *yang* influences. If one cannot balance the *yin* and *yang* influences, he will do harm to his life. Therefore, the treatise *Pao-ming ch'üan-hsing p'ien* comments: "Man emerges through the influence of heaven and earth."[132] It further states: "Heaven and earth allow their influences to combine, and man emerges."[133] That is possible because [what is categorized as] *yang* transforms itself into finest influences, and [what is categorized as] *yin* materializes itself into a shape. The transformation of the ethereal soul[134] corresponds to the change of *yang* [aspects] into finest influences. The transformation of finest matter influences into items corresponds to the materialization of *yin* [aspects]. When the *yin* and *yang* influences unite, the spirit will be in their midst. Therefore the treatise *Yin-yang ying-hsiang ta-lun* says: "Movement and motionlessness of heaven and earth are regulated by the spirit-brilliance."[135] This shows that the spirit-brilliance cannot be grasped with [the categories of] *yin* and *yang*. That corresponds to the statement in the *I[-ching]*: "That which cannot be measured by [the categories of] *yin* or *yang* is called spirit." Therefore it is said: The spirit must not be taxed excessively, otherwise it will be exhausted. The physical form must not be burdened excessively, otherwise it perishes. Consequently, finest essence, finest influences, and the spirit are the most important foundations of human [existence]. One must carefully maintain these foundations. Those who possess knowledge nourish their spirit and economize on their influences in order to strengthen their foundations.

There are scriptures in the world that disregard the rules of the protection of life. If [their advice were] put into action, each and every one of them would represent a violation [of the true principles of the nourishment of life]. Now, because they violate the prohibitions set up to nourish life, [people who have followed the advice in such scriptures] have no choice but to rely on external processes for their deliverance, for one cannot simply sit there and wait for death. The classic of *pen-ts'ao* [knowledge] was created out of this [necessity]. In order to understand the principles of deliverance [by external means], one must completely master the practical requirements. The [*Pen-ts'ao*] *yen-i* was created out of this [necessity]. It is true that the names [of the *Pen-ts'ao ching* and the *Pen-ts'ao yen-i*] are different, but their principles are in complete agreement. The point [in both works] is that knowledgeable as well as ignorant people are led into the Golden Age of Longevity and into the realm of peace and joy. Those who share this idea will explore the meaning [of this book] and therefore will be able [to achieve peace and joy].[136]

cicada *(tse-shan)*—Ch'ung-hsiu cheng-ho pen-ts'ao

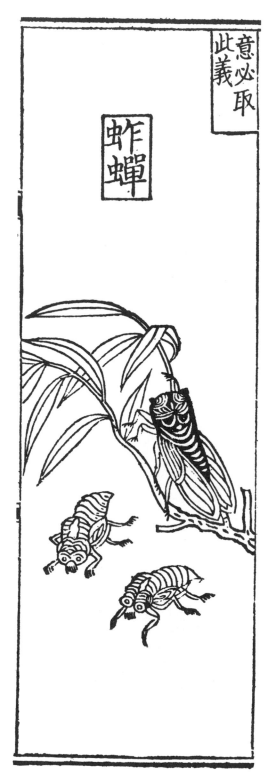

The last paragraph I wish to present here points out again the necessity of viewing people as highly differing individuals who must be treated differently in all cases of illness:

There are rich and poor, young and old people, and their respective illnesses must be considered separately. There are illnesses that have just begun and those that have lasted a long time, as well as [cases of] depletion and repletion, and their respective etiologies, which require different drugs. The hearts of the people, like their faces, differ from individual to individual. Not only are the hearts different but so are the depots and the palaces of the body. And if the depots and the palaces are different [from person to person], how would one manage to cure one [specific] illness in a large number of people with one and the same drug? Therefore, Chang Chung-ching said: There is a difference between high locations and low-lying regions. The nature of things may be soft or hard. There are differences in eating and living. For this reason, Huang-ti posed the question about the four cardinal points, and Ch'i Po mentioned the four therapeutic possibilities. In order to attain successes against illnesses, one must take both of these into consideration.

Consequently, it is crude negligence to combine drugs according to [fixed] prescriptions and then to use them on a broad basis. Wealthy people, for example, appear outwardly happy, but their minds suffer. If clothes and food are available in sufficient amounts, one seems outwardly content. But if, at the same time, the thoughts are burdened by too many reflections, one's mind suffers. Ch'i Po said: The illnesses originate in the vessels. If someone is outwardly happy, there is external repletion. If someone's mind suffers, there is an inner depletion. Therefore, the illnesses originate in the vessels. The lives [of the rich and] of the poor are marked by different nourishment. Sadness, joy, and thoughts are also different. In every case, treatment must be oriented toward the individual person. The medical men of later times really did not pay any attention to this rule; they cut it off and did not follow it. The loss suffered in this manner is considerable![137]

With repeated criticism, K'ou Tsung-shih turned against the former therapeutic practice that was based on the experience of the individual. This is expressed in his determined position against the use of individual effective drugs, and also in his condemnation of the practice of "relying on what one sees." K'ou Tsung-shih thus advocated a use of drugs corroborated by theory.

But if one looks for the theoretical system of K'ou Tsung-shih, only fragments of it are found—as we have seen—in the general sections in the three chapters preceding the monographs. To be sure, an explanation of the entire system would be neither meaningful nor possible in a work on materia medica. But K'ou seems to have consciously restricted himself to allusions, since even the themes suited for a materia medica, such as preparation of drugs and guidelines for the production of medicinal forms, have been given only in the form of excerpts.

Even the fact that K'ou Tsung-shih called the *Pen-ts'ao yen-i* a supplement to the *Chia-yu pen-ts'ao* and the *T'u-ching pen-ts'ao* cannot alter this judgment. This "supplement" is arbitrary and only seems to constitute a well-devised literary form in which K'ou Tsung-shih could express his thoughts. The three general chapters of the *Pen-ts'ao yen-i* might, as a consequence, carry merely a symbolic function. The author referred to all areas in which he was interested. He connected formerly heterogeneous currents on two levels, when he combined medical theory and pharmaceutical practice on the one hand, and Confucian, Taoist, and Buddhist elements on the other.

1.2.2. The monograph section of the *Pen-ts'ao yen-i*

K'ou Tsung-shih discussed 500 drugs in 466 monographs. The descriptions are generally not very detailed, especially in comparison with the works of the advanced main tradition. However, K'ou did not claim completeness, but rather—as the title of the work indicates—an "expanded meaning." Thus, the system of description varies from drug to drug; in most cases the author merely points out some characteristics of a specific drug that had not been mentioned in the latest pen-ts'ao works, or he quoted a statement from earlier authors which he considered false and, then, corrected it. Not all of his comments were based on his own studies; K'ou Tsung-shih frequently quoted other literary sources, such as the *Jih-hua tzu pen-ts'ao*, the *Yao-hsing lun*, and also the *Su-wen*. He described drugs according to origin, physiological effects, indication, appropriate form of medication, incompatibilities, external appearance, and similar technical criteria but, as mentioned before, he did so unsystematically. One also finds scattered Taoist stories which, as K'ou wrote, were meant to reinforce doubts. Only rarely is an explanation according to medical-theoretical considerations found in the monographs. One example of such theoretical reasoning can be seen in K'ou Tsung-shih's discussion of human milk:

> Human milk: It has many good effects in treatments of the eyes. What is the reason? The human heart produces the blood, and the liver stores the blood. When the liver has received the blood, then one is able to see. Thus, when water enters the conduits, the blood is generated from it. It is said further: when it moves upwards, it becomes milk; when it moves downwards, it becomes menstrual water. From this one knows that milk is blood. If one uses it as eye drops, shouldn't the two be suited for each other? Blood is *yin*; thus its nature is cold. People who store cold in their body's depots must not eat too much cheese and similar [food]. Although one speaks of cow's and sheep's milk, these are not exempt from the *yin* and *yang* [categories] of creation! The Western barbarians produce cheese from camel's and horse's milk. Old people who suffer from oral abscesses cannot eat this. For them it is good to drink hot human milk.[138]

K'ou Tsung-shih's remarks on the fishing cormorant provide an example of his critical attitude towards some of the information passed on through the literature for many centuries:

> The Fishing Cormorant. T'ao Yin-chü said: "This bird does not produce eggs. It spits its brood out of its mouth. Today the people call this

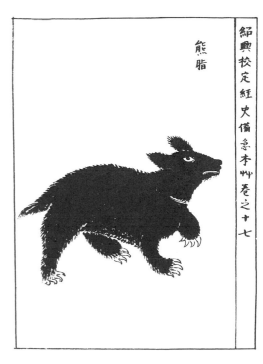

bear fat (*hsiung-chih*)—*Shao-hsing pen-ts'ao*

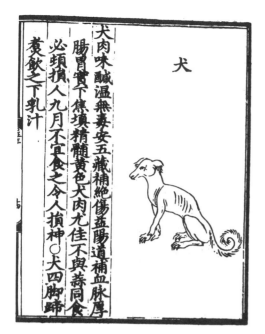

犬肉味鹹溫無毒安五藏補絕傷益陽道補血脉厚腸胃實下焦填精髓黃色犬肉尤佳不與蒜同食必頓損人九月不宜食之令人損神〇犬四腳蹄煮飲之下乳汁

dog *(ch'üan)*—Yin-shan cheng-yao

[bird] 'old water crow.' It nests on big trees in large crowds. The [cormorants] have regular places where they rest, and after a long time the trees wither because the droppings [of these birds] are poisonous. Pregnant [women] do not dare eat them because they spit their brood out of their mouth." Ch'en Ts'ang-ch'i, however, stated: "In order to achieve an easy delivery, when the time has come the delivering woman should hold one [of these birds]." This contradicts T'ao's comments. When I served as an official in Li-chou, a large tree stood behind my office. In its top there were some thirty to forty nests [of these birds]. I observed them day and night. Obviously they had intercourse and there were egg-grains spread all over the place. Their color was greenish. How could they spit their brood out of their mouth? This has never been questioned and investigated. Apparently, former [authors] have listened to somebody's erroneous talk.[139]

In the arrangement of the monographs, K'ou Tsung-shih followed the *Hsin-hsiu pen-ts'ao* of the T'ang period. There is, however, no reference to the old three-class division.

1.3. The theorization of drug knowledge

The description of K'ou Tsung-shih's *Pen-ts'ao yen-i* allows one to recognize the symbolic syncretism—characteristic of this work—which was the mark of the first part of the second phase of Neoconfucian influence on medical thinking in the Sung period. One can also see here the beginnings of the inclusion of practical pharmaceutical knowledge in the medical theory of the old classic *Huang-ti nei-ching*.

Attempts to perfect the theorization of pharmaceutical knowledge by means of a terminology based on the theories of yinyang and the Five Phases (*wu-hsing*) marks the second part of the second phase of the effects of the Sung doctrines on medicine. This endeavor, reflected in the pen-ts'ao literature of the Chin-Yüan period, consisted in building a structure for health care as a whole that would so thoroughly integrate medical theory and pharmaceutical practice that prevention, illness, diagnosis, drug qualities, and drug effects as well as pharmaceutical therapy would all be interdependent and interrelated within one single conceptual system.[140]

To this end, it was necessary to combine the subtly elaborated theory of how the organism was structured and how its functions could be influenced by certain drug qualities—the basis of which was supplied by the *Huang-ti nei-ching*—with the pragmatical values of therapeutic practice as it had been gathered in a centuries-old tradition and reflected in the *pen-ts'ao* and prescription literature.

2. The Pharmaceutical Literature of the Chin-Yüan Period

2.1. The *Chen-chu nang*

Li Shih-chen (1518–1593) recognized in the author of this little treatise—the complete original of which has, unfortunately, not been preserved—the originator of the so-called Chin-Yüan medicine. He described work and author in the following words:

[Chang Yüan-su] declared "Old instructions are not suited for today's illnesses," and developed his own doctrine. He distinguished the qualities of the drugs according to their [thermo-]influence and taste, their *yin* and *yang* [affiliation], their strength or weakness [in taste and thermo-influence], their [ability] to rise or descend [in the body], to float or to dive, to replenish depletions or drain repletions, according to [their relations to the] six climatic influences, and [their ability] to penetrate the twelve conduits. In addition, [he differentiated] the process of drug use according to the symptoms [of an illness]. [On the basis of these conceptions,] he created the "Secret Instructions for Treatment with the Main Therapeutic Effects" in connection with the "Essence of the Method of Experience," and called his work *Chen-chu nang*. With this work, he contributed much to the spread of medical principles. He is, after the [author of the] *Ling-shu*, absolutely the only man who can hold his own. Authors of a later time put the work into verse to facilitate its memorization and recitation. They incorrectly called it *Tung-yüan chen-chu nang*. It is unfortunate that the number of described drugs was limited to one hundred, and that he did not extend his comments to the entirety of materia medica![141]

Chen-chu nang
"The Pearl Bag"
1 chapter / 100 drug descriptions
Author: Chang Yüan-su (ca. 1180)
    tzu: Chieh-ku
    hao: I-lao
    from: I-chou
Written: date unknown
Published: date unknown

Further informative references to Chang Yüan-su and the doctrine he initiated are offered in his biography in the official history of the Chin dynasty:

Chang Yüan-su, whose *tzu* was Chieh-ku, came from I-chou. At the age of eight, he passed the boys' examinations. At the age of thirty-seven, he successfully participated in the *chin-shih* exams, in the subjects classics and essay. But since he used a character under taboo [which was part of the name of an emperor], he was stripped of his degree. Thereupon he turned to the study of medicine. He [knew] nothing that could have made him famous. Then, one night, he dreamed that a man, who was striking at his heart with a big axe and a long chisel, opened a cavity and placed a book with several chapters into it. From this time onward, [Chang Yüan-su] understood his art. Liu Wan-su, [whose *tzu*-name was] Ho-chien, once had been suffering for eight days from an illness caused by cold. His head ached and his pulse beat tightly. He suffered from vomiting, was unable to partake of any food, and did not know what to do. [Chang] Yüan-su went to him and wanted to examine him. [Liu] Wan-su lay facing the wall and took no notice [of his visitor]. [Chang] Yüan-su addressed him and said: "Why do you treat me in such a way?" Then he examined the [movement in his] vessels and began to talk about the condition of the [movement in the] vessels and the nature of the illness. [Liu Wan-su] agreed with him. Now [Chang Yüan-su] told him that he had consumed a particular drug with particular ingredients, and [Liu Wan-su] said that this was indeed so. Then [Chang] Yüan-su said: "You have made a mistake! Those ingredients of [your prescription] with cold nature sink [in the body] and penetrate the *great-yin* conduits. This results in a decrease of *yang* [influences], and perspiration cannot escape. As the [movement in your] vessels stands now, you must take such-and-such medications, so that a successful effect may take place." [Liu] Wan-su took a large dose of this prescription and was soon cured, as [Chang Yüan-su] had predicted. After that, [Chang] Yüan-su attained great fame.

When [Chang] Yüan-su treated illnesses, he did not follow old prescriptions. He explained this as follows: "The seasonal phases and the climatic influences are subject to ceaseless changes. Ancient and modern times cannot be compared. In the same way, the old prescriptions are not suited for today's illnesses!" These [thoughts] developed into the rules of a [therapeutic] doctrine.[142]

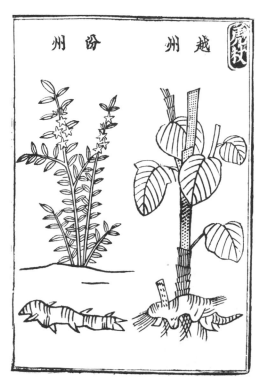

knotgrass root (hu-chang)—Hsin-pien lei-yao
t'u-chu pen-ts'ao

Thus, Chang Yüan-su devoted himself to the study of medicine as an alternative to his unsuccessful career as a Confucian official. The exact dates of his life are unknown; but the fact that he was a contemporary of Liu Wan-su (1120–1200) and the teacher of Li Kao (1180–1251) suggests that he lived in the decades between 1130 and 1210.

In the above-cited biography, an undoubtedly fictive treatment alludes to the contrast that must have existed between Chang Yüan-su and Liu Wan-su, according to all that is known about their differing opinions. Liu Wan-su was one of the "four great medical scholars of the Chin-Yüan period," among which Chang Yüan-su himself is not numbered. However, his pupil, Li Kao, is. In brief, Liu Wan-su was of the opinion that the most important drugs for the treatment of illnesses are those with cool thermo-influence. He ascribed to them the ability to subdue hyperfunctions in the heart and to benefit the level of liquid in the kidneys, and he explained the important functions of these drugs by stating that incongruities in these two depots are the starting point for most illnesses.

In contrast, Chang Yüan-su objected to using treatments for one patient that had been successful in another patient, without first taking the individual differences into account. This attitude is shown quite clearly in the remark, ascribed to Chang Yüan-su, concerning the nonapplicability of old formulas for the conditions of today.

This statement in particular, and thus the whole of Chang Yüan-su's activities, may also be viewed as an accusing metaphor against the outmoded, dogmatized laws of society, which led to the demotion of the young candidate in his bid for an official career. Consequently, this man's striving for a conformation of medical theory and pharmaceutical practice may also be based, to a certain extent, on the personal, bitter experience he was forced to undergo with the narrow-minded "old prescriptions" of the Confucian system and their undifferentiated application to the "conditions of today."

The authors of the biography and Li Shih-chen pointed out that Chang Yüan-su placed drug knowledge in a theoretical framework. At the core of this endeavor were the drug qualities, the thermo-influence, taste, and color, which are primarily perceived through the human sensory organs. From these were to be deduced, secondarily, the associations such as yinyang affiliation and position of the drugs in the system of the Five Phases, and finally, based on these, in a tertiary step, the drugs' modes of effect, such as their ability to rise or descend in the body, to penetrate this or that conduit, to replenish depletion or drain repletion, that is, the so-called secondary qualities. Since every person holds a position in the cosmic system of seasonal and regional influences different from that of his fellow humans, and since all seemingly similar illnesses do not have the same nature, even if their symptoms correspond in several persons, it is irresponsible, according to Chang Yüan-su, just as it was to K'ou Tsung-shih, to compile fixed prescriptions and to proclaim their effect on a specific illness. Only after the etiological background of the illnesses has been recognized in terms of the paradigms of systematic correspondence can one undertake the therapeutic treatment (which is thus different in almost every case) by means of the drugs standardized in the same theoretical system.

The realization of this requirement caused considerable difficulties, which forced concessions to the experiences of practice. When Li-Shih-chen spoke of Chang's "Process of Drug Use According to the Symptoms," he referred to a section that can also be found in later pen-ts'ao works of the Chin-Yüan tradition and which constitutes just such a concession. It lists, in brief directions, drugs that can, for example, cure headaches and many other symptoms, without revealing the theoretical links between the drugs and their effects on the illnesses.

A fragment of the *Chen-chu nang* is preserved as the fifth book of the collection *Chi-sheng pa-ts'ui* by Tu Ssu-ching (fl. 1315). The contents of this fragment, which (as a heading indicates) was chapter five of the original work, contain the following information:[143]

1. A list of 113 drugs with short comments on their respective qualities. For example:

   Pa-tou, acrid, pure *yang* [category]. Eliminates moisture from the stomach and abdomen. Breaks through constipations and congestions. It is a general who cuts open barriers and takes gates. It must not be used carelessly.
   Fang-feng, sweet, pure *yang* [category]. Basic drug for the great-*yang* conduit. Eliminates, from the body, wind moving upwards; slightly eliminates wind moving downwards. In mutual opposition with [the effects of] *kan-chiang*, *li-lu*, *pai-lien*, and *yüan-hua*.

2. A list of twelve conduits with their respective guiding drugs.
3. A list of various illnesses with appropriate drugs. For example:

   In case of repletion of blood, or accumulations of bad blood: *tang-kuei* diminishes [the blood; also] *su-mu*, *hung-hua*.
   In case of ulcers due to excessive [consumption of] wine one must eliminate stagnant heat from the bladder. Use *tse-hsieh*, *fang-i*.

4. Various minor theoretical statements, such as

   If an illness is in the upper [parts of the body], it corresponds to heaven. The [drugs] must be prepared through processes of roasting and washing with wine. When the drugs are boiled [the fire] must be strong, and [the resulting liquids] must be clear. Their intake must be carried out as slow drinking.
   If an illness is in the lower [parts of the body], it corresponds to earth. When the drugs are boiled [the fire] must be gentle, and [the resulting liquids] must be thick. Their intake must be carried out as fast drinking.

2.2. The *Yung-yao fa-hsiang*

The doctrine ascribing fundamental importance to the treatment of the spleen and the stomach is attributed in Chinese literature to Li Kao, another "great medical scholar of the Chin-Yüan period."[144] In view of the misery caused by the political turmoil during the fall of the Sung dynasty and the malnutrition connected with it, Li Kao did

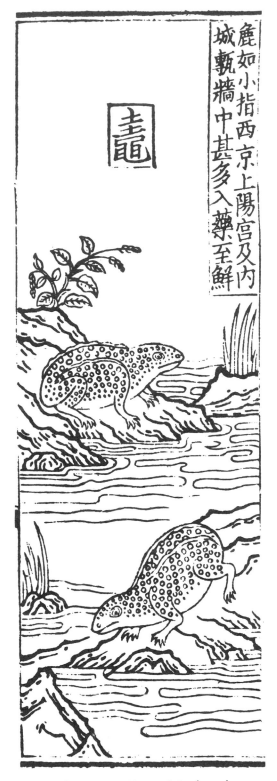

aquatic frog *(wa)*—*Ch-ung-hsiu cheng-ho pen-ts'ao*

Yung-yao fa-hsiang
"Rules and Correspondences in the Use of Drugs"
1 chapter / number of drugs: unknown
Author: Li Kao (1180–1251)
      tzu: Ming-chih
      hao: Tung-yüan
      from: Chen-ting
Written: date unknown
Published: date unknown

indeed stress the problems of digestion, which can become the cause of manifold illnesses.

To judge Li Kao strictly by that, however, is to limit oneself to the superficial. Far more important for Li Kao's position in the history of Chinese medical thinking is the fact that he adopted and expanded the teachings of Chang Yüan-su.

That Li Kao, too, intended to construct a comprehensive therapy system comprising medical theory and pharmaceutical practice is clearly demonstrated by his biography in the official history of the Yüan dynasty. Some excerpts may explain the views of Li Kao:

> Li Kao, whose *tzu*-name was Ming-chih, came from Chen-ting. In his hometown, his family held a powerful position on account of its wealth. Already in his youth, Kao found pleasure in medicine and medications. At that time, Chang Yüan-su from I was well known in the entire region between Yen and Chao for his medical [skills]. Kao paid him a large amount of gold and followed him as a student. After a few years, he had already completely mastered the teachings of [Chang Yüan-su]. Since Kao's family was very wealthy, he did not need to practice such skills professionally. He applied [his knowledge only during his] spare time to increase his personal reputation. Nobody dared to call [Li Kao] a physician. Even if high officials or educated men became ill, it was very rare—because of Li Kao's great wealth and outspoken nature—that he descended to them. They dared even less to consult him for a harmless or nonacute illness. Li Kao possessed extraordinary skills, particularly in the areas of illnesses caused by cold, of abscesses, and of eye diseases.
>
> In Peking lived a man whose name was Wang Shan-fu; he was an official for wine affairs in the capital. [Wang Shan-fu] fell ill with urinary retention, his eyes protruded, his abdomen became swollen like a drum, and his thighs became so hard that one got the impression they would burst immediately. He wanted to partake of neither food nor drink. Sweet and neutral, diuretic and laxative medications were administered to him, but none of them showed any effect. Finally, Li Kao said to the physicians: "The illness has only penetrated deeper [into the patient]. The *Nei-ching* refers to such a case when it states: The bladder is the palace containing the body liquids. It is absolutely necessary that the influences [of these liquids] undergo a transformation; only then can [the liquids] leave [the bladder]. Since you have used diuretic and laxative medications, the illness has only become worse. And that is because the influences were not transformed. Ch'i Hsüan-tzu has said: Where no *yang* [influences] exist, there is nothing from which the *yin* [influences] could arise. If no *yin* [influences] exist, there is nothing available to the *yang* [influences] that could transform them. Sweet and neutral, diuretic and laxative medications are all *yang* medications. But if one offers only *yang* [influences] to the body and no *yin* [influences], how can the [required] transformation take place?" On the following day, Li Kao treated the patient with a number of *yin* preparations. After taking them only once, the patient was cured. . . .
>
> Feng Shu-hsien had a nephew named Li. At the age of fifteen or sixteen, [this nephew] was taken ill with an affliction caused by cold. His eyes were red, and he was plagued by excessive thirst. [During the period of one breath] his pulse beat seven to eight times. Physicians advised him to take a "decoction that supports the influences." The medication had already been prepared when Li Kao entered from outside. Feng informed him of the circumstances, Li Kao checked the [movement in the] vessels [of the patient] and said in alarm: "This medication will almost kill the child! The *Nei-ching* says: 'If the [movement in the]

vessels is too fast, this indicates heat in the body; if the [movement in the] vessels is too slow, this indicates cold.' In our case, the [movement in the] vessels [of the patient arrives] eight to nine times [while he breathes once]. That indicates very great heat in the body of the patient. But the [section *Chih-*]*chen-yao ta-lun* [of the *Nei-ching*] says: 'There are illnesses in the course of which the [movement in the] vessels corresponds to the illness, but the symptoms are contradictory.' What does that mean? In the present case, the [movement in the] vessels corresponds to the illness. If one presses it, it does not [show the] drum [effect]. The other [ostensible] *yang* effects are all similar; they develop into *yin* symptoms." Li Kao then ordered that [the drugs] ginger and aconite be procured [and continued]: "I will prepare a prescription following the rule, 'because an illness is caused by heat, it must be treated with medications with cold (thermo-influence).'" The medication was not even quite ready when the hands and fingernails of the patient began to change. After a single dose of eight *liang*, he perspired heavily and then was cured.[145]

The biography casts a characteristic light on the position of a *ju-i*, a Confucian scholar-physician, who had no need of using his medical knowledge to earn a living. The practical use of these abilities outside of his own family always seems subject to occasions of accidental encounters with the patients. In these situations, the Confucian historians characterize the Confucian medical scholar Li Kao as a virtual *deus ex machina*, who demonstrates true skill to the helpless, apparently professional physicians who commit mistake after mistake.

Li Kao's skills, like the abilities of his teacher Chang Yüan-su, were based on the use of drugs according to theoretical standards. The biography repeatedly ascribes to Li Kao quotations from the *Huang-ti nei-ching su-wen*, which provided the theory that was to be combined with drug knowledge into one system.

The short work *Yung-yao fa-hsiang* has not been preserved in an independent form. In the first chapter of the *T'ang-yeh pen-ts'ao* by Li Kao's student Wang Hao-ku, under the titles "Rules and Correspondences concerning Drugs according to Mr. Tung-yüan" and "Process of Drug Use according to the Experience of Mr. Tung-yüan," we find Li Kao's theoretical doctrine on the application of pharmaceutical knowledge given in a total of twenty-seven essays.

One of the essays is entitled *Yung-yao fa-hsiang;* it cannot be determined to what extent it is identical with Li Kao's work of the same title. I will go into the contents of these twenty-seven essays in the course of my discussion of the *T'ang-yeh pen-ts'ao* (see pp. 108–117), which has been preserved, and which may be considered the most illuminating materia medica of the Chin-Yüan period.

2.3. The *Chen-chu nang chih-chang pu-i yao-hsing fu*

The authorship of this work cannot be definitely established. According to the title, it is supposed to have consisted of the *Chen-chu nang* (by Chang Yüan-su) and the *Yao-hsing fu* (by Li Kao). However, the contents of this particular *Chen-chu nang* are quite different from the *Chen-chu nang* in the *Chi-sheng pa-ts'ui* described above.[146]

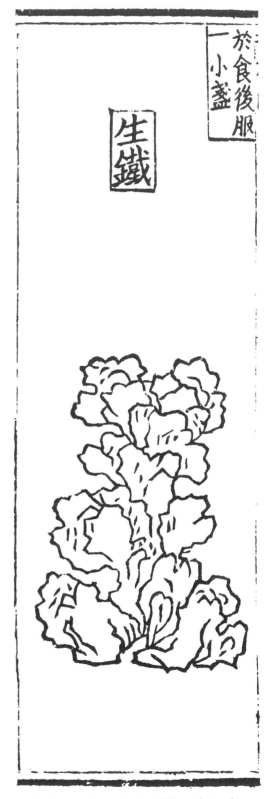

crude iron *(sheng-t'ieh)*—*Ch'ung-hsiu cheng-ho pen-ts'ao*

Chen-chu nang chih-chang pu-i yao-hsing fu
"The Pearl Bag, Expanded and Made Easily Understood [Combined with the] Poem on the Properties of Drugs"
4 chapters // 344/411 drug descriptions
Authors: (?) Chang Yüan-su (ca. 1180);
        tzu: Chieh-ku;
        hao: I-lao;
        from: I-chou
        (?) Li Kao (1180–1251);
        tzu: Ming-chih;
        hao: Tung-yüan;
        from: Cheng-ting
        P'u Li-i (ca. 1700)

The earliest preserved edition of the *Chen-chu nang chih-chang pu-i yao-hsing fu* dates from the time of the *k'ang-hsi* period (1662–1722). It is said to have been revised by a certain P'u Li-i. The work was probably compiled during the late Ming period, or perhaps not until the Ch'ing period; the contents allow a definite classification as a representative of the Chin-Yüan epoch pen-ts'ao tradition, and from the textual correspondences with the first chapter of the *T'ang-yeh pen-ts'ao,* it can be assumed that Li Kao, at least, had a significant share in the authorship.

The *Yao-hsing fu,* which has been lost as an independent work, and the *Chen-chu nang* were said to constitute the first and second chapters of the *Chen-chu nang chih-chang pu-i yao-hsing fu.*[147] The drug monographs follow in the third and fourth chapters. The text was recorded in verse (and will be discussed further during the presentation of drug works in verse; see chap. D. sec. IV).

The outline of contents, reproduced below, shows the differences from the pen-ts'ao works in the main tradition and the authors' method in the construction of a comprehensive therapy system.

Chapter 1

a. Enumeration and description of 248 drugs, subdivided into four classes according to their cold, hot, warm, or neutral nature. Additional information on the taste and medicinal strength of the individual drugs.

b. Explanations concerning the application of drugs:

Treatise on the yin- and yang-related attributes of drugs

Treatise on what is external/secondary and basic/primary

Regulations for the use of drugs

Regulations concerning the rising, descending, floating, diving, replenishing, and draining nature of drugs

(Results) desired in the five depots

Sufferings in the five depots

Enumeration of which five odors penetrate which of the five depots

Table of correlations among the Five Phases, the five colors, the five tastes, and the five depots (as well as a list of those parts of the organism) mastered (by the depots), together with dietetic prohibitions (in case of an illness in one of the depots)

A list of drugs to be used as guiding and main curative drugs in the external and internal sections of the three yang conduits in the hands and feet

A list of drugs for the reduction of fire-evil in all conduits

A list of drugs with mutually opposing effects

A song on 18 drugs with mutually opposing effects

A song on 19 drugs with mutual fear

A song on 6 drugs that must be aged

A list of drugs that develop main curative powers for the restoration of depletion and the reduction of repletion in the five depots

A list of drugs and their use (according to symptoms)

Chapter 2

a. Instructions on the main curative effects of drugs. (A list of 90

drugs and descriptions of the following characteristics, with
varying comprehensiveness and completeness:)
Suitability as ruler-, minister-, assistant-, or aid-drug
Information on mutual compatibility
Information on drug processing and preparation
Appearance
Thermo-influence and taste
Medicinal strength
Rising and descending in the body
Yinyang categorization
Indications
b. Information necessary for the use of drugs:
Rules and correspondences in the use of drugs
Regulations for the use of drugs in connection with the four seasons
(The suitability of) pills and powders in the use of drugs
Song on the origins of the five tastes of drugs
Song on the preparation and further processing of drugs
Song on drugs whose use is contraindicated for pregnancy

Chapters 3 and 4

Monographs on 410 drugs; subdivided into nine sections: precious
stones/minerals, herbs, trees, human, fowl/other animals, worms/
fish, fruits, grains, vegetables (the latter including, for example,
monographs on wine and vinegar). The main emphasis of the
monographs is on the indications, but they also contain descriptions of drug qualities, as in 2a.[148]

2.4. The *T'ang-yeh pen-ts'ao*

Wang Hao-ku, like his teacher Li Kao, belonged to the most distinguished class of medical practitioners, the Confucian scholar physicians. In his writings he referred to Li Kao's, and thus also to Chang
Yüan-su's, teachings in addition to the work of the medical scholar
Ch'eng Wu-i, who was active during the Chin period. Among other
things, Ch'eng Wu-i strove for a new interpretation of Chang Chi's
works on illnesses caused by cold, in light of the theories of the *Huang-
ti nei-ching*.[149]

In combining the teachings of the above-mentioned medical authors
and his own commentaries, Wang Hao-ku created the *T'ang-yeh pen-
ts'ao*, which, consequently, can be viewed as a typical product of the
Chin-Yüan period pen-ts'ao tradition. This work, which has been
preserved, is not particularly extensive and is introduced by three (in
some editions two or only one) prefaces by Wang Hao-ku. The first
chapter contains 37 general treatises; 224 drug monographs are collected in the second and third chapters.

T'ang-yeh pen-ts'ao
"Medications Administered as Decoctions"
3 chapters / 224 drug descriptions
Author: Wang Hao-ku (mid-13th century)
   tzu: Chin-chih
   hao: Hai-tsang
   from: Chao-chou
Written: ca. 1246–1248
Published: date unknown

2.4.1. The second preface of the *T'ang-yeh pen-ts'ao*

Shen-nung tested all herbs and determined the nine indicators [of the
movement in the vessels], in order [to enable mankind] to adjust itself

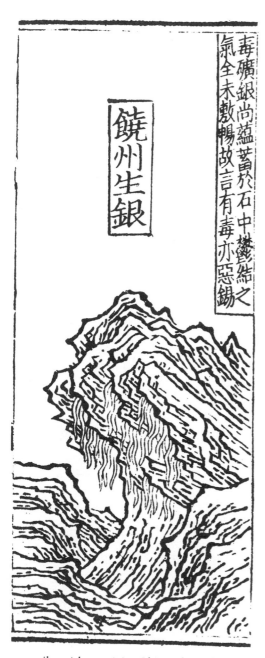

饒州生銀

毒礦銀尚藴蓄於石中欝結之
氣全未敷暢故言有毒亦惡錫

pure silver (sheng-yin)—Ch'ung-hsiu cheng-ho
pen-ts'ao

correctly to the changes and transformations of the *yin* and *yang* [influences] and to provide assistance in case of disturbances and against the premature termination of life. He thus established regulations for all time, which were, at the same time, easily recognizable and important. He was followed [in this endeavor] by I Yin from the Yin period. I Yin doubled [the number of drugs] of Shen-nung and recognized the importance of establishing [medical] regulations. Thus, not causing any harm [to Shen-nung's original work] he compiled the "[Scripture on] Decoctions" (*T'ang-yeh*). This work was expanded by Chang Chung-ching during the Han period; he, in turn, doubled [the number of drugs described by] I Yin. [Chang Chung-ching] also recognized the importance of establishing [medical] regulations. Consequently, not causing any harm [to Shen-nung's original work] he composed the "Real Treatise" (*Ch'üeh-lun*).[150] Chieh-ku Lao-jen, from the Chin empire, continued this line and, in turn, doubled it in comparison with Chang Chung-ching. He also recognized the importance of all the [theoretical] regulations. [His work] was therefore of no harm [to Shen-nung's original work] when he wrote his "Unique Commentary" (*Ch'i-chu*). Chieh-ku's doubling [of the material], compared with Chung-ching's, was in no way different from Chung-ching's expansion [of the material of] I Yin. When Chung-ching doubled [the contents] compared with I Yin, this was in no way different from I Yin's expansion of Shen-nung's material. There were, to be sure, differences in the dimensions of the expansions and continuations [of the works of the respective predecessors]. All of them, however, recognized the importance of establishing [theoretical] regulations. If one examines the words of Chung-ching, the views of I Yin can be recognized. None of them deviated from [the original intentions of] Shen-nung. [For this reason, anyone concerned with medicine] must first study the *Pen-ts'ao*, then the *T'ang-yeh*, then the *Shang-han lun*, and also the *Pao-ming shu*.[151] None of these works may be neglected. In Ch'eng Wu-i's work *Ming-li fang-li* it is written: "All prescriptions that have come down to us from ancient times have become more and more foreign over the years, and it is difficult to check [the criteria] according to which [they were compiled]." The prescriptions of [Chang] Chung-ching constitute the earliest collection. Now, [the work] of Chung-ching goes back to the regulations established by I Yin, and I Yin's [work] has its origins in the prescriptions of Shen-nung. Among the medical writings, these scriptures were especially closely related. The [later works] adhered to the ancient regulations and did not deviate in the least from them! Indeed, the work of the great sages [of antiquity] lies here before us! In Wen Lu-kung's *Yao-chun* it is written: "All prescriptions have their origins solely with [Chang] Chung-ching." However, since olden times—the T'ang and Sung period—there have been [individuals] with a name in medicine, such as Wang Shu-ho [210–285], Ko Hung [281–340], Sun Ssu-mo [581–682?], Fan Wang, Hu Hsia, Chu Feng-i, Wang Ch'ao-feng, Ch'ien Chung-yang [1035–1117], Ch'eng Wu-i, and Ch'en Wu-che. When they discussed the rules of structuring a prescription, they added and took away and applied all kinds of changes [to the original formulas of Chang Chung-ching]. In this manner originated a thousand different works and ten thousand diverging opinions. None of them coincided with the [work and conceptions of] Chung-ching. There were more than a hundred alleged paradises! Chang Yüan-su, [whose *tzu*-name was] Chieh-ku lao-jen, once met a wise man who taught him secret prescriptions that had been handed down from ancestors, which were not supposed to be given [to outsiders]. Chieh-ku later [passed on] these prescriptions to his son, Chang Pi, [whose *hao*-name was] Yün Ch'i-tzu, and to Li Kao, [whose *hao*-name was] Tung-yüan [and whose *tzu*-name was] Ming-chih. All [of these prescriptions] originate in the *T'ang-yeh* of Chang Chung-ching from Ch'ang-sha. Unfortunately, there is no one else in the world who could know of them. I myself learned them from the old Tung-yüan, and, therefore, I dare to make them known.

Written by Wang Hao-ku in the year *ping-wu* [1246], summer, sixth month.[152]

In the prefaces to his materia medica, Wang Hao-ku elucidated, among other things, the medical-historical position claimed by representatives of the Chin-Yüan period doctrine. In the second preface of the *T'ang-yeh pen-ts'ao*, reproduced above, this claim is expressed in two ways: first of all, it is evident in the assertion, introduced in the first preface and continued in the second, that the efforts to "establish regulations," that is, to combine effectively medical theory and pharmaceutical practice, concerned a "renewed accord" between the two components. Second, Wang Hao-ku constructed a tradition that ran visibly from Shen-nung in ancient times to Chang Chi (i.e., Chang Chung-ching) during the Han period and then apparently broke off, continuing somewhere underground; and only now, through the efforts of Chang Yüan-su, had it been restored to its rightful, dominant position.

These assertions correspond strikingly to similar constructions in other areas of literature. Neoconfucians, such as Han Yü (768–824), Li Ao (died 844), and Chu Hsi (1130–1200), referred to a tradition in which they saw the transmission of the true principle tao continued only as far as Mencius (372–289 B.C.), and now claimed for themselves the renewed continuation of the genuine tradition, following a long hiatus.

Like Neoconfucianism itself, the Chin-Yüan period trend of medical thought did not actually mean a resumption of an old tradition that had been buried for centuries—this becomes exceedingly evident in the field of pharmaceutical literature. Rather, it can be viewed as an attempt at reform, which had as its goal the overcoming of obsolete, impractical structures. The authors of the Chin-Yüan tradition of pen-ts'ao literature presented their reforms as a reaction, as a resumption of a tradition unjustly thrust aside. Under this cover they were able to achieve a large following.

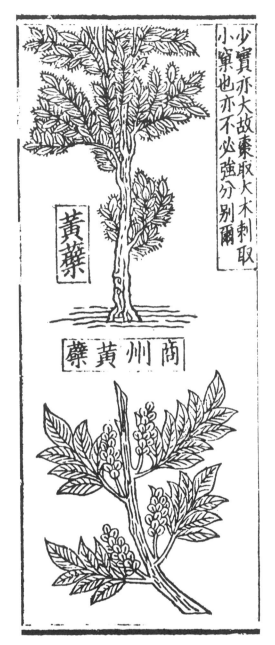

phellodendron bark *(huang-po)*—Ch'ung-hsiu cheng-ho pen-ts'ao

2.4.2. The first chapter of the *T'ang-yeh pen-ts'ao*

The efforts of the Chin-Yüan pen-ts'ao authors to theorize pharmaceutics made it necessary to acquaint the reader with the basics of the relevant theories for the use of medications. In a manner similar to the ten general sections of the *Pen-ching* (which, of course, were concerned with practical use) and the commentaries of T'ao Hung-ching, as well as, to a lesser extent, the *T'ang pen-ts'ao*, Chang Yüan-su, Li Kao, Wang Hao-ku, and the successors to this tradition usually arranged treatises devoted mainly to theory before the monograph section of their drug works.

In the *T'ang-yeh pen-ts'ao* this involves thirty-seven treatises, of which only a few are devoted to purely practical pharmaceutical questions. These can be subdivided into three sections, their distinctive features being the following.

The first section begins with the fundamental treatise "The tastes of drugs one may wish to employ for replenishing [depletions] or draining [repletions] in case of sufferings in the body's five depots." Here Wang Hao-ku presented the system of treating certain conditions in the five depots by means of drug qualities which had been, in each case, derived from theory. His arguments are based on a treatise from the *Su-wen*, in which the theoretical connections between drug qualities and the treatment of symptoms of depletion and repletion are suggested—that is, according to the Five Phases with which the five depots are associated. Wang Hao-ku expanded the purely theoretical statements of the *Su-wen* both by adding annotations to the theory itself and by including concrete drug names as examples of a transformation of theory into practice.

An excerpt from this first treatise is given below. I have underlined the citation from the *Su-wen*, not only to make it visible but also to show its integration into Wang Hao-ku's own assertions. A short graphic summary of the correspondences and interdependencies alluded to in Wang Hao-ku's argumentation may clarify the underlying paradigm before I quote Wang Hao-ku's own words.

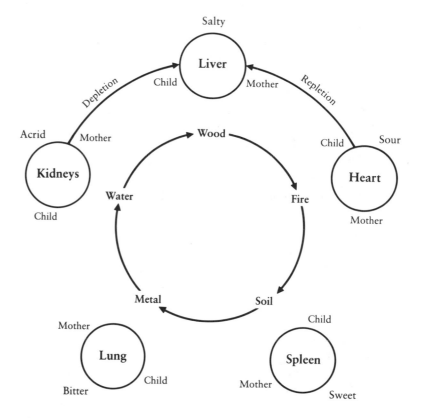

The tastes of drugs one may wish to employ for replenishing [depletions] or draining [repletions] in case of sufferings in the body's five depots.

If the liver suffers from tensions, sweet [drugs] should quickly be taken in order to relieve [these tensions]. [The drug] *kan-ts'ao* [is advisable in this case]. If one wishes to disperse [obstructions within the normal course of influence flow in the liver] acrid [drugs] <u>should be taken quickly</u>. [The drug] *ch'uan-hsiung* [is advisable in this case]. With <u>acrid</u> (drugs) one <u>replenishes</u> the [liver]; *hsi-hsin* [is appropriate]. With sour [drugs] one <u>drains</u> [the liver]; [the drug] *shao-yao* [is appropriate in such a case]. In the case of depletions, drugs such as *sheng-chiang* and *ch'en-p'i* are used for restoration. In the classic it is said: In case of depletion the mother [depot] must be strengthened. Water can produce wood. The kidneys are the mother [depot] of the liver, since the kidneys are the water. Bitter [drugs] replenish [depletions] in the kidneys. Thus, in order to replenish the kidneys [drugs like] *shou-ti-huang* and *huang-po* are appropriate. In case symptoms for other illnesses are not present, the *ti-huang* pills [according to the prescription suggested] by Ch'ien (I) will master [this task]. If there is repletion, [the drug] *pai-shao-yao* drains it. If no symptoms of other illnesses are present, the *hsieh-ch'ing* pills of Mr. Ch'ien will master [this task]. If there is repletion, drain the child [depot]. The heart is the child [depot] of the liver. One takes [the drug] *kan-ts'ao* in order to drain [the heart].[153]

The essential part of the general statements in the first chapter of the *T'ang-yeh pen-ts'ao* is found in the treatises of the second section. Under the headings "Rules and Correspondences concerning Drugs According to Tung-yüan" and "Methods for the Use of Drugs According to the Experience of Tung-yüan," the theoretical and practical teachings of the medical scholars Chang Yüan-su, Li Kao, and Wang Hao-ku himself are collected in twenty-seven treatises.

At this point, for the first time in the pharmaceutical literature, we encounter the pharmacology of systematic correspondence, an innovative doctrine concerning the activities of drugs in the organism. This doctrine established a subtle connection between the central phenomena of illness and medicinal therapy—that is, between organism, illness, diagnosis, drug qualities, and drug effects. As admirable as this system was from the theoretical point of view, however, it nevertheless formed a construction whose application in daily medical practice was considerably limited, if not, considering the requirements, impossible.

A first crucial problem discussed in detail in this section is the standardization of drug qualities. Such a standardization was necessary in order to arrange drug effects into an accepted mechanism of effects. Since it was not possible to examine the effects of drugs within the organism itself, one was limited to assigning to given or assumed characteristics of drugs a certain positional value in the system of the yinyang and Five Phases theories relevant to the organism and its functions.

The subjectivity of human sensory organs, however, hindered this process; for instance, not all drugs described by an author as being "sour" were so distinctly characterized by taste that every other author would necessarily follow this assertion. In this manner, considerable differences arose, resulting from the varying interpretations of, for example, an external characteristic, and the differing values ascribed to the drug in question that such interpretations brought about.

The formation of an objectively reconstructable referential system was further hindered by certain inherent contradictions (and by the compromises necessitated by these contradictions). Since in some cases obvious attributes and characteristics of drugs (for instance, a strong taste) did not agree with the obvious effects resulting from an intake of these drugs (that is, the observed effects contradicted those that were to be expected, through theoretical deduction, from such obvious attributes and characteristics), various constructs were introduced, which increasingly complicated the entire system.

The contradictions could be explained easily by maintaining that the yang contained yin and that the yin contained yang, an ideal possibility for turning black into white. In addition, the distinctness of drug qualities was subjected to various gradations—for example, weak-bitter, normal-bitter, and markedly-bitter—with each of these gradations allowing for a different position of a drug in the system of correspondences and, hence, for a theoretical agreement between quality and effect.

A second crucial problem that considerably hindered the application of the pharmacology of systematic correspondence in actual therapeutic practice is to be seen in the diagnosis of the medicine of systematic correspondence. One should keep in mind the complexity of a system in which all known and hypothetical processes in the organism and their disturbances were assigned, by means of rather complicated constructions, to the categories of the yinyang and Five Phases theories. Mainly by examining the movement in the vessels, a patient's condition was now to be diagnosed so accurately that the drug effects suitable for treatment, which were associated with the above-mentioned theories in a similarly complicated system, could be designated exactly and supplied for the effective application.

In an earlier investigation, I demonstrated how uncertain, even today, the mass of practitioners of the traditional Chinese curative system on Taiwan are, with respect to their diagnostic abilities. This does not include the considerable skills of observation, based upon long experience, that such medical practitioners are able to acquire. These skills always contain, however, a strongly subjective element; the uncertainty of the practitioner is based upon the lack of a standardizable system.[154]

In the middle of the second section of the first chapter of the *T'ang-yeh pen-ts'ao,* we find a treatise entitled "Drugs for the Treatment of Illnesses, in Accordance with the Symptoms." It is found under the heading "Techniques for the Use of Drugs According to the Experience of Tung-yüan" and differs from the preceding treatise in that the presentation of the recommended treatments with drugs is not based upon theoretical considerations, but rather in accordance with the observations of actual symptoms and successful cures: "The [drug] *shao-yao* should be taken for abdominal pains; for bad cold and pains add [the drug] *kuei*; for bad heat, add [the drug] *huang-po*."[155]

The instructions in this treatise represent an obvious advance with respect to medical practice. The traditional system of diagnosis required decades of study to master, if that were even possible. As long as diagnosis based upon theory and its appropriate treatments is not possible, the medical practitioner is forced to rely upon experience. By far the greatest portion of prescription literature, which itself characteristically forms the most extensive genre within traditional Chinese medical literature, contains such "experience" prescriptions. Far re-

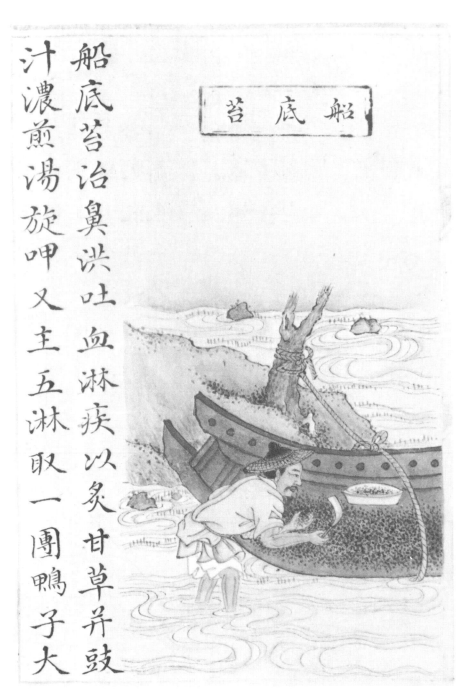

船底苔治鼻洪吐血淋疾以灸甘草并豉

汁濃煎湯旋呷又主五淋取一團鴨子大

苔底船

gathering moss from the bottom of boats
(ch-uan-ti t'ai)—Pen-ts'ao p'in-hui ching-yao

Illustrations depicting the preparation of "powder frost" (fen-shuang) from epsom salt, table salt, alum, and quicksilver (upper left and right, lower left); "spiritual sand" (ling-sha: lower right), artificial cinnabar prepared with honey—Pen-ts'ao p'in-hui ching-yao

114

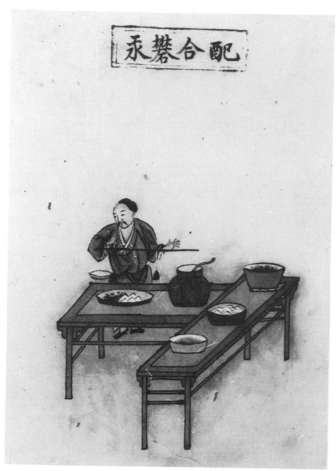

配合礬汞

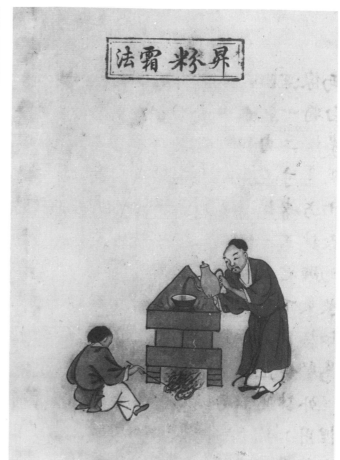

昇粉霜法

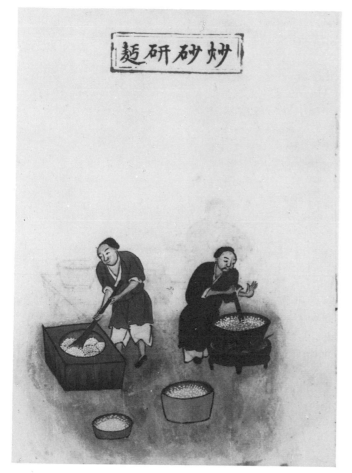

炒砂研麪

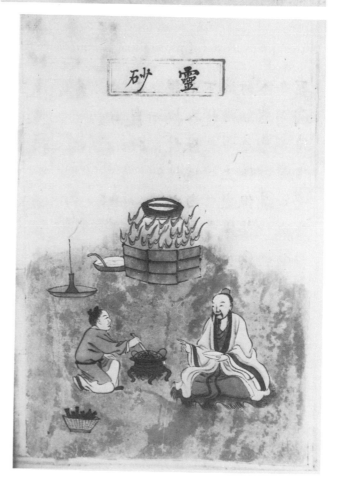

靈砂石

moved from any theory, the mass of medical practitioners could make use of such sources for their requirements.

The subsequent treatises in the middle section of the first chapter of the *T'ang-yeh pen-ts'ao* are devoted in part to the preparation of drugs. Here are found, often justified by theory, information on the preparation of prescriptions, on relative quantities and units of measurement, and instructions for the preparation of drugs and their processing into medicinal forms.

The third section in the general discussions of the first chapter mentions, among other topics, the handling of potent medications, demonstrated by a quotation from the *Su-wen*. The authors of that period were thoroughly acquainted with the problem of secondary effects, a problem that became acute when illnesses were treated inappropriately with potent drugs. Other treatises in this section are based upon the doctrine of the five seasonal phases and six climatic influences (*wu yün liu ch'i*), the beginnings of which were already 五運六氣 contained in the *Su-wen* but which had gained wide attention only after the publication of the *Yün-ch'i lun* by Liu Wen-shu in 1099.

2.4.3. The drug monographs in the *T'ang-yeh pen-ts'ao*

In the second and third chapters of his materia medica, Wang Hao-ku describes 242 drugs, 128 of which he had taken from the prescription works of Chang Chi.[156] These monographs were not arranged in accordance with the main tradition of pen-ts'ao works. Wang Hao-ku placed the extensive sections dealing with the frequently used herbs and tree drugs at the beginning; the sections on fruits, vegetables, grains, precious stones/minerals, fowl, quadrupeds, and worm drugs followed.

The oldest subdivision of drugs—into upper, middle, and lower classes—is absent in these monographs. Nevertheless, Wang Hao-ku's work includes a valuation of drugs utilizing the *chün-ch'en-tso-shih* 君臣佐使 terminology; this terminology, however, was no longer used in the sense of the first general section of the *Pen-ching*, but rather was based upon the passage from the *Su-wen* which had been quoted for the first time in the second of the general sections in the *Pen-ching*, (see C, I, 1.1.1) and which read: "Rulers (*chün*) are those drugs that conquer illnesses. Ministers (*ch'en*) assist the rulers. Aides (*shih*) help the ministers."[157]

The meaning of the three classes (*tso* and *shih* drugs combined) was thus reversed for pen-ts'ao literature. Beginning with the Taoist-influenced *Pen-ching* and throughout the main tradition, the class of ruler drugs had been considered as a collection of rather preventive drugs lacking a pronounced medicinal efficacy. Now, in accordance with the *Su-wen*, the concept of "rulers" included those drugs supposed to develop the main effect in a prescription. The reinterpretation of the remaining concepts developed accordingly.

Moreover, the concept *shih* ("aide," "envoy") received a completely new meaning: "conduit-guiding drug." This designates those drugs capable of guiding other drugs through the corresponding conduits in the body to the intended location.

The individual monographs in the *T'ang-yeh pen-ts'ao* begin—like the drug works of the main tradition—with information on taste, thermo-influence, and medicinal effectiveness. Advice on contraindications, place of origin, collection time, drying methods, incompatibilities, and drug preparations is almost completely lacking.

New is the assignment of drugs, based upon respective taste and thermo-influence, to the three yin and three yang depots and to the twelve conduits in the body. In addition, possible use as a "guiding drug" is specified.

Wang Hao-ku also cited earlier works and authors, although the quotations are usually not presented word for word, but rather in an abridgment faithful to the original sense. He made a special effort to include the main effects on each drug, rejecting the simple listing of drug effects with no evaluation, which had been customary in the works of the main tradition. The *T'ang-yeh pen-ts'ao* contained no illustrations.

The *T'ang-yeh pen-ts'ao* was subsequently the object of never-ending interest in all centuries as the most representative work of this new direction. For this reason, it has been preserved in sixteen Chinese editions from the Yüan, Ming, and Ch'ing epochs, and also from the period of the national Republic and People's Republic, as well as in one Korean and four Japanese editions.

2.5. The *Pen-ts'ao yen-i pu-i*

Pen-ts'ao yen-i pu-i
"Additions to the Elucidation of the Meaning of Pharmaceutics"
1 chapter / 153 drug descriptions
Author: Chu Chen-heng (1282–1358)
    tzu: Yen-hsiu
    hao: Tan-hsi
    from: I-wu in Che-chiang
Written: date unknown
Remained unpublished as an individual work; in 1536 it was included in the collection *Tan-hsi hsin-fa*

Chu Chen-heng became known as the fourth, and also last, in the series of "four great medical scholars of the Chin-Yüan period." He had studied Confucian literature intensively since his early years, so report his chroniclers, and had prepared ambitiously for the exams required for a career in government service. His poor performance in the exams for the rank of *chü-jen* ended all these hopes. As a consequence, Chu first devoted himself to the study of Neoconfucianism and only later, when he was already thirty-six, turned his special attention to the acquisition of medical knowledge. Supposedly, this step was the result of a pious attitude toward his mother who, like Chu himself, suffered from chronic indigestion.[158]

Chu Chen-heng combined the teaching of his three predecessors Liu Wan-su (1120–1200), Chang Ts'ung-cheng (1156–1228) and Li Kao (1180–1251) and developed the theory of frequent depletion of yin influences and surplus of yang influences as a cause of illness.

Numerous case histories from Chu Chen-heng have come down to us; as in the case of Li Kao, they depict him as a physician who towered above all other medical practitioners of his time. After all, because of his education and demeanor he could be included in the class of the Confucian scholar-physicians.

Chu Chen-heng left several works. In the preface to this best-known book, the *Ke chih yü-lun* ("Further Discussion of the Study of Things and of the Acquisition of Knowledge"), one can once more find the usual conceptions of the Chin-Yüan authors, to whom the *Su-wen* supplied the medical theory, the *Pen-ts'ao* provided the pharmaceutics, and Chang Chi's works, the prescriptions.

The *Pen-ts'ao yen-i pu-i,* whose title can be understood as a reminiscence of K'ou Tsung-shih's drug work, is the final *Pen-ts'ao* of the Chin-Yüan epoch. Its contents elucidate Chu Chen-heng's contribution to the theorization of drug knowledge. Chu continued to undermine the system of standardization of drug qualities by adding a new variant to the concessions already inherent in this system. For example, if a red drug had previously been assigned to the element fire, including all additional associations of fire, and if all effects of the drug in question that did not conform with those expected from these associations were explained, for instance, by the varied influences in the interplay of yin and yang, Chu Chen-heng would assign some drugs to two or three categories of the Five Phases theory at the same time, possibly in order to resolve those effects in contradiction with theory. In so doing, he expanded the possible associations and correspondences to such an extent that the system of standardization thoroughly lost its definitive power.

The *Pen-ts'ao yen-i pu-i* was never published as an individual work; perhaps it was not even conceived as such. It does not contain any general treatises, but rather 153 drug monographs in which, above all, the author attempted to provide the prescriptions of the Han period pragmatist, Chang Chi, with a theoretical reference.

Following the primary works of the Chin-Yüan tradition, all of which have been discussed here, there came a long series of secondary works whose authors adopted Chin-Yüan ideas, continuing them for centuries without providing any new impulses. I shall present some representative products of this subsequent tradition—no claim of completeness is made. The comprehensiveness of my characterization will correspond to the significance of the work.

3.1. The *Pen-ts'ao fa-hui*

The author of the *Pen-ts'ao fa-hui,* the earliest pen-ts'ao work of the Ming period, was a student of Chu Chen-heng. In a preface to an edition of the *Pen-ts'ao fa-hui* prepared by Hsüeh K'ai (ca. 1500) and his son, Hsüeh Chi (ca. 1505–1566), included in their compilation *Hsüeh-shih i-an ch'üan-shu,* Hsü Yung-ch'eng's work is clearly characterized as a sequel to the Chin-Yüan epoch:

> In later times when prescriptions and drugs were discussed, the *Pen-ts'ao* of Shen-nung was considered to be the origin. The authors Chang Chieh-ku, Li Tung-yüan, and Wang Hai-tsang elucidated the meaning [of this work]. During the *chih-cheng* period of the Yüan dynasty [1341–1367], Hsü Yung-ch'eng from Shan-yin once again collected the thoughts of Chu Tan-hsi and Ch'eng [Wu-i] from Liao-she and wrote a work in which he revised their teachings, supplied information that had been lacking, and undertook classifications.[159]

Hsü Yung-ch'eng began his work with three chapters of drug monographs; the theoretical treatises were placed in a fourth chapter at the conclusion. The description of the individual drugs followed the pat-

3. Later Works in the Chin-Yüan Tradition of Pen-ts'ao Literature

Pen-ts'ao fa-hui
"Elucidation of Pharmaceutics"
4 chapters
Author: Hsü Yung-ch'eng (?–1384)
    tzu: Yen-ch'un
    from: Hui-chi in Che-chiang
Written: ca. 1341–1367
Published: date unknown

tern: metals/minerals, herbs, trees, man, quadrupeds, fowl, worms/ fish, fruits, rice/grains, and vegetables.

The monographs are introduced by two- to three-line references to the characteristics and qualities of the drugs, in which taste, thermo-influence, medicinal strength, and main indications are stressed. Quotations from earlier works of Chang Yüan-su, Li Kao, Chu Chen-heng, Ch'eng Wu-i, Wang Hao-ku, K'ou Tsung-shih, and from the *Su-wen* then follow. The theoretical treatises in the fourth chapter are frequently based upon exact quotations, slightly expanded, from Chin-Yüan authors. Li Shih-chen, in a critique of this work, stated that the author did nothing but "bind together" excerpts from Chin-Yüan authors, without adding any contributions of his own.

This work, preserved in several editions from the Ming and Ch'ing epochs, as well as from the period of the republic, was not illustrated.[160]

3.2. The *Pen-ts'ao chi-yao*

Pen-ts'ao chi-yao
"A Collection of the Important Elements in Pharmaceutics"
8 chapters / 545 drug descriptions
Author: Wang Lun (ca. 1500)
    tzu: Ju-yen
    hao: Chieh-chai
    from: Tz'u-chi in Che-chiang
Written: 1492–1496
Published: 1496

The author, Wang Lun, portrays the structure of the *Pen-ts'ao chi-yao* and his own intentions in the preface:

In my free time I undertook comparative studies of the *Pen-ts'ao* and of the work of [Li] Tung-yüan and [Chu] Tan-hsi. I eliminated superfluous material and retained what was important. I limited this material to five chapters which [constituted] a middle section [of my own work]. Furthermore, I took over all information from the first chapter of the *Pen-ts'ao,* as well as statements from the *Nei-ching* and from Tung-yüan, insofar as they were related to the *Pen-ts'ao.* The result was a chapter which I placed at the beginning. It presents the source of pharmaceutics and constitutes the first section. I then arranged, in twelve groups, curative properties of drugs according to their natural characteristics, comprising a total of two chapters. This constituted the third section, which I consider a simplification of prescription arrangement, if, as a result of illness, one is faced with the necessity of using drugs. I changed the manuscript three times; after four winters and summers the work was completed. It contains a total of eight chapters. The title reads *Pen-ts'ao chi-yao* simply because I have selected what was most important, in order to facilitate the work of beginners and Confucians like myself, who would like to pursue this art as a sideline. Specialists gifted with great intelligence will, of course, have to consult the complete works [of pharmaceutics]. They cannot disregard so much material and be satisfied with such a simplification.[161]

When Wang Lun mentioned the *Pen-ts'ao,* he meant the *Cheng-lei pen-ts'ao* from the main tradition. Although Wang's own work, in terms of content, can clearly be included among the sequels to the Chin-Yüan tradition, it nevertheless shows the increasingly intensifying trend towards uniting elements of both traditions, creating, in the process, a new doctrine which valued as equal the purely pragmatic and theorizing tendencies. Wang Lun's work shows the beginnings of this effort, which may have resulted from an inapplicability of the pure Chin-Yüan system for practical use. Only a short time later, a separate tradition in this direction can be ascertained—the eclectic pen-ts'ao tradition (see C, IV).

Apparently, Wang Lun was not a physician by profession, but rather had become interested in medical questions because of the ethical obligations of the educated Confucian. He had passed the *chin-shih* exams and had risen through the ranks in governmental service. His work opened with an introduction in which he referred to his esteem for the works of Li Kao and for the information in the *Su-wen*. The preface, excerpts of which have been given above, and the first chapter (which is preceded by a table of contents) follow this introduction. The first chapter begins with the first ten general sections of the *Pen-ching* followed by numerous quotations from the *Su-wen*, to which the author added his own remarks.

Monographs comprise the second through sixth chapters. The arrangement is similar to that in the *T'ang-yeh pen-ts'ao;* descriptions of drugs from the following areas are provided: herbs, trees, vegetables, fruits, grains, minerals, quadrupeds, worms/fish, and man.

The characterization of the individual drugs begins with information on taste, thermo-influence, medicinal strength, and conduit affinity. This is followed by a description of the main effects and finally—here the influence of the main pen-ts'ao tradition is recognizable again—by directions on suitable medicinal forms, drug dosage, and time for the administration of medication.

In the final two chapters (seven and eight) which constitute the third section of his work, Wang Lun arranged all drugs into twelve groups, in accordance with their effective properties. In so doing, he partially resumed the tradition of T'ao Hung-ching, who had begun his materia medica with drugs listed according to the illnesses and symptoms they were capable of curing. While T'ao, however, had subdivided his list into eighty-three groups of concrete symptoms, Wang Lun undertook a classification into twelve groups determined mostly by theoretical considerations of drug effects. He differentiated the following groups:

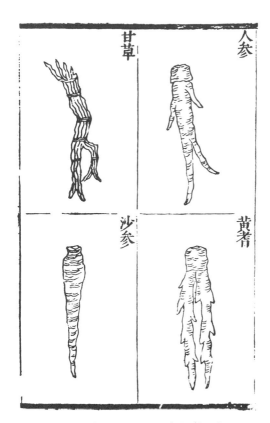

ginseng (*jen-shen:* upper right), licorice root (*kan-ts'ao:* upper left), astragalus root (*huang-ch'i:* lower right), and adenophora root (*sha-shen:* lower left)—*Pen-ts'ao hui*

Drugs for the treatment
  of the influence balance   of the influence of wind
  of the influence of cold   of dryness in the body
  of the blood   of abscesses
  of the influences of heat   of poisonings
  of mucous afflictions   of women's complaints
  of the influences of moisture of childhood diseases

The *Pen-ts'ao chi-yao* was not illustrated; it has been preserved in several Ming editions, the earliest of which is dated 1529. It was not reprinted after the Ming period.[162]

3.3. The *Pen-ts'ao hui*

The writing of the *Pen-ts'ao hui* and of subsequent works in the later Chin-Yüan tradition had been preceded by an extremely incisive turning point in the development of pen-ts'ao literature. In 1596, the

Pen-ts'ao hui
"Collected Pharmaceutical Knowledge"
18 chapters / 488 drug descriptions
Author: Kuo P'ei-lan (seventeenth century)
    tzu: Chang-i
    from: Wu-hsien in Chiang-su
Written: date unknown
Published: 1666

Pen-ts'ao kang mu by Li Shih-chen had been published. This gigantic work influenced almost all of the later pen-ts'ao authors; numerous drug works of the following period must be understood as immediate reactions to the *Pen-ts'ao kang mu.*

The *Pen-ts'ao hui,* written by Kuo P'ei-lan, was also subjected to such an influence, and it would probably be appropriate to undertake its discussion only after an analysis of the *Pen-ts'ao kang mu.* However, since I wish to give priority to the description of continuous traditions, I will place the discussion of the last three selected representatives of the later Chin-Yüan tradition before the section dealing with the *Pen-ts'ao kang mu.*

The *Pen-ts'ao hui* was published only in the two editions that have been preserved: a Chinese edition from 1666 and a Japanese from 1693. The Chinese edition was published by the author himself.

Kuo P'ei-lan was a pupil of one of the best-known medical writers of the Ming period, Li Chung-tzu (died 1655), who edited this work and supplied a preface. Two other prefaces were written by Kuo P'ei-lan.

Following the prefaces, 208 illustrations to the drugs are presented together. There are four illustrations per page; some portray the drugs, others the original plants or other materials in simple sketches that, nevertheless, emphasize the major characteristics. There is one illustration per drug. Differences in drug development owing to geographic conditions were not taken into consideration.

The table of contents is followed by a preliminary chapter containing a list of forty-seven earlier *pen-ts'ao* works and relevant information concerning their authors, number of chapters, number of drugs, as well as brief critical characterizations.

In an introduction, also contained in the preliminary chapter, the author wrote that he considered his work to be a supplement to the *Pen-ts'ao kang mu,* particularly in the areas of drug qualities, the four methods of diagnosis, and the theories of the seasonal phases and climatic influences (*wu yün liu ch'i*), as well as in the area of conduits, all of which had been neglected in the *Pen-ts'ao kang mu.* Otherwise, the *Pen-ts'ao kang mu* had served as the foundation of his work. However, he had not adopted any superfluous material.

The first chapter of the *Pen-ts'ao hui* begins with a treatise on all conduits and also contains illustrations otherwise known only from handbooks on acupuncture. These are followed by theoretical introductions which continue through the eighth chapter. In these introductions the author discussed very thoroughly the Chin-Yüan theories. Many quotations bear the names of Li Kao, Chu Chen-heng, K'ou Tsung-shih, or the *Su-wen,* and have been provided with new commentaries for better understanding.

Among other things, we find here a list of drug effects, which have been borrowed from the theories of the Five Phases and yinyang, as, for example, "divert in the child [depot]," "strengthen in the mother [depot]," or "stimulate the influences into flowing." In each case, suitable drugs are cited.

In addition, we find a list of guiding drugs and an enumeration of specific illnesses, including the drugs suitable for treatment. For various categories of illness, contraindications are also given. An important section here contains the description of the course of illnesses, such as those caused by cold, and women's and children's diseases.

The drug monographs are collected in chapters nine through eighteen. The structural pattern is independent, but it shows the influence of the *Pen-ts'ao kang mu:* herbs, grains, vegetables, trees, worms, scaly animals, crustaceans, fowl, quadrupeds, humans, metals/minerals, pieces of clothing/household utensils, waters, fires, and soils.

The monographs begin with the usual information on thermo-influence and taste. This is followed by remarks concerning the ability to penetrate specific conduits and to cure specific illnesses. All this information is theoretical; remarks about, for example, methods of preparation or measurements are missing. In some cases, the geographical areas producing the best-developed drug types are noted. To avoid adulteration, Kuo P'ei-lan occasionally also described the appearance, size, and color of drugs.[163]

3.4. The *Pen-ts'ao shu*

In 1625, Liu Jo-chin successfully completed the *chin-shih* exams and entered into a career as a Confucian official. Later, he withdrew for some time into seclusion; and in thirty years he wrote what is probably the most extensive sequel to the Chin-Yüan tradition of pen-ts'ao literature. After a minor revision of the original manuscript, this drug work appeared in three printings from the years 1700, 1810, and 1876, all of which have been preserved.

Among the five to six prefaces that introduced each of the various editions, the one by a man named Kao Yu, dated 1699, is particularly striking. It represents a late excursion into the Sung philosophy of Chou Tun-i (1017–1073) and Chu Hsi (1130–1200) and classifies Liu Jo-chin's *Pen-ts'ao shu* in the Chin-Yüan tradition:

Pen-ts'ao shu
"A Presentation of Pharmaceutics"
32 chapters / 512 drug descriptions
Author: Liu Jo-chin (1584–1665)
      tzu: Yün-mi
      hao: Li-yüan i-sou
      from: Ch'ien-chiang in Hu-pei
Written: ca. 1635–1665
Published: 1700

太極

> The principle of the highest point of reference (*t'ai-chi*) is fulfilled by the *yin* and *yang* [categories of all phenomena]. One of the latter is always idle or moving and, alternately, one is the origin of the other. [The *yin* and *yang* categories] themselves are therefore fulfilled by *yin*-in-*yang* and by *yang*-in-*yin* [subcategories]. The *yin* and *yang* [influences] of heaven had to disperse, and they formed the Five Phases of Change. When it is said that the [concrete] substance collected in the earth, that [subtle] influences rose into heaven, and that nothing remained exempt [from being made up of either *yin* or *yang* influences], then this shows the ubiquity [of these categories] in the universe. Is not this also the reason that man's reception of *yin* and *yang* [influences] is reflected in the formation of his body's depots and palaces, of his [subtle-matter] influences and blood and of his body's construction and protection facilities? And if we assume all that as given, is it not also the reason why the reception [of *yin* and *yang* influences] in herbs, trees, worms, fish, birds, quadrupeds, metals, minerals, waters and soils [is reflected] in their warm, cool, cold, and hot [thermo-influence], in their dryness or humidity, as well as in their quality of rising or descending

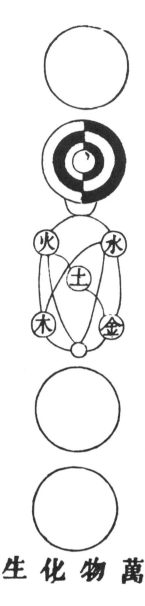

萬 物 化 生

[in the human body]? Even if the *yin* and *yang* [category of a phenomenon] can be easily distinguished, the so-called *yin-in-yang* and *yang-in-yin* [subcategories] are subtle and mysterious and difficult to put into words. When of the two sages Shen-nung and Huang-ti [the former] chewed [drugs] in his mouth and observed their internal [effects] and [the latter] used stones to punctuate [the skin], they endeavored to discover the doses and the limits [in the use of medications] and to recognize the vessels and their connections. Only after [such investigative efforts] they arrived at their knowledge [about the *yin-in-yang* and *yang-in-yin* subcategories]. In contrast, the common practitioners and dilettantes occupy themselves only very superficially with these things; what errors are the result! When one strives to examine thoroughly the *yin-in-yang* and the *yang-in-yin*, one should investigate the entirety of things. Here [one will find that] the one highest point of reference and every individual thing contain the principle of the highest point of reference. And this implies the knowledge that the characteristics of man correspond to the four seasons just as the effective properties of drugs correspond to the body's five depots and six palaces. The underlying principle is the same. The correspondence of man's characteristics to the four seasons, and of the effective properties of drugs to the body's five depots and six palaces, is based on the fact that they are affected by the influences of heaven and earth, which take shape, assume their characteristics, and through this turn into the respective concrete [phenomena]. Thus, movement and rest are opposites, but each is the origin of the other. *Yin* and *yang* are separate and lie, nevertheless, next to each other. When it is said that the Five Phases of Change form the one [duality of the] *yin* and *yang* [categories], that the *yin* and *yang* [categories] form the highest point of reference, and that the highest point of reference, in turn, constitutes that which is without reference [*wu-chi*], then this means that ten thousand diversities go back to one origin. The foundation of the great creation lies in the transformation of the [*yin* and *yang*] influences; the genesis of men and of things is not excluded from this [process]. For man this implies that the *yin* and *yang* [categories] of the highest point of reference are materialized as the body's five depots and six palaces. For things this implies that everything is divided as belonging to one of the *yin* and *yang* [categories] of the highest point of reference; the [thermo-]influences and the tastes are, of course, distinguished accordingly. That means that one origin produces ten thousand variations. If one traces back all [variations to their origin], one arrives at the single essential element. And of [this essential element's] ten thousand possible applications, there is not one that is not realized. The one essential element disperses into ten thousand applications. This one essential element has always been present. Therefore, the sages Hsüan [Yüan] and Ch'i [Po] partook of this knowledge from the time of birth on; the exemplary Chang Chieh-ku, Li Tung-yüan, Wang Hai-tsang, and Chu Tan-hsi explained and clarified it.[164]

The external form of the *Pen-ts'ao shu* has been influenced to a much greater degree by the *Pen-ts'ao kang mu* than was the case with the *Pen-ts'ao hui*. The subtle structural pattern is oriented entirely on that of the *Pen-ts'ao kang mu*, and it will be discussed with that work.

The individual monographs are very detailed. Numerous submonographs are added to the 512 major headings, bringing the total number of described drugs to 691. The drug descriptions all contain Liu Jo-chin's own explanations, and many also provide precisely marked quotations from earlier works, from the *Huai-nan tzu* to the Chin-Yüan authors, and, finally, to Miu Hsi-yung.

In the spirit of the Chin-Yüan teachings, great value is placed on the description of theoretical relationships. In addition, the monographs contain references to prescriptions and frequently, in an appendix introduced by the designation "Preparation," information on the preparation of the drugs.[165]

3.5. The *Pen-ts'ao shu kou-yüan*

As indicated by the title of the *Pen-ts'ao shu kou-yüan*, and as stated in one of its prefaces, Yang Shih-t'ai intended to revise the *Pen-ts'ao shu*. Therefore, almost every monograph in his work contains longer or shorter sections that correspond to the text of the *Pen-ts'ao shu*. The format of both works is also very similar; the arrangement of the drugs is nearly the same, and the main monographs are also divided into several submonographs. Thus, for example, the monograph "pig" is divided into individual descriptions of stomach, spleen, heart, heart blood, tail blood, gall [bladder], liver, lung, intestines, kidneys, lard, sow's milk, and pork, so that far more drugs are discussed than one would assume from the number of main monographs.

In spite of the fact that large portions of the text were taken over from the *Pen-ts'ao shu*, the contents of the monographs are different in the *Pen-ts'ao shu kou-yüan*. Following the names of the drugs, Yang Shih-t'ai described—although not systematically—their origin, occurrence, seasons of growth and of origin, time of gathering, appearance, method of preparation, and other things. This is followed in the monographs by information concerning the taste, thermo-influence, suitability as guiding drug, and the yinyang associations. This information has been taken mainly from the *Pen-ts'ao shu*. Whereas Liu Jo-chin had clearly marked each of the quotations from earlier authors by introductory words such as "Hai-tsang wrote," similar care cannot be discerned in Yang Shih-t'ai's efforts. Only sporadically does he insert the author's name at the end of some quotations, in small print. In comparison with the *Pen-ts'ao shu*, it is also striking that Yang Shih-t'ai always omitted the references to the strength of medicinal efficacy (*tu*).

Further on in the text we find information on the indications and examples for the use of the drug by earlier authorities. In a section entitled "Discussions" (*lun*), which was not added to all the monographs, the author dealt with, in the spirit of the Chin-Yüan theories, the physiological connections of the drug's effects.

As in the *Pen-ts'ao shu*, some of the monographs also contain an additional section entitled "Preparation," in which problems of pharmaceutical technology, such as the preparation of suitable forms of medication, are addressed.

One of the prefaces of the *Pen-ts'ao shu kou-yüan* is dated 1842, and was written by Tsou Shu (1790–1844), the author of another pen-ts'ao work which we will encounter during the discussion of the pen-ts'ao literature in the *Han-hsüeh* tradition. Tsou Shu was an avowed opponent of the Chin-Yüan tendencies in medical thought, a fact that

Pen-ts'ao shu kou-yüan
"A Study of the Origins of the Presentation of Pharmaceutics"
32 chapters / 495 drug descriptions
Author: Yang Shih-t'ai (?–ca. 1832)
　　tzu: Mu-ju
　　from: Wu-chin-hsien in Chiang-su
Written: ca. 1830–1832
Published: 1842

毒

論

漢學

he also pointed out, though in a cautious manner, in his preface to the *Pen-ts'ao shu kou-yüan:*

> The *tao* is expressed ten-thousandfold in all things, yet all things are not sufficient to reflect the *tao* adequately. The [principle] *li* is expressed [ten-thousandfold in all] words, yet all words do not suffice to describe the *li* adequately. Because those who speak about medical themes are hindered by [the insufficiency of] language, they do harm to [the principle] *li*. It is generally claimed that specific drugs cure specific illnesses, and further, that the treatment [of illnesses] must proceed according to rigid regulations. That may be successful in one case, but in nine out of ten cases [the treatment undertaken according to such principles] remains ineffective. As a result, thorough investigations of the actual [relationships between drugs and successful cures] and, furthermore, of the hypothetical [connections are conducted. The outcomes of these investigations] are written down in great detail and at extreme length. It thus occurs that the simplicity of the old literature is confronted with the complexity of contemporary works. The simple [literature] is difficult to understand, whereas the complex [literature] easily leads to mistakes. If one wants to find the suitable [mean] between complexity and simplicity, one must understand the origin of the *tao* and not diverge from it. One must penetrate to that which corresponds to the [principle] *li* and make one's decisions accordingly. Therefore, Mr. Yang Mu-ju has written a *kou-yüan* for the *Pen-ts'ao shu*. The *pen-ts'ao* [knowledge] is profound, simple, and old. In the Han period, Chung-ching and Yüan-hua had taken up [the tradition] that had been handed down orally by teachers and pupils since the three epochs of antiquity. Chen-pai curbed the flow [of the tradition]. Chen Ch'üan and Jih Hua-[tzu] supported the waves [of the tradition] and [T'ang] Shen-wei, finally, clarified the origin [of the tradition]. They all just pointed out the facts as far as the correspondence of application to substance of all things is concerned. The four scholars of the Chin-Yüan period subsequently wanted to clarify the reasons for these facts. They did not compare the suitability of specific drug qualities and specific drug effects for the treatment of [specific] processes and peculiarities of illnesses, but they relied on abstracts, and, for systematizations, collected all theories in which something is classified, for example, as a metal or as wood, and is therefore able to penetrate the lung or the liver. They claimed that there were wondrous peculiarities of separation and combination.
>
> I fear that the verbosity in which people were lost in later times has contributed in no slight degree to the spreading of mistakes.
>
> Mr. Liu Jo-chin from Ch'ien-chiang wrote the *Pen-ts'ao shu*. In it, he explained the [constant] up and down of *yin* and *yang* by means of a temporal arrangement of the genesis and maturation of drugs, as well as by means of their five [thermo-]influences, five tastes, and five colors. He apparently intended to combine the [teachings of the] four scholars into one sequence. Unfortunately, his explanations are convoluted and far too voluminous. The reader has almost no chance of discovering their meaning.
>
> Mr. Yang is an extensively educated Confucian scholar who has comprehended what is essential in the pure principle. He removed the superfluous portions [of the *Pen-ts'ao shu*] and thus attained an [original] simplicity [of expression].[166]

The elimination of "superfluous material" referred to by Tsou Shu did not include any discarding of Chin-Yüan theorization. Yang Shih-t'ai quoted the Chin-Yüan authors exactly; he also made extensive use in his own commentaries of the theories of the Five Phases and yinyang, as well as of the abilities of the drugs, deduced from these theories, of balancing surfeits and deficiencies or of penetrating into a certain conduit.

Yang was unable to witness the publication of his work. It did not appear until ten years after his death, published by one of his pupils, Wu Chung-ch'ang.[167]

Through the subdivision into "Drug Works of the Actual Chin-Yüan Epoch" and "Later Works in the Chin-Yüan Tradition," I have already pointed out that, following the passing away of the original authors of the Chin-Yüan period, only epigonic works were created,

4. Concluding Observations on the Chin-Yüan Tradition of Pen-ts'ao Literature

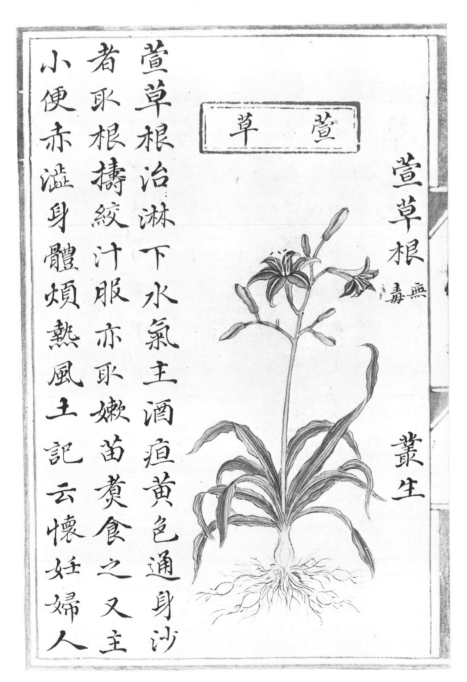

the "lily of forgetting" (hsüan-ts'ao)—Pen-ts'ao p'in-hui ching-yao

which took over the new thoughts but could no longer provide further impulses. Two major reasons may have contributed to the fact that the original impetus of the Chin-Yüan tendency exhausted itself so soon. One reason may be seen in changes in the sociopolitical climate coinciding with the establishment of the Ming dynasty. Although Neo-confucianism was adopted by the Ming and also by the Ch'ing administrations as the official doctrine, it is not difficult to recognize that the Sung concepts had lost their attractiveness for a majority of Chinese intellectuals. Chinese thinkers turned their attention away from solutions proposed by Sung authors to remedy the ills of society; intellectual eclecticism and the school of Han-learning (Han-hsüeh) emerged as alternatives. Both of these two intellectual currents exerted their own impact on medical and pharmaceutical literature and will be discussed in later sections of this present work. Thus, it should not be surprising that the attempts to link the application of drugs to the concepts of the Huang-ti nei-ching were not pursued any further. But aside from this external condition there may have been another, more immanent reason for the apparent lack of innovative Chin-Yüan thinking after the time of Chu Chen-heng. One might simply assume that the sophistication of theorization of drug knowledge reached in Chu Chen-heng's materia medica served its purpose well. It was possible now to explain every detail of drug effects on the basis of concepts borrowed from the Huang-ti nei-ching. Interviewing contemporary practitioners of traditional Chinese medicine in Taiwan and recording their conversation with patients, I found, for the most part, that they were satisfied with the utility provided by the conceptual framework of the yinyang and Five Phases theories in understanding drug efficacy.[168] As an outsider, though, one may legitimately point out that these theories, while suitable for providing a posteriori explanations, appear to lack the basis for developing objective criteria needed for predicting drug efficacy. The emphasis on taste, thermo-influence, and color as basic parameters appears, from today's perspective, insufficient for a generation of a standardized pharmacological science.

III. TWO OUTSTANDING DRUG WORKS OF THE SIXTEENTH CENTURY

As we have seen, the main pen-ts'ao tradition had broken off in the thirteenth century for at least one major reason. The drug works that appeared during the final phase of that tradition suffocated from their own structure, which permitted no meaningful development beyond the point already reached. The *Pen-ts'ao p'in-hui ching-yao* might have become the nucleus of crystallization for a new productive development. At the time it was written, two circumstances coincided which appeared favorable. The authors of the *Pen-ts'ao p'in-hui ching-yao* were able to overcome the structural crisis of the old tradition; and simultaneously, for the first time in several centuries, an imperial order was issued for the revision of a drug work—the *Cheng-lei pen-ts'ao*.

Various sources give us a fairly detailed description of the history of the origin of the *Pen-ts'ao p'in-hui ching-yao*. Apparently out of personal interest, the scholar and official Ch'iu Chün (1420–1495) had taken the trouble to prepare a fundamentally revised version of the *Cheng-lei pen-ts'ao*.[169] He succeeded in recognizing and removing the main obstacle for a practical application of the overly long Sung-period works in the main *Pen-ts'ao* tradition: his merit lies in the restructuring of the individual drug monographs. While each encyclopedic pen-ts'ao work of the Sung period chronologically cited all statements of previous authors and added its own commentary as a conclusion, Ch'iu Chün took numerous individual statements from the total oeuvre of earlier authors and arranged them according to thirteen technical aspects. If a medical practitioner wanted to inform himself about a specific characteristic of a drug, such as its origin or main therapeutic effect, he was no longer compelled to read the gigantic monographs from cover to cover in order to arrive at a comprehensive overview and judgment. He now had the means of obtaining specific information by one glance under the appropriate rubric. In this manner, Ch'iu Chün saved a great deal of space and paper, because, for example, if all previous information concerning the thermo-influence and taste of a specific drug was in agreement, it was necessary to record it only once. Only for rubrics such as "indications," "place of origin," and some others did it seem advisable to identify by name individual statements of previous authors and to present them in sequence. This differentiated method of quotation contributed significantly to the practicality of the work.

Ch'iu Chün died before he was able to complete his work. The overall plan had been finished, but he had been able to write down only one single monograph as an example for all the others. These records came into the hands of an official of the Imperial Medical Office, Liu Wen-t'ai, who, it is believed, intended to pass the work off as his own achievement. It is thought that he wanted to attract the favor of the emperor, Hsiao-tsung (1470–1505), whose great interest in questions of medicine and pharmaceutics was well known. Tradition tells us that this ruler personally made pills in a pharmacy in the southern part of the capital, in order to pass them out to officials and to the people.

1. *The Yü-chih pen-ts'ao p'in-hui ching-yao*

Yü-chih pen-ts'ao p'in-hui ching-yao
"Materia Medica Written on Imperial Order, Containing Essential and Important Material Arranged in Systematic Order"
Short title: *Pen-ts'ao p'in-hui ching-yao*
42 chapters / 1815 drug descriptions
Author: Ch'iu Chün (1420–1495)
    tzu: Chung-shen;
    from: Hai-nan
    Liu Wen-t'ai (ca. 1500) and others
Written: 1503–1505
Published: 1937

In the sixteenth year of the governmental period *hung-chih* (1503), Emperor Hsiao-tsung ordered the eunuch Hsiao Ching (1438–1528) to deliver the following decree to the Grand Secretary Liu Chien (1434–1527):

> Since [the statements in] the old editions of the Materia medica do not seem to be uniformly detailed or brief, two officials of the Han-lin Academy, in collaboration with the officials of the Imperial Medical Office, are to eliminate the superfluous, rectify deficiencies, and thus create a [new] work, in order to facilitate the use [of the Materia medica].[170]

A severe dispute arose over the responsibility for carrying out this decree. Liu Chien suggested the officials Shen Tao (1452–1515) and Ch'en Chi (1465–1539) as representatives of the Han-lin Academy. This was granted. A petition, signed by Shih Ch'in, was sent from the Imperial Medical Office to the emperor requesting that the execution of the task be entrusted to the colleague Liu Wen-t'ai. This request was also granted. But Liu Chien objected, giving the following arguments: the writing of books requires literary knowledge and bibliographical skills. Only with such skills can one make selections and cuts in accordance with appropriate criteria, without committing any mistakes. The pen-ts'ao works had formerly been revised by wise men and were related in many respects to the classical and historical works. This makes these works difficult to understand. The officials of the Imperial Medical Office were competent only in the handling of drugs, Liu argued; they did not have any knowledge in the field of literature. Therefore, one could reasonably fear that a revision of the materia medica undertaken by these people would contain numerous mistakes that could bring only harm to subsequent readers. Consequently, Liu Chien asked the emperor to charge the Ministry of Rites with the testing of all people concerned. Only those who really possessed pharmaceutical as well as literary training should participate in the work. Under no circumstances should unqualified people, concerned only with the emperor's favor, be included. Liu Chien concluded by demanding that the two Han-lin officials who had already received the order be entrusted with the responsibility. They should be urged to give all instructions and to check on their fulfillment, so that the result would not fall short of previous works in any way. Only then should the work be presented to the emperor for his perusal. Besides, Liu continued, one could not justify the lower official Liu Wen-t'ai being given control while the high officials of the Han-lin Academy were accorded lower functions. This hierarchy, Liu Chien claimed, did not correspond to the customary rules.

Liu Wen-t'ai was among those who, in Liu Chien's opinion, were unqualified and only speculated on tokens of the emperor's favor. He had intended to infiltrate the editorial committee with a clique dependent on him. Apparently, there was no expert within this clique who could master such tasks, for when Liu Wen-t'ai and his followers heard about the test plans, they wanted to withdraw hurriedly. They submitted a petition deploring their incompetence and requested their discharge. Thereupon, the emperor issued the directive that it was solely the task of the Han-lin Academy to carry out the editorial work. The officials of the Imperial Medical Office should neither participate nor take an examination.

Surprisingly, Liu Chien changed his standpoint again—we do not know his reasons—and, in a new petition, told the emperor that drug works and prescription books fell under the authority of the Imperial Medical Office. He stated that the task of his own office was the discussion and consideration of problems, so that participation in the planned project could be viewed as an infringement of authority. There were so many officials in the Imperial Medical Office; surely one could find among them some who had literary training and who would be capable of carrying out the completion of the drug work. Liu Chien requested that the previous decree be canceled and the Imperial Medical Office, as originally intended, be entrusted with the execution of the work. Shen Tao and Ch'en Chi should also be withdrawn, so that jurisdiction would remain clear and order be maintained. In response, the emperor stated that the works of pharmaceutics could not be compared with normal medical books. He had wanted to entrust the compilation to Liu Chien and his office because people there were so well educated. But he would accede to the new request, and he now charged the Imperial Medical Office to carry out the project.[171]

Liu Wen-t'ai had reached the object of his desire. Shih Ch'in submitted a list with the names of forty-seven persons who were to make up the editorial committee. Not only members of the Imperial Medical Office, but also Confucian scholars from other offices were listed. In the southern districts of the capital, a special Materia Medica Office was established, in which the authors were to devote themselves to their task. The eunuch Chang Yü was appointed office director. The editorial committee consisted of three chief editors (among them Liu Wen-t'ai), three vice-chief editors, two editors, three vice-editors, fourteen copiers, five controllers for the appearance and quality of the drugs, and two assistants to the director (among them Shih Ch'in). In addition, there were eight painters for the drug illustrations, including Wang Shih-ch'ang, who must be mentioned as a famous artist.

Already two years later, in the eighteenth year of the governmental period *hung-chih* (1505), Liu Wen-t'ai was able to present the completed work to the emperor. He received the large rewards, and the emperor's favor was secured for him. Emperor Hsiao-tsung himself determined the title of the work and personally wrote a brief preface. Since this drug work had been written "by the order of the emperor," the appropriate term *Yü-chih* was placed before the actual title of the *Pen-ts'ao p'in-hui ching-yao*. Okanishi also mentioned the term *Yü-tsuan*.[172]

御製

御纂

Two months later, the emperor died. His successors apparently did not share his interest in pharmaceutics and medicine. Unpublished, the completed manuscript disappeared in an archive. Two hundred years later, a Ch'ing period emperor became aware of it again and ordered a copy and expansion to be made (C, III, 1.2). Thus, there was no new start for the fruitful tradition of a *pen-ts'ao* literature constantly being brought up to the latest and most comprehensive state of pharmaceutics by governmental order. Governmental initiative was lacking; suitable authors could have been found, as we see from Ch'iu Chün and, a few decades later, from Li Shih-chen.

1.1. Structure and contents of the work

The beginning of the *Pen-ts'ao p'in-hui ching-yao* is composed of the two-line preface by the emperor, an accompanying letter signed by Liu Wen-t'ai, with which he presented the work to the emperor, a list of the names and ranks of all collaborators, with the exception of the eight painters, as well as another preface, and explanations of individual questions.

The second preface provides an interesting insight into the motives and methodology of the authors of the *Pen-ts'ao p'in-hui ching-yao*, and it clearly points out which position in Chinese pharmaceutical literature they aspired to:

> Pharmaceutical knowledge was initiated by Shen-nung. He distinguished the tastes of the drugs and, as a result, a list [of suitable med-

the production of tin "ashes" *(hsi-hui)*—*Pen-ts'ao p'in-hui ching-yao*

axle grease *(kung-chung kao)*—*Pen-ts'ao p'in-hui ching-yao*

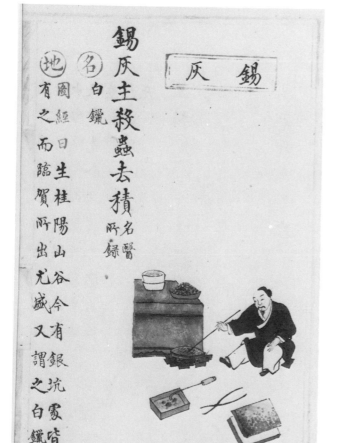

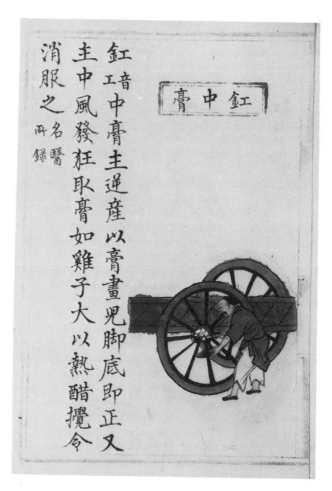

ications] existed. This is probably the reason why [this knowledge] is recorded in one of the Three Sacred Writings of Antiquity. Shen-nung selected 365 drugs to correspond to the number of degrees [of a solar year]. They constituted the Original Classic of Shen-nung. [Within this classic, he arranged] 120 drugs into an upper class: the rulers. They master the nourishment of life, and correspond to heaven. They have no distinct medical effectiveness, and it does not harm man to take them often or over a long period of time. Therefore, it is said that they are suited to free the body from its material weight, to replenish influences, and to prolong life without aging. Into a middle class [Shen-nung also grouped] 120 [drugs]; these are the ministers. They master the nourishment of one's nature and correspond to man. Some have a distinct medicinal effectiveness, others do not. It is therefore necessary to choose the type suitable [for a specific treatment]. Consequently [the minister drugs] are used to suppress illnesses, to compensate for deficiencies, and to hasten [the healing of] injuries. [Shen-nung grouped another] 125 drugs into a lower class; these are the assistants and aides. They master the cure of illnesses and thus correspond to earth. They often possess a distinct medicinal effectiveness, and it is therefore not possible to take them over a longer period of time. Thus, their success lies in driving away hot and cold and [other] evil influences [that have penetrated the body from outside], in breaking through obstructions of various kinds, and in curing illnesses.

All authors who in subsequent times evaluated and classified [drugs] were guided by this [classic]. The "[Prescription Work for] Drugs Prepared by Boiling" *(T'ang-yeh)* by I Yin originated in the work [of Shen-nung]. And the "Discussion of Illnesses Caused by Cold" *(Shang han lun)* by Chung-ching was written on the basis of the *T'ang-yeh.* During the Liang period, T'ao Yin-chü was the first to introduce "Additional Notes by Renowned Medical Men" *(Ming-i pieh-lu)* into the work [of Shen-nung], that is, another 365 drugs. During the T'ang era, in the period *hsien-ch'ing* (656–660), an order was issued to Su Kung, Li Shih-chi, and others to correct mistakes and deficiencies in this work and to examine its advantages and disadvantages. [The authors] added 114 drugs and called the new edition "T'ang Materia Medica" (T'ang *pen-ts'ao*). In the Sung era, during the period *k'ai-pao* (968–975), the emperor charged Liu Han, Ma Chih, Lu To-hsün, Li Fang, Wang Yu, and Hu Meng [with a new revision of the materia medica. The committee] added to the work 133 drugs frequently used by medical practitioners which had proven to be effective, and designated them "First included in the Sung edition." [Emperor] Meng Ch'ang of the Shu dynasty ordered Han Pao-sheng and others to undertake an expansion of the T'ang edition and of the commentaries to its illustrations. [The resulting edition] is generally called *Shu Materia Medica (Shu pen-ts'ao).*

Thus, during the one thousand years from the Han period, and through the T'ang to the Sung period, three revisions and expansions [of the pharmaceutical classic originally written by Shen-nung] had been carried out; still, [the work] did not yet meet all requirements. Later, in the second year of the period *chia-yu* (1056–1063) of the Sung era, a new order was issued to Chang Yü-hsi and others to examine the pharmaceutical works of all kinds of authors. [Chang Yü-hsi and his colleagues] expanded, compared, corrected, supplemented, and annotated, completing in this manner a further edition which was entitled "Materia Medica of the Cheng-ho period, Which Has Its Sources in Classics and Historical Works, and Whose Material is Explained and Classified by Types" *(Cheng-ho ching-shih cheng lei pen-ts'ao).*[173] This work was handed down for a long period of time; its evaluation shows that it contains much exemplary wisdom. But the learned were constantly annoyed by its greatly overloaded scope and the disorganized [contents]. This could by no means be regarded as proper.

[The work] "Elaboration of the Meaning of Pharmaceutics" (*Pen-ts'ao yen-i*) was published; but in it, too, mistakes and truth remained side by side, and could be distinguished for a [flawless] use [of pharmaceutical instructions] only with difficulty. Subsequently, Wang Hao-ku, Li Ming-chih, Chu Yen-hsiu, and others wrote pharmaceutical treatises, but they all turned out equally superficial and sketchy.

The [present] emperor then followed in the succession of rulers. In the sixteenth year of his administration, after he had—during the time he was free from imperial duties—personally taken a look at this [situation, the emperor] issued a special order to us officials to eliminate the superfluous matter [from these works], to supplement what was missing, and to compose a [new work] that would considerably facilitate practical use. This attitude of humanity and love for all living beings was an expression of the attitude of Shen-nung and Huang-ti! As those responsible in the Imperial Medical Office, we—Shih Ch'in and Wang Yü, the officials responsible for the submission of memoranda, the secretaries Liu Wen-t'ai and Wang P'an, Kao T'ing-ho, the Imperial Personal Physician, and others—together with the eunuch Chang Yü, who held the rank of editorial director, [worked] day and night with extreme diligence, after the [emperor's] order had been issued. How could we have dared not to exhaust completely our dilettante and superficial knowledge! We examined the statements of all [previous] authors, eliminated material, produced definitions, supplemented, and compiled, in order to comply with the wise intention [of the order]. We are medical men, and we consider the fulfillment of this order, if only because of our profession, a duty. But if we had not been appointed by the emperor's order, one must fear that the talk of our alleged one-sidedness could have been brought to no end at all. And then what should we have handed down to later, distant generations?

The authors [of pharmaceutical works] in earlier centuries were indeed artists of literary style, but we are afraid that they were not very proficient in the principles of drug use. However, our abilities and our knowledge are also shallow and mediocre; they scarcely suffice to fulfill our duty.

Yin and *yang* and the Five Phases are abstract concepts. Fowl, aquatic animals, land animals, and plants—these are concrete things. The section "Contemplation of Things" (*Kuan-wu*) of the "Book on the Sublime Principle which Governs All Things in the World" (*Huang-chi ching-shih shu*) states: "All [those things in which] the Five Phases have become materialized are related to one another." Therefore, even herbs and trees harbor the desire to fly and walk; minerals are divided into water [-like] and fire[-like]. Among the waters, one distinguishes wood[-like] and mineral[-like]. One must be informed about the origin of the classification of things for all these types. One must distinguish especially among birds, quadrupeds, worms, and fish, and also between the viviparous and oviparous modes of origin, and between genesis out of moisture and genesis through transformation. With herbs and trees, fruits and vegetables, one must distinguish among dense growth, cultivated growth, sparse growth, and dependent growth.

[In our work] we have placed the sections from the Original Classic of Shen-nung at the beginnings [of the appropriate monographs] and designated them with red characters; after these, we have placed the "Additional Notes of Renowned Medical Men" in black ink. In this manner, we have also published the old versions for comparison.

In works of former times, the words of T'ao Yin-chü were placed first, followed by the comments made by Jih Hua-tzu; then [were added statements from] the *T'u-ching,* from Sung comments, from the Shu-edition, and from Ch'en Ts'ang-ch'i. The name of one single object was discussed two or three times, and the properties of one single item were listed four times. Already in the "T'ang edition" errors [of the preceding

work] were pointed out; the "Elaboration of the Meaning of Pharmaceutics" was then written in order to establish certain statements of
the [T'ang-edition] as being false. Although some of T'ao's words were
known to be quite wrong, they were not eliminated. [K'ou] Tsung-shih
had also recognized previous mistakes, but he was unable to dissociate
himself completely from them.

If, therefore, those who make the statements are in doubt about the
facts, from where shall those who examine these [statements] for practical use take the criteria for their action? Thus, we have established
twenty-four criteria [for the description of the individual drugs], we
have selected [and arranged] all the factual information [from the statements of previous] authors, and have divided it according to individual
criteria. We have taken over what is essential in the old editions and
have placed it at the beginning of present and previous [statements] for
comparison. The discussion, in the *T'u-ching*, of investigations carried
out by earlier people appear to be quite reasonable in many respects.
Therefore, we have written them down at the beginning. To that we
have added the explanations of T'ao. These are followed by the statements of Jih Hua-tzu, of the T'ang edition, and of the Shu edition, in
this order. We have cited the important sections from the "Discussions
of Drug Qualities" (*Yao-hsing-lun*) and the "Elaboration of the Meaning
[of Pharmaceutics]," as well as from [the work] of Ch'en Ts'ang-ch'i,
and have omitted what was superfluous or repetitious. When no decision
had been made concerning correctness or falseness, we have conducted
appropriate examinations and selected what was suitable for use. As to
the statements of, for example, Wu P'u, [Chang] Yü-hsi, and Shen-kua,
as well as the quotations from the prescription literature, such as the
"[Prescriptions] from the Sluice-Gate" (*Tou-men fang*), the "[Prescrip-
tions] for Comprehensive Assistance" (*Po-chi an-chung fang*), or the
"Handbook [of Prescriptions] for Urgent Cases" (*Chou-hou pei-chi
fang*), it appeared unnecessary to mention all the individual authors.
We have called them collectively "Additional Notes." Furthermore, we
have [included in the work those drugs] which in contemporary application have proven effective and about which there is clear information,
and have designated them [with the words] "carefully evaluated." [Drugs
that] had not yet been separated in old editions, such as *tu-huo* and
ch'iang-huo, *ch'ing-p'i* and *ch'en-p'i*, *pai-shu* and *ts'ang-shu*, or *ch'ing-
mu-hsiang* and *kuang-mu-hsiang*, but whose effects differ greatly and
also do not correspond in terms of outward appearance and quality,
have been discussed in separate monographs. [For drugs that] were
omitted in old editions, such as *ts'ao-kuo*, *san-lai*, *pa-chiao-hui-hsiang*,
chang-nao and *lu-kan-shih*, we have also prepared illustrations and have
included them here. These are drugs frequently used by physicians which
should not remain concealed from the public. Concerning the modes
of origin and growth, blossoms, leaves, appearance, and quality, as well
as nature and tastes [of the drugs], we have first gathered information
from the people who use [these drugs] and from those who deal in
them. We have made further inquiries with the natives in the places of
origin [of the drugs]. Our object was to trace back each individual
statement to its source! Thus, we have not undertaken the enlargement
and elimination of material according to our own opinions.

We asked His Majesty to determine the name of the work. He entitled
it "The Essential and the Important in Pharmaceutics, in a Classified
Arrangement."

We have fulfilled our tasks with reverence. The book is now completed. We would by no means dare to wish to surpass [the authors of]
past centuries. But [we do want to point out one difference:] Formerly,
one had to be an outstanding scholar to be able to weigh what was
correct or false in [the statements of] the old editions. The new edition

[prepared by us] enables even the beginning student, whose knowledge is still mediocre, to understand things immediately, without having to consult [this and other works] in great detail. After all, for what purpose does the literature on drug use need so much profound theory? What makes [this book] valuable for the treatment of illness is [the fact] that it allows for easy [information] on the effects [of drugs].

This is how superficial our knowledge is; we have presented it in the arrangement that follows."[174]

In the subsequent explanations on the structure and contents of their work, the authors discussed issues concerning, for example, the arrangement, information on place of origin, and the illustrations. Of particular interest in these explanations are the references to various beginnings of a systematization of the mineralogical, zoological, and botanical origins of the individual drugs. As the authors themselves wrote, they took over, in part, suggestions from the *Huang-chi ching-shih shu* by Shao Yung (1011–1077), a philosopher of the Sung period. Shao Yung tended strongly toward Taoism; nevertheless, he was also on very friendly terms with the leaders of the Neoconfucian movement, such as Chou Tun-i (1017–1073). He conducted extensive cosmological studies and, among other things, published the following schema for the comprehension of all human and nonhuman creatures:[175]

The great heaven:	sun	moon	stars	twilight
To it belong the creatures:	flying (animals)	land (animals)	herbs	trees
These are determined by:	nature	desires	form	substance
The wise human beings:	ruler	emperor	king	nobleman
To these belong the humans:	scholars	peasants	laborers	merchants
They are determined by:	humanity	rites	righteousness	wisdom

The authors of the *Pen-ts'ao p'in-hui ching-yao* were influenced by this arrangement and other statements of Shao Yung when they wrote:

According to the *Huang-chi ching-shih shu,* precious stones and minerals must be divided into those that are natural and those that were artificially created by man. Metals and minerals, for instance, are natural substances; salts and alums are examples of products artificially created by man. We follow the [*Huang-chi*] *ching-shih shu* [further] and subdivide each of [the sections on precious stones and minerals] into the four groups of mineral[-like], water[-like], fire[-like], and metal[-like]; in this way, everything can probably be recorded in its entirety.

Herbs, trees, grains, vegetables, and fruits are all subdivided into the four groups of herb[-like], tree[-like], flying animal[-like], and land animal[-like] according to the *Huang-chi ching-shih* [shu]. Thus, there are among the herbs, herb[-like] herbs, tree[-like] herbs, flying animal[-like] herbs, and land animal[-like] herbs. It is similar for trees, grains, fruits, and vegetables. By means of these characteristics, the outward appearance is defined.[176]

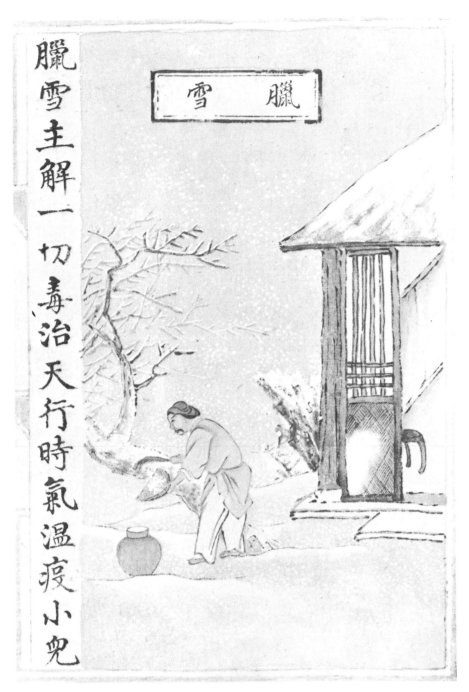

臘雪主解一切毒治天行時氣溫疫小兒

gathering snow in the twelfth month (*la-hsüeh*)—*Pen-ts'ao p'in-hui ching-yao*

The production of genuine camphor (*chang-nao:* above and lower left) and Borneo camphor (*lung-nao-hsiang:* lower right)—*Pen-ts'ao p'in-hui ching-yao*

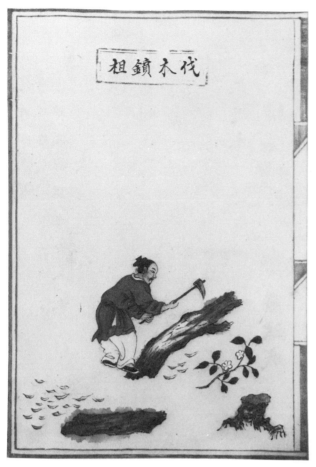

伐木鎮租

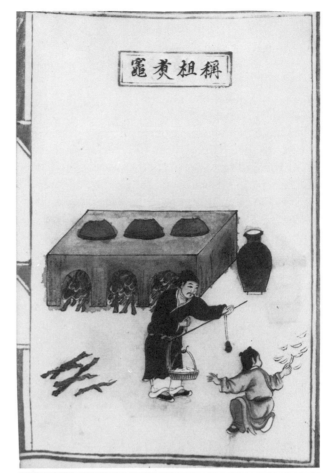

稱租煑罷

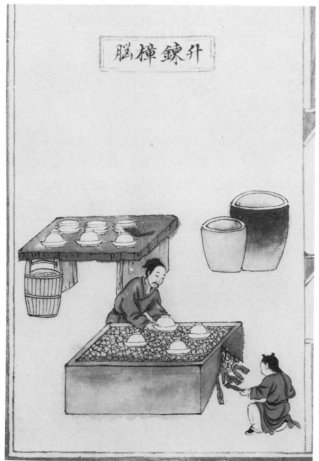

升鍊樟腦

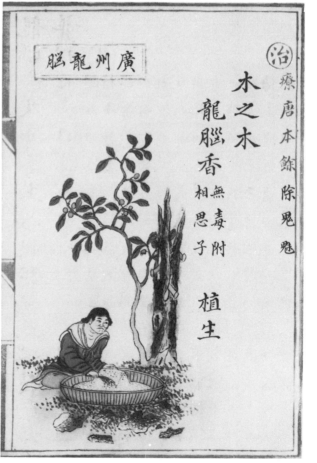

廣州龍腦

治

療唐本餘除鬼魅

水之木

龍腦香 無毒附

相思子

植生

The following examples may explain these brief indications: stalactites are an earth-like mineral, realgar is a mineral-like mineral,
mercury is a water-like mineral, sulphur is a fire-like mineral, and
gold sand is a metal-like mineral.

The "outward appearance" was chosen as the criterion for these
classifications. Thus, an important step was made in the development
toward a detailed natural order of types. As we remember, drugs were
arranged according to the properties ascribed to them in the *Pen-ching*
of the Han period. Since T'ao Hung-ching, the overall structural principle was the natural origin of the drugs, generally according to the
pattern: precious stones/minerals, herbs, trees, man, quadrupeds, fowl,
worms/fish, fruits, rice/grains, and vegetables. Each of these ten sections was then subdivided according to the three classes of the
Pen-ching. Shao Yung's explanation now resulted in an additional
classification of drugs which, however, was restricted in the *Pen-ts'ao
p'in-hui ching-yao* to an individual designation of a great number of
drugs. The authors did not go so far as to combine, for example, all
monographs of the tree-like, flying animal-like, or land animal-like
herbs into groups.

Of particular interest in this context are also the authors' explanations in which further criteria for the systematization of flora and
fauna are alluded to:

> The modes of growth of trees and herbs are by no means uniform.
> Those that grow vertically we will now call "vertically growing" (*t'e-
> sheng*). Those that show sparse and disorderly growth we will call
> "sparsely growing" (*san-sheng*). Those that grow through cultivation
> we will call "growing from cultivation" (*chih-sheng*). Green climbing
> plants will be called "convolvulous" (*man-sheng*). Those that grow on
> other trees will be called "growing dependently" (*chi-sheng*). Those that
> grow luxuriantly on walls will be called "growing without indepen-
> dence" (*li-sheng*). Those that grow on muddy ground we will call "grow-
> ing in mud" (*ni-sheng*). In each case, the outward appearance [of the
> plants] was taken into account, in order to facilitate their selection for
> [medicinal] application.
>
> Fowl, quadrupeds, worms, and fish are all divided into the five types
> of feathered, fur[-bearing], scaly, and crustaceous, as well as bare-skinned.
> Each of these types is further subdivided according to the possibilities
> of origin [of living beings], into viviparous, oviparous, and genesis through
> humidity or through transformation.[177]

Unmentioned in these preliminary remarks was the differentiation
of soils, minerals, metals, and precious stones according to their respective "mode of growth and origin." The reason may be that the
classifications were so varied here. In this section we find, among
others, the designations "originated from earth and minerals," "originated from earth (or minerals)," "grown in earth caves," "grown in
mountain caves," or "produced through a forging- or melting-process"
and "produced by minting"; the last designation applied to the drug
"old coins." In all, fifteen modes of origin were distinguished here.

Finally, I would like to mention two longer treatises in the general
preliminary remarks, which demonstrate the main features of the connections between pharmaceutics, on the one hand, and the theories

of yinyang and of the Five Phases, on the other hand. They indicate that the Chin-Yüan tendencies in pharmaceutical literature were taken into account.

The general preliminary remarks are followed by some attempts of the authors of the *Pen-ts'ao p'in-hui ching-yao* to renew the old main tradition: the entire general sections of the *Pen-ching*, a selection (changed only slightly) from T'ao Hung-ching's guidelines for pharmaceutical practice, and finally, the preface to the "Discussion of Drug Preparation According to Lei-kung" (*Lei-kung p'ao-chih lun*). The subsequent table of contents shows the structure of the *Pen-ts'ao p'in-hui ching-yao*. It largely resembles the pattern introduced by T'ao Hung-ching—that is, the grouping of the drugs into one of the sections of precious stones/minerals, herbs, trees, man, fowl, other animals, worms/fish, fruits, grains, and vegetables. Within these groups, drugs are classified as belonging to the upper, middle, or lower class. Following the old example, the beginning of each chapter states how many of the drugs discussed in the following were taken from the *Pen-ching* and the *Ming-i pieh-lu*, and how many came from other sources. At the end of the table of contents, we find the following information:

"Old and new drugs total   1815
    of these, newly included   46
newly listed in individual monographs   21
newly defined   2
rearranged   31
not included   2"

But a count of the table of contents yields a total of 1,786 drugs; the actual contents do not agree with either of these numbers.[178]

Most of the monographs are preceded by an illustration of the original material of the drug in question; there are a total of 1,358 illustrations.[179] In particular, the illustrations of plants often resemble those in the "Materia Medica of the *Ta-kuan* Period" (*Ta-kuan pen-ts'ao*), but they are executed more imaginatively and a great deal more precisely, and are done in color. As in the *Ta-kuan pen-ts'ao*, geographical variations of one and the same plant were represented by different illustrations. Extremely well-done and detailed paintings can be found, particularly in the sections on precious stones and minerals but also scattered among the illustrations of later chapters. The artists here were not satisfied with a representation of the drugs but drew them in their natural surroundings or illustrated the exact process of their artificial production. Utilizing bright colors, they portrayed chemical-pharmaceutical utensils and the people who used them. If a drug came from a foreign country, we see it in the hands of foreigners clothed in exotic garb. The illustration of a carrot, for example, is so true to life that one can hardly imagine it more perfect. When the drug "swallow's nest herb" had to be shown, the artists drew a house, above whose gable the swallows are flying back and forth—on account of the fact that, from a ladder leaning against the roof, some men are busy removing the nests from the beams. Thus, these illustrations convey more to us than merely a description of the appearance of the drugs; they are also a bequest of cultural-historical value, from which we can gather extensive information on pharmaceutical technology, garb, work, clothes, and many other things.

The main text following the illustrations clarifies the most fundamental difference between the *Pen-ts'ao p'in-hui ching-yao* and the *Cheng-lei pen-ts'ao*. For each chapter, all of the monographs were divided into "proper articles" (*cheng-p'in*) and "additional articles" (*fu-p'in*). Among the former were the drugs from the works of the main tradition; the second group consists of drugs from Ch'en Ts'ang-ch'i's "Supplement to the Materia Medica" (*Pen-ts'ao shih-i*) and a work entitled "The Book of Drugs from the Southern Ocean" (*Nan-hai yao-p'u*). In the area of the "proper drugs," the authors took over, from the early works of the main pen-ts'ao tradition, the custom of separating, by means of red and black ink, the portions of the *Pen-ching* from those of other sources.

正品
附品

The title of each monograph is the name of the drug discussed. The texts of most monographs are also preceded by information on the systematization according to Shao Yung, the strength of medicinal efficacy (*yu-tu, wu-tu,* etc.), and on the various modes of growth and origin of the original plants or other materials of the drugs. Whenever possible, the text begins with the original monograph of the *Pen-ching* or of the *Ming-i pieh-lu*. Only then do the descriptions of the drugs follow, subdivided into technical rubrics and based on the statements of previous authors and more recent commentators. Ch'iu Chün had established thirteen criteria; the authors' committee expanded these into the following twenty-four criteria:

有毒　無毒

名	*ming*	listing of the various names of the drug
苗	*miao*	description of the morphology of the original plants and other basic materials, and indications of differences from similar plants, etc.
地	*ti*	information concerning the drugs' places of origin
時	*shih*	information on the time for gathering the drug
收	*shou*	information concerning drying and storage
用	*yung*	information concerning the usable parts—for example, of an original plant—and their characteristics
質	*chih*	information on the external appearance of the drugs
色	*se*	information on the color of the drugs
味	*wei*	information on the taste of the drugs
性	*hsing*	information concerning thermo-influence and mode of effect of drugs in the body (i.e., cold, hot, warm, cool; gathering, dispersing, retarding, hardening, softening)
氣	*ch'i*	information concerning the strong or weak development of the effective properties, the yinyang associations, the rising or descending effect of drugs in the body
臭	*ch'ou*	information on the odor of the drugs
主	*chu*	information on main indications
行	*hsing*	information on the conduits that the drug is able to penetrate
助	*chu*	information on drugs that support the effect of a specific drug

反	*fan*	information on drugs whose effects are directly opposed to those of a specific drug
製	*chih*	information on the pharmaceutical processing of drugs
治	*chih*	information on the entire spectrum of drug effects; divided into "healing" and "strengthening"
合治	*ho-chih*	information on mutual efficacy when used with other drugs
禁	*chin*	information on side effects and contraindications
代	*tai*	information on substitute drugs
忌	*chi*	information on foodstuffs and other drugs that are not allowed to be taken during treatment with the drug in question, and also information on utensils with which this drug must not come into contact (for example, iron pots)
解	*chieh*	information concerning the ability of the drug to serve as an antidote
贗	*yen*	information on the distinction between genuine and spurious samples of a particular drug

Not every monograph needed all twenty-four rubrics. If a drug could not serve as an antidote, for example, or if there were no known contraindications, the corresponding rubrics were omitted altogether.

The thousandfold ladling of "sweet softened water" *(kan-lan-shui)—Pen-ts'ao p'in-hui ching-yao*

Clay from the floor of a fireplace *(fu-lung-kan)—Pen-ts'ao p'in-hui ching-yao*

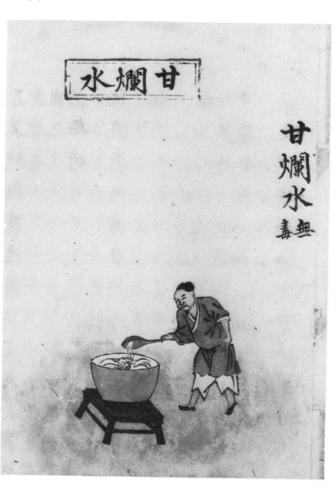

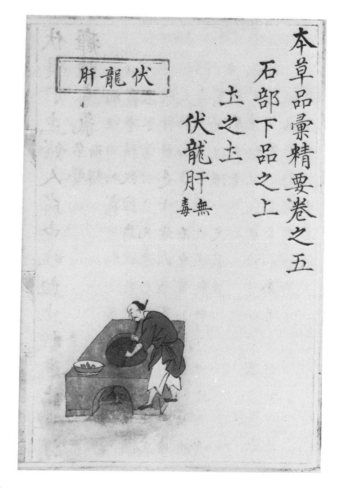

The system of twenty-four criteria was not applied at all to the so-called additional drugs. They are briefly described, separated only by a punctuation mark, at the end of each chapter, following the "proper drugs."

In the work's appendix, five sections are added to the monograph part:

1. List of possible poisonings and antidotes
2. List of drugs that must not be boiled or processed into wines
3. Enumeration of reciprocal effects of drugs when taken simultaneously
4. List of drugs that must not be taken by pregnant women
5. Information concerning differences between former and present place names

The table of contents does not mention the first section, but gives a "List of secondary names" which is missing in the appendix, apparently because the secondary names are mentioned in each individual monograph.[180]

The authors were aware of the need for a new form for the old main tradition. The work they created, however, was not carried out consistently enough with respect to this perception. The renewed use of the division of drugs into the three classes and the distinction between "proper drugs" and "additional drugs" considerably diminished the value of the *Pen-ts'ao p'in-hui ching-yao*. Li Shih-chen, who during his employment in the Imperial Medical Office (ca. 1558) may have become acquainted with the *Pen-ts'ao p'in-hui ching-yao*, eliminated these deficiencies with his experience as a practicing physician and pharmacist, and, a few decades later, created the best-known work of the pen-ts'ao literature with his "Materia Medica Arranged According to Monographs and Technical Criteria" (*Pen-ts'ao kang mu*).

1.2. The transmission of the *Pen-ts'ao p'in-hui ching-yao* and the *Pen-ts'ao p'in-hui ching-yao hsü-chi*

For nearly two centuries, the *Pen-ts'ao p'in-hui ching-yao* was kept in the imperial collection, hidden from the public. No Ming or Ch'ing bibliography mentions this work. Emperor K'ang-hsi (1655–1723), who developed great literary enthusiasm and had well-known and extensive encyclopedias, dictionaries, and concordances produced under his personal supervision, was the first to pay some attention to the hitherto unpublished manuscript. In 1700, he instructed the two officials Ho Shih-heng and Chang Ch'ang-chu to copy part of the drug illustrations of the original. Simultaneously, the medical official Wang Tao-ch'un and the physician Chiang Chao-yüan were ordered to prepare a revised version of the Ming period manuscript by rectifying omissions and correcting mistakes. The two medical men and their colleagues revised the existing forty-two chapters accordingly and expanded the original by an appendix of ten additional chapters containing a total of 534 drug monographs, as well as by two chapters which contain a work on the pulse, "The Most Important from the Instructions Concerning the [Movement in the] Vessels, Written in [Sentences of] Four Characters" (*Mai-chüeh ssu-yen chü-yao*). The twelve new chapters, as a whole, were designated by the title "Continued Collection for the Materia Medica Which Contains the Essential and Important in a Classified Arrangement" (*Pen-ts'ao p'in-hui ching-yao hsü-chi*). The *Hsü-chi*, as this supplement is also called, is preceded by the written presentation of the completed work to the throne, dated 1701 and signed by Wang Tao-ch'un and Chiang Chao-yüan. The structure of the drug monographs in the *Hsü-chi* follows that of the main text. These monographs come mainly from the *Pen-ts'so kang mu*, which had appeared in the meantime; numerous other sources extended from the *Pen-ching* into the seventeenth century; some drugs are listed for the first time. The work entitled *Mai-chüeh ssu-yen chü-yao* was written in the Sung period by Ts'ui Chia-yen. The text in the *Hsü-chi*, however, does not correspond to that of the original. The authors took it from a version, changed by Li Yen-wen (ca. 1500), of the Chiang-hsi edition of the *Pen-ts'ao kang mu* of 1603.[181] The entire revised and expanded work, which now comprised fifty-two chapters, did not contain any of its own drug illustrations.

1.3. The further fate of the known versions of the *Pen-ts'ao p'in-hui ching-yao*

The following three versions existed, as we know, in the imperial collections:

1. the original manuscript of 1505
2. the copy of the drug illustrations, produced in 1700
3. the revised and expanded text of 1701

Versions 1 and 2 disappeared either in 1923, when part of the palace buildings went up in flames, or during the unrest of the year 1924, when Feng Yü-hsiang drove the last emperor from the palace; in each case, looting took place. It was assumed that the manuscripts were completely lost. Version 3 was preserved and was printed in lead type by the Commercial Press in 1937.[182] Thus, almost four-and-a-half centuries after its original completion, and almost 250 years after its revision, the *Pen-ts'ao p'in-hui ching-yao* reached the public for the first time—although, unfortunately, in the nonillustrated version. Perhaps the refined artistic execution of the drug illustrations had been a reason why there had been no immediate publication; they would have required a complicated color printing not yet possible at that time. It is difficult to agree with the assumption, expressed by G. Bertuccioli, that the original had been prepared solely for the emperor's use.[183] No such indication can be found anywhere; besides, such a restriction would have contradicted the main tradition, which the authors resumed in a sense, as well as the medical-pharmaceutical intentions of Emperor Hsiao-tsung, which were not aimed at his own needs.

Later, in the thirties of our century, it was discovered that versions 1 and 2 had not been lost after all but were in private hands in Peking. Via intermediate stations, the original manuscript 1 came into other private hands in Hong Kong. In the early fifties, the Italian chargé d'affairs in the British Crown colony at that time, Bertuccioli, had an opportunity to examine this work thoroughly. From that time on, it was referred to as the "Hong Kong edition" in publications on the subject. That term is now out of date, as the manuscript was bought in the meantime by the library of the Japanese pharmaceutical company Takeda in Osaka. Therefore, we will have to speak of the "Takeda edition" from now on.

In 1936, a publication by Wang Chung-min pointed out that a manuscript of the *Pen-ts'ao p'in-hui ching-yao* was also located in a Roman library.[184] It bears a mark indicating that it comes from the collection An-lo t'ang of Yün-hsiang (1686–1720), the twenty-second son of Emperor K'ang-hsi (1655–1723). Lodovico de Besi, a Veronese monk and missionary who first came to China in 1835, was mission leader of the region of Nanking from 1840 to 1847, and died as a bishop in 1870 after his return to Italy, brought this manuscript to Europe. It is an exact copy of the Ming manuscript of 1505, though not quite its equal in regard to the drug illustrations; it is not known whether it was made during the Ch'ing period or already in the Ming period.

A third specimen of the manuscript of the *Pen-ts'ao p'in-hui ching-yao* came from the private collection of the German Sinologist F. Hirth (1845–1927) into the Staatsbibliothek Preussischer Kulturbesitz in Berlin, where it is still located today. It was perhaps acquired by Hirth during his activity as customs official in China during the years 1870–1899.

The Berlin manuscript is apparently also a copy of the original *Pen-ts'ao p'in-hui ching-yao* of 1505. As W. Fuchs realized, its preparation should be dated to the governmental period *ch'ien-lung* in the Ch'ing period (1736–1795) because of the taboo placed on the character *hung*.[185] Unfortunately, this manuscript is incomplete. Of the original thirty-five Chinese-style volumes, only twenty-three are preserved; chapters 7, 8, 18–21 and 24–33 are missing.[186]

A fourth copy of the *Pen-ts'ao p'in-hui ching-yao* was kept by the London Library at St. James Square in London, England, until 1972. The manuscript was misidentified as Li Shih-chen's *Pen-ts'ao kang mu* and was sold as a double to Quaritch, a firm dealing in antique books. It was then offered at a book fair in Tokyo, where it was acquired by the Japanese physician and medical historian Otsuka Yasuo, in whose private collection it has remained. The Otsuka edition, as we will call it, was acquired by the London Library from an undocumented source in 1841. It measures 33.9 by 20.9 centimeters and, therefore, corresponds closely in size to the Takeda edition. It may be older than the Berlin edition because the character *hung* appears in its original form. The Otsuka edition is bound in Western style; its ten volumes carry, on their back, the designation "Li Shih Chen Chinese Materia Medica."[187]

As mentioned above, a copy of the drug illustrations of the *Pen-ts'ao p'in-hui ching-yao* had been produced in 1700; its current whereabouts are unknown to this author. However, in the National Central Library in Taipei, another copy of just the drug illustrations was discovered recently. It had escaped prior attention possibly because of its title which reads *Chin shih k'un ch'ung ts'ao mu chuang* ("The Appearance of Metals, Stones, Insects, Herbs, and Trees"). This copy was produced by a female painter, named Wen Shu (1594–1634), during the years 1617–1620. It consists of twenty-seven chapters in twelve Chinese-style volumes, bound in yellow silk brocade, measuring 31 by 21 centimeters each. Except for the three prefaces, the tables of content, and the names of the drugs written (by Wen Shu's painter-father Wen Ts'ung-chien) in the upper right corner of each respective illustration, this version does not include any texts. The illustrations depict 1,070 different drugs in 1,316 colored drawings, only forty-two fewer than in the original 1505 edition. Most of the drawings, though, lack the sophistication of the original and, in comparison, appear as rather crude copies.[188]

2. The *Pen-ts'ao kang mu*

Pen-ts'ao kang mu
"Materia Medica, Arranged according to Drug Descriptions and Technical Aspects"
52 chapters / 1893 drug descriptions
Author: Li Shih-chen (1518–1593)
   tzu: Tung-pi
   hao: P'in-hu lao-jen
   from: Wa-hsiao-pa in Hupei
Written: ca. 1547–1580
Published: 1596

On his own initiative, Li Shih-chen created a work in the long tradition of *pen-ts'ao* literature that proved to posterity that he was one of the most important naturalists of imperial China. In China, as well as in other parts of the world, the *Pen-ts'ao kang mu* is the best-known and most respected description of traditional Chinese pharmaceutics. The value of this enormous achievement, however, written by one person, goes far beyond the scope of a pharmaceutical-medical drug work, and, in fact, constitutes an extensive encyclopedia of knowledge concerning nature and the technology required for the medicinal use of nature.

2.1. Life and works of Li Shih-chen

Li Shih-chen came from Wa-hsiao-pa, a place north of Ch'i-chou in the province of Hupei.[189] It is known that Li Shih-chen's grandfather was a medical practitioner of the class of "bell physicians" (*ling-i*), that is, he offered his services and abilities, wandering from town to town. On the traditional scale of values of medical practitioners, the bell physicians, who were also called "physicians who go across rivers and lakes [to sell their services]" (*chiang-hu i*), held the lowest rank, because—in contrast to the *ju-i,* the Confucian medical scholars—they considered their medical knowledge an object of trade, with whose sale they made their living.

Already Li Shih-chen's father, Li Yen-wen, was able to dissociate himself from this little-esteemed class; the family acquired some farmland, so that the practice of medical activities was no longer required as the professional basis of their lives. Li Yen-wen had passed the central state exams and attained the rank of *hsiu-ts'ai*. On the strength of his medical skills, he was employed for a time as an official in the Imperial Medical Office. He made a name for himself not only as a

鈴醫

江湖醫
儒醫

秀才

practicing physician but also as an author of medical works. Five works written by him are known; they deal with such themes as technique of diagnosis, smallpox, and the doctrine of the pulse, as well as with the drugs ginseng and mugwort. Thus, Li Shih-chen grew up in an environment which, in terms of family tradition, possessed all requirements favorable for his own successful activity as a medical practitioner.

Li Yen-wen introduced his weak and frequently ailing son, Li Shih-chen, to literature at an early age and planned a career in government service for him. But when Li Shih-chen, at the age of seventeen, was unable to pass the decisive exams after three attempts, he subsequently devoted himself, with his father's consent, solely to the study of medicine; this is an interesting parallel to the start of several renowned medical authors, especially Chang Yüan-su, the founder of the Chin-Yüan tradition.

Li Shih-chen is said to have become so engrossed in his studies that he did not leave his parents' house for over ten years and worked through all obtainable books, even nonmedical texts. In this manner, he developed into a well-known physician, whose exact diagnoses and effective treatments were widely esteemed.

During the course of time, Li Shih-chen wrote eleven purely medical studies; three of them have been preserved,[190] and we can see from these that he followed closely the Chin-Yüan teachings of Chang Yüan-su and others. His special ambition was to develop prescriptions in which one drug dominated as the "ruler," developing the main effectiveness. The fact is, however, that Li Shih-chen did not devote himself exclusively to medical problems, as is proven by collections of poetry and prose that he compiled, as well as by a study of the rules of prosody.

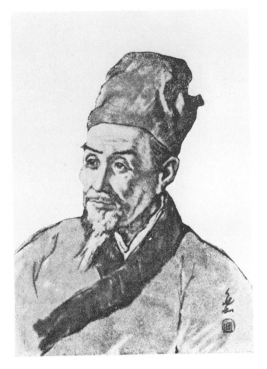

Li Shih-chen (1518–1593)—author of the *Pen-ts'ao kang mu*

His abilities resulted in, among other things, a call to the Court of the King of Ch'u, where he was named head of the temple of ancestors, and later, a call to the Imperial Medical Office of the capital. During these appointments, none of which lasted very long, Li Shih-chen had the unique opportunity to become acquainted with and to study otherwise inaccessible works from the princely and imperial collections.

Approximately twelve years after failing the civil service exams, when he was not quite thirty years old, Li Shih-chen began a task whose completion required enormous devotion of an individual: a comprehensive revision of pharmaceutical knowledge recorded in the pen-ts'ao works which would present this knowledge completely and with the greatest responsibility. Almost all comparable undertakings of the T'ang period, the Sung period, and the compilation, fifty years before, of the *Pen-ts'ao p'in-hui ching-yao* had been carried out by large committees with about twenty to fifty members, composed of experts and scholars. Li Shih-chen believed that he had sufficient ambition and abilities to master such a task on his own.

After about forty years' work, of which thirty were devoted to the compilation itself, he achieved his goal with the completion of the *Pen-ts'ao kang mu*. Li Shih-chen mastered source material that seemed nearly boundless. In the *Pen-ts'ao kang mu*, he quotes 952 previous authors. From the pen-ts'ao literature he took as his starting point the most comprehensive work up to that time, the *Cheng-lei pen-ts'ao*. Of course, he did not limit himself to medical-pharmaceutical literature; he also made full use of all kinds of other genres, as can be seen from the bibliography at the beginning of his work.

Thus, he expanded the *Pen-ts'ao* from a work on drugs to a comprehensive and detailed encyclopedia of medicine, pharmaceutics, mineralogy, metallurgy, botany, and zoology, which contained not only the expert knowledge of its own author and of other authors but also critical statements on the historical developments in various areas of the knowledge of nature.

Since he, unlike the pen-ts'ao committees of the T'ang and Sung periods, had no imperially ordered, empire-wide collection drives at his disposal, Li Shih-chen was forced to travel extensively in order to acquaint himself with, for example, the origin, the original appearance, or the processes of collecting and preparing the original plant, animal, and mineral substances of the drugs. Thus, Li Shih-chen visited the provinces of China that were most important for drugs. He traveled through Honan, Kiangsu, Kianghsi, and Anhui, but not through Szechwan, which was, and still is, especially well-known for its wealth of drugs.

Despite the greatest care and most responsible studies, however, even Li Shih-chen was not free of errors. As Watanabe Kōzo put it, he too frequently made the mistake common to all pen-ts'ao works, namely, he overemphasized the value of older literature.[191] Li Shih-chen wrote, for example, that glowworms develop from the roots of certain types of grass, and he did not realize that two drugs that he described separately are actually synonyms for the *nux vomica*. But such deficiencies are insignificant compared with the new understanding of the nature of many things that Li Shih-chen attained and which he recorded in the *Pen-ts'ao kang mu*.

As Lu Gwei-djen has pointed out, outstanding examples of this new understanding include Shih-chen's recognition of how some living beings adapt to their environment and how the environment influences the characteristics of living beings.[192] Li Shih-chen described unchangeable types and pursued genetic peculiarities, as in lotus plants and domestic fowl. He recognized hereditary influences and family characteristics, and described artificial selection by the examples of grain plants and goldfish. Li Shih-chen's experiments resulted in statements concerning the spontaneous genesis of organisms, the nutrition of anteaters, and the reciprocal effects of drugs taken simultaneously. He discovered the erroneous classification of gall-nuts under tree drugs and criticized the belief that worms in the intestines were useful for digestion. Instead, he pointed out the pathological appetite that can be caused by such "guests."

Li Shih-chen also collected knowledge of similar value outside the areas of flora and fauna. He demonstrated the connection between the consumption of candy and tooth decay and described occupational illnesses, such as lead poisoning. His descriptions of hygienic practices are noteworthy: he recommended a fumigation of sick rooms and treatment of patients' clothing by means of steam, in order to prevent a spreading of diseases.[193]

This brief and, of course, extremely incomplete suggestion of the achievements of Li Shih-chen may indicate why this man and his work are still regarded today with such great esteem. Recognition by his contemporaries, however, was largely denied to the great work that Li Shih-chen had created during the course of decades. I have already pointed out that Emperor Hsiao-tsung, at the beginning of the six-teenth century, was the only Ming ruler who initiated any activity in the medical-pharmaceutical area, and that the unpublished *Pen-ts'ao p'in-hui ching-yao* remained the only pen-ts'ao work compiled under governmental order during the Ming period. Li Shih-chen and, after his death, his son, Li Chien-yüan, applied in vain for assistance in the publication of the completed work. A copy of the manuscript sub-mitted to the court by Li Chien-yüan received the following notation by Emperor Shen-tsung (1563–1620) who, as historians report, ex-celled in countless extravagances but not in the care for the people's welfare: "Taken notice of; to be kept in the Ministry of Rites."[194] A passage in Li Shih-chen's biography in the official history of the Ming dynasty that contains the opposite sense is quite obviously character-ized by embellished wishful thinking: "Shen-tsung ordered the printing [of the work] and its circulation in the entire empire. Henceforth it was found everywhere in the homes of scholars and officials."[195]

Li Shih-chen himself had revised the manuscript three times. In 1580 and again in 1587, as a man of almost seventy years, he had to travel to Nanking to seek the printing and publication of his volu-minous work on a private basis. In 1580, he was able to persuade a friend, the poet and man of letters Wang Shih-chen (1526–1593), to write the first preface. As we learn from Wang's words, Li Shih-chen appeared at his house "with an emaciated face and body." He had been "an enthusiastic debater and a unique man under the sign of the Great Bear."

Ten years later, in 1590, the publisher Hu Ch'eng-lung in Nanking gave his consent and financial assistance for the publication. Sons and grandsons of Li Shih-chen all assisted in the completion of the texts. Li Shih-chen was probably no longer able to supervise the preparation of the illustrations; they were compiled by his son Li Chien-chung and drawn by the above-mentioned son, Li Chien-yüan.

But Li Shih-chen did not live to see his great life's work printed and published. The first edition was not finished until three years after his death, in the year 1596.

2.2. Structure and contents of the *Pen-ts'ao kang mu*

Li Shih-chen found the source richest in material, and thus the starting point for his work, in the *Cheng-lei pen-ts'ao*. Since its first edition, it had been reprinted almost forty times and enjoyed a wide circulation. Li Shih-chen took from it 1,479 drugs. He supplemented these with 39 drugs that had been included in the drug compendia of the Chin-Yüan period, as well as with 374 drugs that he himself described for the first time, so that the *Pen-ts'ao kang mu* contains a total of 1,892 drugs. This number is confirmed by the table of contents. The actual

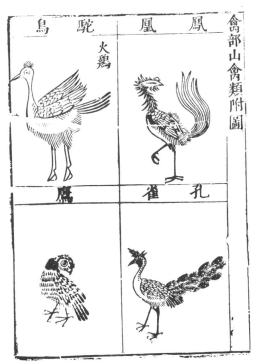

A page from the section "fowl," subdivision "mountain fowl" in the second edition of the *Pen-ts'ao kang mu* (1603). Pictured are a phoe-nix (upper right), peacock (lower right), ostrich (upper left), and eagle (lower left)

number, however, should be 1,898. To continue the statistics: the number of drug illustrations is 1,160; that of the recorded prescriptions is 11,096, of which Li Shih-chen collected or newly compiled 8,161 himself. [196]

The entire work was divided into two—in some later editions three—chapters of illustrations and another fifty-two chapters containing the texts. The first four text chapters are of a general nature; chapters five through fifty-two contain the monographs.

In a preliminary chapter, we find the prefaces and an introduction, in which the author discusses some differences between his work and earlier pen-ts'ao editions, explains the structure of the drug monographs he has introduced, and, above all, familiarizes us with his new classification of the drugs as a whole.

To enable the reader of the present work to compare for himself the extent to which Li Shih-chen took over or omitted traditional elements or introduced innovations in the structure of his work, I have listed below the titles of the individual text sections and treatises:
Chapter 1:

1. Enumeration of forty earlier pen-ts'ao works, with brief commentaries by other authors and also by Li Shih-chen. The list is concluded by the *Pen-ts'ao kang mu* itself.
2. Enumeration of all sources used.
   a. Older and newer medical/pharmaceutical works: 277
   b. Classics, historical works, others: 591
3. Enumeration of all earlier pen-ts'ao works from which drug descriptions were taken for the *Pen-ts'ao kang mu*, with a precise classification of the drugs according to the sections to which they belong.
4. Text of the general preliminary sections of the *Pen-ching* with the designated commentaries by T'ao Hung-ching and other authors.
5. The treatises of T'ao Hung-ching that contain pharmaceutical references.
6. A quotation from the *Su-wen* concerning the influence of climatic factors on drugs.
7. "The seven ways of compiling a prescription," with commentaries by Ch'i Po (legendary), Wang Ping (eighth century), and various Chin-Yüan authors.
8. "The effects of the ten kinds of prescriptions," with commentaries by Hsü Chih-ts'ai (sixth century), Chin-Yüan authors, and Li Shih-chen himself.
9. Ten treatises on the medical-theoretical teachings of the Chin-Yüan period.

Chapter 2:
1. Enumeration of drugs known with up to five synonyms.
2. Enumeration of drugs according to their reciprocal effects when taken simultaneously.
3. Enumeration of foodstuffs whose consumption is forbidden during the period when specific drugs are being taken.

4. Enumeration of drugs that must not be taken by pregnant women.
5. Enumeration of beverages and foods that must not be consumed together.
6. "The use of drugs suitable for the symptoms, according to Li Tung-yüan."
7. "Enumeration of all drugs that, according to Ch'en Ts'ang-ch'i, are used in the treatment of depletions."
8. "The three processes of perspiring, vomiting, and purging, according to Chang Tzu-ho."
9. "In case of illness there are eight important points, six [possible] mistakes, and six [conditions under which] no treatment [is successful]."
10. The five sections from the *Yao-tui,* already quoted in the *Pen-ching.*
11. The table of contents of the *Pen-ching.*
12. The table of contents of the *Cheng-lei pen-ts'ao.*

Chapters 3 and 4:

Enumeration of all illnesses and symptoms, with the appropriate therapeutic drugs and information concerning their preparation and administration. Here, Li Shih-chen continued the double classification introduced by T'ao Hung-ching. T'ao had divided the drugs according to 83 illnesses and symptoms for whose treatment they appeared suited; Li expanded this number to 493.

Chapter 5:

The beginning of the monograph section of the *Pen-ts'ao kang mu.* Li Shih-chen divided the total number of drugs into sixteen groups 部 (*pu*). These constitute a further refinement of the classification of the materia medica. Almost exactly one thousand years earlier, T'ao Hung-ching had introduced the classification of drugs according to their natural origin. He started with six groups. The Sung period works of the main tradition usually distinguished nine drug groups, and the manuscript of the *Pen-ts'ao p'in-hui ching-yao,* completed a few decades before Li Shih-chen's work, contained ten groups. Like the authors of that work, Li Shih-chen, too, described the motives for his innovative structural pattern. He wrote in his introduction:

> In the old [pharmaceutical] works, precious stones, minerals, waters, and soils were [described] in total confusion. The [groups of] worms, scaly animals, and crustaceans were not separated. In addition [drugs from the group of] worms were found among the tree [drugs], and tree [drugs] appeared among the herbs. I have now established individual groups. At the beginning, I have placed the waters and fires, followed by the soils. For water and fire are the beginning of all things, and the earth is the mother of all things. Next, I have added the metals and the minerals; they emerge from the earth. These are followed by the herbs, grains, vegetables, fruits, and trees. I have proceeded from the insignificant to the eminent.
>
> Then come the clothes and commodities, because they are made of herbs and wood. They are followed by the worms, scaly animals and

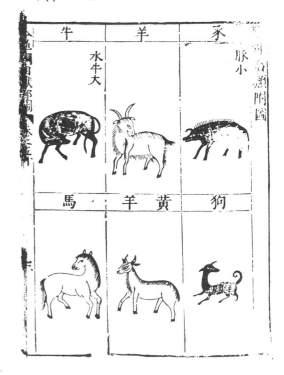

A page from the section "quadrupeds," subdivision "breeding animals" in the second edition of the *Pen-ts'ao kang mu* (1603). Pictured are a pig (upper right), dog (lower right), goat (upper middle), "yellow goat" (lower middle), ox (upper left), and horse (lower left)

crustaceans, fowl and quadrupeds; and man concludes the list. From the low I have ascended to the noble.[197]

For thirteen of the sixteen groups Li Shih-chen mentions in his introduction, it proved appropriate to establish subgroups *(fen)*. Thus, for example, he divided the "waters" into "waters of the heavens" (which included rain, snow, frost, dew, and hail) and "waters of the earth" (which included well water, river water, and others). The group of "herbs" was divided into the subgroups of "mountain herbs," "aromatic herbs," "swamp herbs," "poisonous herbs," "convolvulous herbs," "water herbs," "stone herbs," "moss and lichen herbs," and finally, "various herbs." The "utensils" were divided into two subgroups, "clothes/silk" (with drugs such as rope of a suicide victim, clothes of sick people, deathbed, head-scarf) and "frequently used articles" (including paper, printed paper, pot lid, cart grease, fish hooks, and chamber pot). Li Shih-chen divided the group of "worms" into three subgroups, namely "originating from eggs," "originating through transformation," and "originating from moisture." In the group "scaly animals," we find the subdivisions "dragons," "snakes," "fish," and "fish without scales." The "crustaceans" are divided into "turtles" and "shellfish."

Each group is preceded by an exact definition. This is followed by a list of the earlier works from which the drugs described in the group were taken and from which commentaries were borrowed.

The monographs are presented after another table of contents. Li Shih-chen grouped them according to the mutual affinity or interdependence of the original drug substances. This corresponds to the system practiced in the *Pen-ts'ao p'in-hui ching-yao,* and indicates a systematization into, for example, botanical groups, resembling today's families, genera, and so forth. For Li Shih-chen, additional criteria for classification were external appearance and "internal" effective properties of the drugs.

Each monograph bears as title that name of the drug under which its earliest description appeared. This also corresponds to the system used today for certain scientific nomenclatures, such as in zoology and botany. Since, in each case, Li Shih-chen also stated the titles of these oldest sources, it is easy to see when a drug first appeared in a drug work or some other book. If the source was the *Pen-ching,* brief mention is also made as to whether the drug was classified in the upper, middle, or lower class. In his introduction, Li Shih-chen justified this information, of little actual use, as a "preservation of old traces." That is the only reminiscence in the *Pen-ts'ao kang mu* of the old three-class system.

綱

日

Li Shih-chen called the individual monographs *kang.* The technical criteria within these monographs, according to which he arranged the descriptions of the drugs, were called *mu.* These terms and, consequently, the title of the *Pen-ts'ao kang mu,* reflect the respect Li Shih-chen felt for the Sung period scholar, scientist and Neoconfucian Chu Hsi, the author of the *T'ung-chien kang mu.*

In the *Pen-ts'ao p'in-hui ching-yao,* the authors had, for the first
time, replaced the traditional arrangement according to sources with
a division of the monographs according to technical criteria. They
introduced, as we have seen, twenty-four rubrics. Li Shih-chen found
the following ten criteria sufficient. They were used as needed, so that
not all are contained in each monograph.

校正	*chiao-cheng*	Information concerning a previously false classification of the drug
釋名	*shih-ming*	Information on secondary names of the drug, including the sources of these names
集解	*chi-chieh*	"Collected explanations"; here, in chronological order, various commentaries are quoted, from earlier authors to Li Shih-chen himself, in which origin, occurrence, appearance, time of collection, medicinally usable parts of the basic substances, and similarities with other drugs are discussed.
修製	*hsiu-chih*	Information concerning the pharmaceutical-technological preparation of the drug
辯疑	*pien-i*	"Explanation of doubtful points"
正誤	*cheng-wu*	"Correction of mistakes"
氣味	*ch'i wei*	Information on the thermo-influence and taste of the drug
主治	*chu-chih*	Enumeration of the main indications of the drug
發明	*fa-ming*	Explanations concerning the effects of the drug
附方	*fu-fang*	Enumeration of prescriptions in which the drug is used, and information on the preparation of the medicinal form and on the dosage.

The prescriptions of the *Pen-ts'ao kang mu* are composed of four
groups. So-called *ching-fang* prescriptions come from the works of
Chang Chi. Usually, they consist of three, five, or seven drugs and,
theoretically, after one dose the patient must either be cured or die.
The *shih-fang* prescriptions had become more and more popular since
the T'ang period, since harsh penalties had been introduced for medical
errors. These prescriptions are also prepared according to a system
and contain numerous ingredients; there may be up to a hundred or
more drugs that are supposed to control and secure the effect of the
main drugs. *Tan-fang* prescriptions provide a contrast to this; they
generally contain only one single drug. Finally, the *yen-fang,* "experience prescriptions," must be mentioned, which contain several ingredients and originated in the practical experience of individual
physicians or in family traditions. 經方 時方 單方 驗方

Li Shih-chen differentiated between an external and an internal
application. Here he had in mind not only the place of application
but also the place of the effect of the medication. He included sudorific,
purgative, mucus-removing, diuretic, pain-relieving, sedative, blood-
strengthening, anthelmintic, and other medications among those meant
for internal use. For external use, he intended eyedrops, eye washings,

blowing powders into the nose, inhaling, sticking in of needles, moxa, ointments, rubbing of teeth, plasters, washings, and other methods.

2.2.1. The monograph of the drug *pa-tou* in the *Pen-ts'ao kang mu*

The following translation of two monographs from the *Pen-ts'ao kang mu* demonstrates Li Shih-chen's method of drug description even better than the schematic overview presented above. First, I will give most of the monograph on the drug pa-tou, with which we are by now familiar:

> *Pa-tou* [bean from Pa], [from the] *Pen-ching*, [there:] lower class of drugs.
> Explanations concerning the name *(shih-ming)*:
> *Pa-shu* [in the] *Pen-ching; kang-tzu* [in the] *P'ao-chih* [lun]; *lao-yang-tzu.* [Li] Shih-chen says: This drug comes from [the district of] Pa Shu and looks like the *shu* bean. This was the reason for its name. The designation *pa-chiao* in the *Sung pen-ts'ao* is based on an incorrect writing of *shu.* Lei Hsü, in his work *P'ao chih-lun*, differentiates hard, small, yellow [specimens of this bean] as *pa*, and triangular, black ones as *tou.* Those that are small and pointed at both ends he calls *kang-tzu.* He wrote: "The *pa* and the *tou* are usable. The *kang-tzu* must not be used; their effect is fatal to man." This statement is completely false. The hard and small specimens are the female, the angular ones and those pointed at both ends are the male forms. The male ones are extremely effective, the female ones have a milder influence. When the drug is applied according to appropriate criteria, its effect is always positive. But if in the administration [of drugs] the necessary criteria are disregarded, even the [otherwise harmless drugs] *shen* and *shu* may have a harmful effect! This is all the more true in the case of the *pa-tou!*
> Collected explanations *(chi-chieh)*:
> [In the] *Pieh-lu* it is written: "*Pa-tou* grows in the district of Pa, in river valleys. It is gathered in the eighth month. It is dried in the shade. The seed coat is removed before use." [Su] Sung says: "Today [this drug] is found in Chia-chou, Mei-chou, and in Chiai-chou. It [originates from] a tree, which attains a height of one to two *chang.* Its leaves are a little thicker and larger than those of the *ying-t'ao* [trees]. In their early stage, they are greenish; later they change to colors ranging from yellow to red. By the twelfth month at the latest, the leaves have withered. In the second month, new leaves grow again gradually. While the new leaves are growing, all the old ones fall off by the fourth month. Then, spike-shaped pale-yellow inflorescences develop. In the fifth and sixth months, fruits with chambers develop. They are greenish during their growing stage. In the eighth month, when they ripen, they turn yellow and resemble the *pai-tou-k'ou.* Gradually, they drop off and are then gathered. Each [fruit-]chamber has two lids. Each lid yields one, perhaps even three seeds. The seeds are surrounded by a shell, which is removed [before medicinal] use. The seed-shell of the [pa-tou] specimens that come from Jung-chou has a pattern of lines that stand out like threads; there may be a single line, or two or three. The natives call this type gold-thread-*pa-tou.* It is considered the best type of all. It is said to occur in other areas as well." [Li] Shih-chen says: "The [fruit-]chambers of the *pa-tou* are similar to the [seed-]shells of *ta-feng-tzu*, only a little thinner

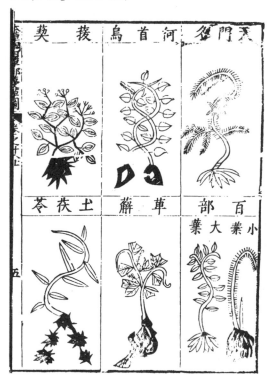

A page from the section "herbs," subdivision "twining plants" in the second edition of the *Pen-ts'ao kang mu* (1603). Pictured are the asparagus plant (*t'ien-men-tung:* upper right), stemona plant (*pai-pu:* lower right), knot-grass root (*ho-shou-wu:* upper middle), dioscorea plant (*pei-hsieh:* lower middle), smilax plant (*pa-ch'ia:* upper left), and the heterosmilax plant (*t'u-fu-ling:* lower left)

and more fragile. The seeds and the [seed-]kernels both resemble the seeds of *hai-sung*. A resemblance to *pai-tou-k'ou* has been reported but it does not exist."

Preparation (*hsiu-chih*):

[T'ao] Hung-ching says: "*Pa-tou* has a strong laxative effect on man. Fresh [drugs] are to be preferred. For [medicinal] use, the peel and the heart [of the bean] must be removed. Then [the drug] is boiled until its color turns yellow-black; it is crushed to a pulp and processed into pills or powders." [Lei] Hsü says: "For [medicinal] use, *pa* and *tou* are first crushed, then heated with hemp-seed oil and wine until dry, and, finally, pounded to a pulp. For each *liang* [of drugs] one should use seven *ko* each of oil and wine." Ta Ming says: "For [medicinal] use [of the drug] in a roasted form, as pills or powder, it is advantageous to remove the seed-skin and then heat [the drug] to a boil five to seven times, using fresh water each time." [Li] Shih-chen says: "[From the raw drug] *pa-tou*, the seed, the seed-coat, and the [seed-]oil are used [medicinally]. [The seed and the seed-coat] can be used fresh or [according to the type of illness to be treated] after roasting over low heat, after boiling in vinegar, or even after burning them, but preserving their qualities. [The raw drug] can also be crushed to a pulp, wrapped in paper, the oil can be extracted and the [residue called] *pa-tou-shuang* can be used."

[Thermo-]influence and taste (*ch'i wei*):

Acrid, warm, distinct medicinal effectiveness. [In the] "Additional Notes [of Renowned Medical Men]" it is written: "[In a] fresh condition [the drug possesses] a warm [thermo-influence; in a] prepared condition, a cold [thermo-influence]. It develops strong medicinal effectiveness." [Wu] P'u says: "Shen-nung, Ch'i Po, and Mr. T'ung [ascribe to the drug *pa-tou*] acrid [taste and] distinct medicinal effectiveness. [According to] Huang-ti [the drug has a] sweet [taste] and distinct medicinal effectiveness. Li Tang-chih [ascribes to it a] hot [thermo-influence]." [Chang] Yüan-su says: "The nature [of the drug] is hot; the taste is bitter. [Its] influences are weak, its taste is strong. The drug is heavy and descends [in the body]. It is *yin*." [Li] Kao says: "The effectiveness is distinct. [The drug] remains at the surface [of the body] and constitutes the *yang* in the *yang*." [Li] Shih-chen says: "*Pa-tou* has a hot [thermo-]influence and acrid taste. When fresh [the drug] shows an intense effect; when prepared, the effect is mild. *Pa-tou* can induce vomiting and can purge, halt [bodily influences] but also stimulate [them], and it is a drug that can rise and descend [in the body]. When it says in the 'Additional Notes [of Renowned Medical Men]' that the nature of the prepared drug is cold, or when Chang Yüan-su says [the drug] descends [in the body], and when Li [Kao] claims it remains at the surface [of the body], all [these authors] narrow-mindedly cling to only one [of the many properties of this drug]. For if one does not remove the seed-skin [of the drug], it is harmful to the stomach. If the heart [of the seed] is not removed [the drug] induces vomiting. After a long soaking in aromatic water it is able to rise as well as descend [in the body]. The laxative effect on man is retarded when *ta-huang* is administered at the same time, because [the effect of] both drugs decreases when they are taken simultaneously. Wang Ch'ung says [in his work] *Lun-heng:* 'All things that come into existence containing the influence of fire from the sun have a distinct medicinal effectiveness.' For this reason, *pa-tou* has a bitter [taste], hot [thermo-influence], and possesses distinct medicinal effectiveness." [Hsü] Chih-ts'ai says: "*Yüan-hua* assists [*pa-tou* in delivering its effects when used simultaneously]. [*Pa-tou*] fears *ta-huang, huang-lien, lu-sun, ku-sun, li-lu, chiang-ch'ih,* and cold water. The influence of heat has a positive effect [on the drug]. It hates *jang-*

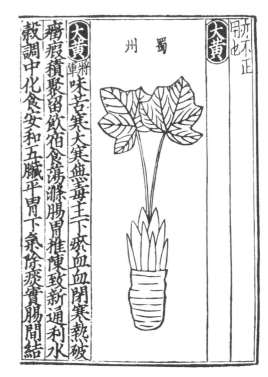

rhubarb root *(ta-huang)—Hsin-pien lei-yao t'u-chu pen-ts'ao*

ts'ao and is opposed to *ch'ien-niu*. For poisonings [through *pa-tou*], cold water, *huang-lien* juice, and *ta-tou* juice should be taken as antidotes."

Main indications (*chu-chih*):

Illnesses caused by cold; malaria fevers; fits of cold and heat; breaks through intestinal obstructions of various kinds; hardenings in the abdomen, stagnation of drinking liquids, mucous congestions, abdominal edema; cleanses the five depots and the six palaces; opens and penetrates obstructions; it clears the ways for waters and grains, removes spoiled meat, expels poisonings caused by demons, [removes] possessions by the *ku* and [other] evil things; kills worms and fish. [These indications are taken from the] *Pen-ching*. Cures stagnation of the monthly period and [induces] an overdue fetus [to leave the womb. Further it cures] cuts, and viscous blood in women; sexual weakness in men; kills the poison of *pan-mao* and snakes. One can also take [this drug] after subjecting it to a process of [alchemical] refining. It has a beneficial effect on the blood vessels, gives a good coloring to humans, and helps them to transform themselves, and to associate with demonic spirits. [These indications are taken from the] "Additional Notes [of Renowned Medical Men]." Cures ten kinds of water-swellings, paralyses; [leads to] miscarriages. [These indications are taken from the] *Yao-hsing* [*pen-ts'ao*]. Reaches all illnesses; dissolves obstructions; purges foods and has a restorative effect in cases of exhaustion; strengthens the spleen and opens the stomach; loosens phlegm and breaks blood [clottings]; drives out pus and removes swellings; poisons and kills worms in the palaces and depots of the body; heals malignant abscesses and flesh-tumors, itching skin ailments and swelling. [These indications are taken from the] *Ji-hua* [*tzu pen-ts'ao*]. It leads away influences and dissolves congestions; removes concentrations of cold in the depots and in the palaces; heals damage caused by raw, cold, and hard things. [These indications are taken from the work of Chang] Yüan-su. Cures diarrhea, shock and seizures, heart and abdominal pains, influence accumulations, and dry mouth caused by wind, deafness, numbness in the throat, toothaches; penetrates all internal paths and openings. [These indications come from Li] Shih-chen.

Explanations (*fa-ming*):

[Chang] Yüan-su says: "*Pa-tou* resembles a general who breaks through barriers and opens gates. [This drug] must not be administered carelessly." [Chu] Chen-heng says: "*Pa-tou* removes concentrations of cold in the stomach. [The drug] should not be used when no concentrations of cold are present." [Chang] Yüan-su says: "*Pa-tou* has long been used as a drug with a hot [thermo-influence], in order to treat illnesses resulting from [the consumption of] wine and also [in order to treat] influences [pressing against the] diaphragm. Because of its acrid [taste] and hot [thermo-influence] this drug is able to open congestions in the bowels and in the stomach. This, however, causes blood loss, damaging the real *yin* [influences]." [Chang] Ts'ung-cheng says: "This [drug] is used for afflictions caused by cold, wind, and moisture, for abscesses in infants, and for women after giving birth to drive out the membrane [of the placenta]. Even though [the patient] does not necessarily die [the treatment with *pa-tou*] is nevertheless dangerous. Why do the common people fear [the administration of] *ta-huang* but not [the administration of] *pa-tou*? Because its nature is hot and because it is used in small amounts only! They do not know that the administration [of *pa-tou*] as a laxative, even with a coating of wax, causes man's water balance to dry out, the chest to become heated, and the mouth to become parched, and damages the original [endowment supplied by] heaven. The poison [that causes

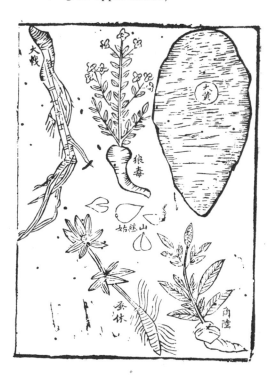

Illustrations from the *Pen-ts'ao hui-yen*—rhubarb root (*ta-huang:* upper right) and wolfsbane (*lang-tu:* upper middle)

the illness] remains in the body and is not removed; on the contrary, secondary illnesses are caused! Therefore, *pa-tou* should not be used as a laxative." [Ch'en] Ts'ang-ch'i says: "*Pa-tou* controls [the cure of] obstructions and congestions of various kinds, influence of cold, blood clots, digestive trouble, accumulations of liquids and water-spitting. [One should select] greenish-black, large [specimens of the drug] and take one [seed] daily on an empty stomach. [First] the seed-shell must be removed. The white seed-membrane, however, must not be damaged. Then [the drug] is taken with a liquid and, after a brief period of time, develops a fire-like heat in the stomach. All bad things are purged. Nevertheless, this does not result in any depletions. After the drug has been taken for a long time, its purging effect on man is lost. Specimens whose white seed-membrane has been damaged must not be used." [Wang] Hao-ku says: "In situations where a quick treatment [is appropriate], it [is used for] preparations [affecting] the passageways of water and grains. In this case [the drug] is applied fresh, after the removal of the skin, the membrane of the kernel, and the oil. If one wishes to achieve mild effects, one should make preparations that dissolve indurations and remove obstructions. For this purpose, the drug is roasted until no more smoke rises and a violet-black color has been obtained. It is not widely known that this drug is able to penetrate the bowels, as well as end diarrhea. Chang Chung-ching uses it in his 'Pills prepared for urgent cases to treat the hundred illnesses and possessions by the malevolent.'" [Li] Shih-chen says: "When one applies *pa-tou* heroically, one is able to remove the worst illnesses. Even with careful use [the drug is] wonderful for soothing and harmonizing one's center. Thus, it can be compared to the brave and ferocious warriors Hsiao Ho, Ts'ao Ts'ao, Chou Po, and Kuan Ying, who—appointed as ministers—were able to bring about a great peace. When Wang Hai-tsang points out that (*pa-tou*) is able to penetrate the intestines as well as stop diarrhea, he discloses a secret from ancient times. A woman over sixty years old had already been suffering from diarrhea for five years. Meats, oily, raw, and cold foods did her harm and caused pain. She took all sorts of medications that were supposed to bring her spleen back into harmony, medications which [have a] rising [effect in the body], others which cause constipation, and which retain or constrict. When these medications reached her stomach, her diarrhea only became worse. Finally, she came to me and I examined her. [The movement in] her vessels felt deep and smooth. That meant that the spleen and the stomach had been damaged for a long time, resulting in extensive concentrations of cold and in obstructions. In Wang T'ai-p'u's work it says: If a great cold has concentrated inside, and if diarrhea has already lasted for quite a while, one can achieve [only an apparent] cure, for [the illness] will return again and again! In old people it is recommended that such [concentrations] be drained with hot drugs. This removes the cold and ends the diarrhea. Thus, I had [the patient] take fifty wax-coated *pa-tou* pills. After two days, her bowels were obstructed and the diarrhea was gone. Since that time, I have been able to eliminate the diarrhea in all treatments of such diarrheic illnesses, concentrations, and obstructions; the number of people cured is close to a hundred. [This drug] is really wonderful when used at the appropriate moment, and when it is directly opposed to the illness. If [the drug] is used in inappropriate cases, however, that is a violation of the warning against careless administration, leading to a damage of *yin*(-influences)."

Correction of mistakes (*cheng-wu*):

[T'ao] Hung-ching says: "The Taoists possess an alchemical process for preparing [this drug]. It is said that one could become immortal after taking [the drug prepared in this manner]. One man took a dose of it, and he died immediately; a rat consumed it for over three years and became thirty *chin* heavier. This shows how the natures of things can tolerate one another." [Li] Shih-chen says: "In the Han period, the prescription masters stated that the [drug] *pa-tou* prepared through a melting process could have the effect of improving the appearance of people [who have taken it] and that these people became immortals. This opinion came into the *Pen-ts'ao* via the 'Additional Notes of Renowned Medical Men.' Chang Hua writes in [his work] *Po-wu chih:* 'When rats eat *pa-tou*, they attain a weight of thirty *chin*.' All that is nonsense and false. Mr. T'ao believed in it and considered these stories to be facts. But he was wrong. When, in addition, it says that a man would die after a dose, that is not true either. I now correct all [these errors]."

Prescriptions included (*fu-fang*):

Thirteen [of the following prescriptions] are old, twenty-six [I have] newly [added]. . . . (In the following, only a selection is quoted.)

[Against] all concentrations and obstructions:

pa-tou 1 *liang*, *ko-fen* 2 *liang*, *huang-po* 3 *liang*; pulverize, prepare water pills of the size of green beans, take five pills with water per dose. [From:] *I-hsüeh ch'ieh-wen*.

[Against] concentrations of cold and digestive problems:

[In case of] no digestion and constipation [one may take] 1 *sheng* of *pa-tou* seeds, and 5 *sheng* of clear wine; heat [the *pa-tou*] for three days and three nights, crush, add the wine, and heat over low flame. Prepare pills the size of peas, take one pill with water per dose. In cases of nausea two pills. [From:] *Ch'ien-chin fang*.

[Against possessions by] water-*ku* and enlarged abdomen:

[When the patient] moves or shakes [his body], one can hear the sound of water. The skin is of black color. Take ninety *pa-tou* [seeds], discard the seed-peel and roast until they turn yellow. Take sixty almonds, discard the peel and the pointed ends. Roast until they assume a yellow color. Crush. Prepare pills the size of small beans. Take one pill [after another] with water and stop the intake when success appears. Do not drink wine! [From:] Chang Wen-chung's *Pei-chi fang*.

[Against] attacks by flying corpse-demons:

[If one has been] hit by the malevolent, [if the] heart aches and [if the] abdomen is swollen, [and if one] is constipated, [he should prepare the] Running Horse Decoction [as follows]: One takes two *pa-tou* [seeds], which, after the skin and the heart have been removed, are roasted until they become yellow. Then they are wrapped in silk together with two almonds and crushed to pulp. [The silk bag containing the pulp] is then turned around in one *ko* of hot water and the [resulting] white juice is to be consumed. The intake [of this drug] is immediately followed by the cure of the illness. When using this [medication] one should take the age [of the patient] into consideration. [From:] *Wai-t'ai pi-yao*.

[Against influence of] wind and moisture, and mucous diseases [caused by these influences]:

The patient should sit down in a closed room. At his left, place a bowl of boiling water; at his right, a bowl with a charcoal fire. In front of the patient, place a table and on the table, a book. Before that, one has taken forty-nine oil-free, fresh *pa-tou* grains, which were crushed to a pulp, and from which the oil has been pressed, after being wrapped in paper; this has been divided into three portions. If the illness is in [the patient's] left side, his right hand should be placed on the book, back of the hand down. The medication is placed in the center of the palm, on that a bowl, into which hot water is then poured. When the water has cooled, it is replaced. After [the patient] has perspired for a long time, a miraculous effect sets in. If

the illness is in [the patient's] right side, [everything] is put into the
center of the left palm. It is also said: "[The medication] is to be
placed correspondingly, right or left." [From:] *Pao-shou-t'ang ching-
yen-fang.*
[Against] silk-threats of heaven penetrating the throat:
If one consumed drinks or food with spots of dew and with flying
threads penetrating the surface, ulcers will grow in his throat. *Pai-
fan* and *pa-tou* should quickly be burned to ashes and blown into
[the throat]. The illness will then be cured. [From:] *Suo-sui lu.*
[Against] sudden deafness:
One *pa-tou* seed is wrapped in paper and a hole is pierced into this
with a needle so that air may pass through. With this, then [the ear]
is stopped up and the [desired] effect will be achieved. [From:] *Ching-
yen* [*fang*].
[*Pa-tou*] oil, main indications: . . . [by Li] Shih-chen.
[*Pa-tou*] seed-shell, main indications: . . . [by Li] Shih-chen.
    Prescriptions included:
     . . . Root of the [*pa-tou*] tree, main indications: . . . [by Li] Shih-
    chen, on the basis of the *Yang-ch'eng ching-yen-fang.*[198]

2.2.2. The monograph of the drug *a-fu-jung* in the *Pen-ts'ao kang mu*

Whereas we were able to pursue the development of the *pa-tou* monograph from the *Pen-ching* onward, the following *a-fu-jung* monograph
describes a drug whose listing in the *Pen-ts'ao kang mu* constitutes
its first appearance in a Chinese pharmaceutical work.

A-fu-jung is a Chinese name for poppy and opium. The cultivation
of poppy for the purpose of opium production has existed in China
since the T'ang period. Nothing is known, however, about the use of
the products at that time. Only in the sixteenth century did opium
appear as a therapeutic drug and an aphrodisiac. Around 1600, as far
as we know, opium smoking was indulged in for the first time. In later
works, the drug was also described and recommended for fever.[199]

poppy *(ying-tzu-su)—Shao-hsing pen-ts'ao*

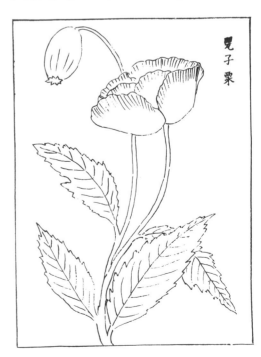

    A-fu-jung [first recorded in the *Pen-ts'ao*] *kang mu*
Explanations concerning the name:
    A-p'ien. [Li] Shih-chen says: "Generally, [the drug] is called *ya-p'ien.*
    The meaning of this name is unclear. Someone has said that, in local
    dialects, the pronunciation of *a* corresponds to *o*. Since the color of
    the blossom [of the original plant] resembles that of *fu-jung*, this term
    has been adopted."
Collected explanations:
    [Li] Shih-chen says: "In earlier generations, one heard very little of
    a-fu-jung. It is used only in modern prescriptions. It is said to be
    poppy juice. When the poppy plant bears green capsules, one must
    scratch the outer green shell [of the capsules] with a large needle late
    in the afternoon. In the process, the hard inner shell must not be
    damaged. Three to five spots should be treated this way. On the
    following morning, the liquid will have emerged from these scratches.
    It is scraped off with a bamboo spatula, collected in an earthenware
    receptacle, and can be used [medicinally] after drying in the shade.
    As a result [of this method of production,] the [*a-fu-jung*] on the
    market today is occasionally contaminated by fragments of the cap-
    sules. In the *I-lin chi-yao* of Mr. Wang [Hsi] it is said that [the original
    plant] 'is the red poppy cultivated in Arabia. The head [of the plant]

must not get too wet. In the seventh or eighth month, after the blossoms have withered, one obtains [the opium] by scratching the green skin.' If we take a closer look at this [statement] we may ask how it can be possible that there are still green skins in the seventh or eighth months with the blossoms producing fruits and withering in the fifth month already? Maybe there are local differences."

[Thermo-]influence and taste:

Sour, astringent; warm; slight medicinal effectiveness.

Main indications:

Incessant diarrhea until the rectum prolapses. [A-fu-jung] is able to halt the outflow of the essential influences of males. [These indications come from Li] Shih-chen.

Explanations:

[Li] Shih-chen says: "The ordinary people use [a-fu-jung] for the art of the bedchamber. In the capital [a-fu-jung] balls are sold as 'gold-pills,' with the claim that they are able to cure all illnesses. All of these usages are based upon the techniques of prescription specialists."

Prescriptions included:

Four newly [introduced prescriptions]:

[Against] chronic diarrhea:

A portion of a-fu-jung, the size of small beans, is taken with warm water on an empty stomach. That is one daily dose. [During the treatment with a-fu-jung, the consumption of] onions, garlic, and starch (?) is not permitted. Thirst is to be quenched with hydromel. [From: I-lin] chi-yao.

[Against] red- and white-colored diarrhea:

[Prepare a powder of] one fen each [of the drugs] ya-p'ien, mu-hsiang, huang-lien, and pai-shu, and make from that rice pills the size of small beans. Strong people receive a dose of one fen, old people and youths, half that amount. One should take the drug on an empty stomach, with rice. [During the treatment with this medication, the consumption of] vinegar dishes, of raw, cold, oily, and fatty things, and of tea, wine, and farinaceous products is not permitted. Each case of diarrhea is brought to an end with this [prescription]. Thirst [during this time is to be quenched] with small amounts of water in which rice has been boiled. Another prescription: Before the blossoms of the poppy have opened, there are, on their outside, two green leaves covering them. When the blossoms open, [these leaves] fall off. They should be gathered and ground to powder. Each dose consists of one ch'ien, to be drunk with rice. Miraculous effects will be achieved. In case of red diarrhea, use the [leaves] from red blossoms; in case of white diarrhea use the [leaves] from white blossoms.

A ball of "gold-pill":

One fen of genuine a-p'ien is crushed with nonglutinous rice and made into three pills. The individual dose is one pill. If it has no effect, a second one should be taken. However, one should not take too many. Vinegar is to be avoided [during the period in which the drug is taken]; otherwise, the intestines of the patient can tear. [These "gold pills"] are to be taken with hot wine in cases of paralysis caused by wind, with boiled ch'iang-huo in cases of dry mouth and evil in the eyes, with tu-huo decoction in case of pain in all joints, with ch'iang-huo decoction in case of straight head wind, with ch'uan-hsiung decoction in case of partial head wind, with fang-feng decoction in case of dizziness, with tou-lin wine in case of poisoning through yin [influences], with a decoction of peach tree and willow branches in case of malaria fevers, with t'ing-li decoction in case of mucous coughing, with kan-chiang and a-chiao decoction in case of chronic coughing, with k'uan-tung-hua decoction in case of exhaustion and coughing, with huo-hsiang decoction in case of vomiting and diarrhea, with huang-lien decoction in case of red diarrhea, with chiang de-

coction in case of white diarrhea, with *pai-shu* decoction in case of
difficulties in swallowing and dysentery, with *mu-hsiang* wine in case
of all kinds of pain caused by the influences, with *chih-tzu* decoction
in case of heat pain, with *teng-hsin* decoction in case of pain below
one's navel, with *ch'uan-lien* and *hui-hsiang* decoction in case of air
in the small intestines, with *ju-hsiang* decoction in case of pain caused
by [problems with the] blood and influences, with hot wine in case
of pain in one's ribs, with *sheng-chiang* and *ting-hsiang* decoction in
case of choking from food, with *wu-ling-chih* decoction in case of
female hemorrhage, with *sha-jen* decoction in case of slow [injury to
the] spleen [apparent in symptoms as caused by] wind in small children. [From:] *Kung Yün-lin i-chien*.[200]

2.3. The Ming editions of the *Pen-ts'ao kang mu*

2.3.1. The Chin-ling edition of the *Pen-ts'ao kang mu*

The Chin-ling edition is the first edition of the *Pen-ts'ao kang mu*. It   金陵
was prepared in the twenty-fourth year of the governmental period
wan-li (1596) by the publisher Hu Ch'eng-lung in Nanking. In twenty-
five volumes there were fifty-two chapters of text and two additional
chapters of drug illustrations, which had been drawn by Li Shih-chen's
son Li Chien-yüan. They generally corresponded to the illustrations
in the *Cheng-lei pen-ts'ao*, as far as the drugs had already been described there; only a few were drawn after actual models.

These illustrations were criticized, on the one hand, because of their
poor quality, and on the other, because only one single drawing had
been prepared for each illustrated drug description. Regional differences or various possible forms of one plant had not been taken into
consideration. New, improved illustrations were later prepared for the
Ch'ien-shih edition of 1640, but the latter deficiency was not remedied.

Each page contained twelve lines of twenty-four characters. Wang
Shih-chen's preface, dated 1590, was placed at the beginning of the
work; it was followed by a "list of the names of people who participated in the compilation of the work"—for the most part, members
of the Li family. Li Shih-chen himself, four of his sons, and four of
his grandsons are listed.

The Chin-ling edition was apparently not suited for establishing Li
Shih-chen's fame. Owing to the rather careless production, it attained
only a small distribution. As far as is known, six copies of the first
edition are extant today, of which two are in China, three in Japan,
and one in the United States Library of Congress. A seventh copy was
lost in Berlin during World War II.

2.3.2. The Chiang-hsi edition of the *Pen-ts'ao kang mu*

The Chiang-hsi edition was published in the thirty-first year of the
period *wan-li* (1603) by Hsia Liang-hsin in Chiang-hsi. This time, the
work appeared in twenty-nine volumes; the illustrations were placed
at the beginnings of the individual chapters to which they belonged.
Each page contained nine lines of twenty characters. This edition was
given an additional preface by Hsia Liang-hsin and Chang Ting-szu;

重刻本草綱目序
夫醫之為道君子用之以衛生而推
之以濟世故稱仁術乃後世以藝視
之縉紳先生多所弗講賈子不云乎
古之聖人不居朝廷必居醫卜之間
醫可以賤簡為哉本草者固醫家之
耰鋤弓矢也洪纖動植最為煩雜散

The beginning of publisher Hsia Liang-hsin's preface to his second edition (1603) of the *Pen-ts'ao kang mu* (Chiang-hsi edition)

the list of Li Shih-chen's collaborators was omitted, replaced by the accompanying letter of the son Li Chien-yüan, which contains Li Shih-chen's text for the planned presentation of the work to the throne, and which Li Chien-yüan had submitted to Emperor Shen-tsung together with a copy of the completed *Pen-ts'ao kang mu*.

The editors added to the *Pen-ts'ao kang mu* three other works by Li Shih-chen: the *Ch'i-ching pa-mai k'ao* ("Studies Concerning the Eight Irregular Conduits"), the *Mai-chüeh k'ao-cheng* ("Verification of Instructions on the [Movement in the] Vessels"), and the *P'in-hu mai-hsüeh* ("The Doctrine of P'in-hu on the [Movement in the] Vessels"). The edition was concluded by the *Ssu-yen chü-yao*. Originally written by Ts'ui Chia-yen in the Sung period, under the title *Mai-chüeh szu-yen chü-yao* ("The Most Important Points from the Instructions on the [Movement in the] Vessels, in Sentences Consisting of Four Words"), this little work appeared here in a version largely changed by Li Yen-wen.

The Chiang-hsi edition was not widely distributed either. Because of the qualitative deficiencies of the Chin-ling edition, however, almost all of the numerous Ch'ing period editions followed the Chiang-hsi edition. Various copies of this edition are still extant today, in China and Japan, in the British Museum in London, in the Staatsbibliothek Preussischer Kulturbesitz in Berlin, and in the United States.

Supplied with an additional, fourth preface by Tung Ch'i-ch'ang, the Chiang-hsi edition was reprinted in 1606 by a man in Hupei named Hsüeh. One copy of this reprint has been preserved and is located in Shanghai.[201]

2.3.3. The Ch'ien-shih edition of the *Pen-ts'ao kang mu*

錢氏

The Ch'ien-shih edition appeared in the thirteenth year of the period *ch'ung-chen* (1640) and was published by Ch'ien Ya in Wu-ling. It constitutes a reprint, expanded by two additional prefaces, of the 1603 Chiang-hsi edition, but differed from the latter through the new and more careful drug illustrations which Ch'ien Ya substituted for the sketches of the first edition. This edition was the first to reach Japan.

The precise number of new editions and reprints of the *Pen-ts'ao kang mu* published during subsequent centuries cannot be determined. The *Hsien-ts'un pen-ts'ao shu-lu* alone lists fifteen Ch'ing editions that have been preserved.[202] The *Pen-ts'ao kang mu* was translated, not only into Japanese but also in a more or less complete form into the Western languages of Latin, Russian, French, German, and English.[203]

2.4. The position of Li Shih-chen in the history of Chinese pharmaceutical literature

The personal situation of Li Shih-chen certainly constitutes an important starting point for the understanding of the man and his work. From the social low of the bell-physician's existence, the family, under Li Shih-chen's father, was able to rise to a respected rank. Agriculture formed the basis of their life. Li Yen-wen was an official for a time;

his study of medicine could be considered an ethical duty. Li Shih-chen had been destined from his earliest years to secure for the family a firm place in the very respected world of Confucian officials. He failed the exams three times; there was little left for him to do except to return to the family tradition—medicine. With incredible ambitiousness, almost obsessed, he attempted to create a work which was to surpass the *Cheng-lei pen-ts'ao,* the last visible manifestation of the former main tradition of pharmaceutical literature. In a sense, he resembled Chang Yüan-su, who, after his failure in the Confucian system, also sought his future in medicine and created a significant work in the field. But the only person whose position approaches that of Li Shih-chen in the course of this description of the pen-ts'ao literature is T'ao Hung-ching. One can recognize parallels in their behavior but differences in their motivation. Possibly as a result of similar traditions in their families, both of them were greatly interested in medical practice and personal experiences connected with their own experiments. Both developed similarly critical consciousnesses, and both endeavored to create newer, more practicable forms and contents—retaining but transforming what existed. They recognized the intolerable disorder of the representative pharmaceutical works extant during their times. They introduced new classifications of drugs and the original materials from which they came and strove for a natural order of things.

T'ao Hung-ching may have acquired the motivation for his actions from his affinity to Taoism. Li Shih-chen was a would-be Confucian, and we cannot but assume that he wanted to compensate, consciously or subconsciously, for this deficiency through his work. Chu Hsi apparently served as a model for him. The latter's school of thought still constituted the official government version of Confucianism during Li Shih-chen's lifetime. To obtain a clear picture of things on one's own—this had been one of the main demands of Chu Hsi. Li Shih-chen conscientiously followed this maxim and thus arrived at new understandings. Title and structure of the *Pen-ts'ao kang mu* clearly refer to Chu Hsi.

It might be interesting to determine which elements in the *Pen-ts'ao kang mu* are original and which derived from outside suggestions. As far as I know, there is no remark anywhere in Li Shih-chen's work indicating that he had known the *Pen-ts'ao p'in-hui ching-yao.* On the basis of his great interest in pen-ts'ao literature and his extensive search for more and more new sources, however, we may assume that he had become acquainted with that unpublished manuscript, possibly during the brief period of his employment in the Imperial Medical Office. Perhaps he did not see the original manuscript but only heard about it; and therefore he would have also known about the new subdivision of the monographs according to individual technical criteria. This is apparently not the only important idea that Li Shih-chen took over from predecessors in his own century.

Watanabe Kōzo suggested that Li Shih-chen's structural pattern was influenced by Wang Chi, who had written the *Pen-ts'ao hui-pien* at the beginning of the period *chia-ching* (1522–1566).[204] In his review of that work, Li Shih-chen wrote: "[Wang] Chi abolished the division

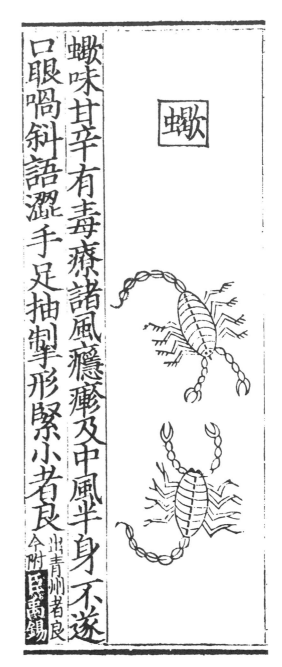

scorpion *(hsieh)—Ch'ung-hsiu cheng-ho pen-ts'ao*

類

of the *Pen-ts'ao* into the upper, middle, and lower classes of the drugs and instead arranged the drugs according to related types (*lei*)."[205]

Finally, one should look at the theoretical foundations presented in Li Shih-chen's work. Apparently, Li Shih-chen did not contribute any original ideas in this area. His comparative study of relevant literature and his own observations of facts in nature enabled him to correct previous mistakes, although of course his own assertions are not free of numerous errors either. Li Shih-chen, then, may have questioned alleged facts, but he did not question basic concepts. As a result, he did not doubt the validity of the paradigms of systematic and magic correspondence, both of which he frequently referred to in his work. Since Li Shih-chen was trained to enter a Confucian civil service career, one might have expected that he would have rejected the concepts of demonology. However, this is not the case. Li Shih-chen believed in possessions by corpse-spirits and demons, and he knew that if a person afflicted by such "guests" died, the evil spirit would immediately enter a bystander as its next host. Consequently he adopted without any critical remarks and even invented himself pertinent prescriptions against such ills, as can be seen, for instance, in his selection of formulas using peach kernels as an effective ingredient.

Criticism of the *Pen-ts'ao kang mu* by subsequent pen-ts'ao authors was directed mainly against the size of the work. This criticism is justified when one judges the work according to its usefulness for the practicing physician. While T'ao Hung-ching in his work had restricted himself to the presentation of a purely medical-pharmaceutical subject, Li Shih-chen created a comprehensive encyclopedia, in which he frequently went beyond the popular pharmaceutical scope.

The size of the work made it expensive as well as unwieldy. The ballast of treatises digressing into marginal areas—of interest perhaps to Confucian medical scholars but not to practicing physicians and pharmacists—therefore became the target of criticism.

In spite of such voices and of initial difficulties, a few decades after its publication the *Pen-ts'ao kang mu* totally replaced the previously most comprehensive *Pen-ts'ao,* the *Cheng-lei pen-ts'ao.* The advantages of the new form succeeded without opposition. And yet, the *Pen-ts'ao kang mu* remained only a remarkable individual work. Only a few of the many smaller pen-ts'ao works that followed remained uninfluenced by this enormous model; but there was nobody who might have revised and further developed the *Pen-ts'ao kang mu* itself. One single work, the *Pen-ts'ao kang mu shih-i,* was written as an immediate supplement to the *Pen-ts'ao kang mu.*

Under Emperor K'ang-hsi (1655–1723), a variety of activities were undertaken in the literary field. Still, the *Pen-ts'ao kang mu* itself remained disregarded; the outdated *Pen-ts'ao p'in-hui ching-yao* was removed from the archives and was expanded by a number of additional drugs, most of which were taken from the *Pen-ts'ao kang mu.* Thus, the *Pen-ts'ao kang mu* must be regarded as the qualitative and quantitative climax in the development of the pen-ts'ao literature and, consequently, of recorded traditional Chinese pharmaceutics. The following three centuries of the empire only brought improvements in some details.

2.5. Supplementary works to the *Pen-ts'ao kang mu*

2.5.1. The *Wan-fang chen-hsien*

"Thread and Needle for Ten Thousand Prescriptions"—this is the title the author Ts'ai Lieh-hsien gave to what may be the earliest Chinese index work. Ts'ai admired the over 11,000 prescriptions scattered throughout the *Pen-ts'ao kang mu,* but he also recognized the great difficulties the practitioner experienced when he wanted to look up the appropriate prescription for a patient and his illness. Therefore, he wrote an index for the prescriptions of the *Pen-ts'ao kang mu,* in which he listed the illnesses as *kang* in eight chapters, and subordinated to these the various manifestations of an illness, *mu.* Under each mu he listed chapter and page numbers for the best-known prescriptions in the *Pen-ts'ao kang mu* and, in this manner, significantly facilitated the practical use of that work. Some subsequent editions of the *Pen-ts'ao kang mu* contain Ts'ai Lieh-hsien's *Wan-fang chen-hsien* as an appendix.[206]

Wan-fang chen-hsien
"Needle and Thread for Ten Thousand Prescriptions"
8 chapters
Author: Ts'ai Lieh-hsien (seventeenth century)
Published: ca. 1652

2.5.2. The *Pen-ts'ao kang mu shih-i*

Only one single author of the following centuries took the trouble to investigate mistakes and deficiencies in the *Pen-ts'ao kang mu* and to write a work that would correct these and also add the drugs that had become known in the meantime or had not been included in the *Pen-ts'ao kang mu.* This was Chao Hsüeh-min, author of the *Pen-ts'ao kang mu shih-i.* All other pen-ts'ao authors of these centuries, when they referred to the *Pen-ts'ao kang mu,* wrote summaries of the work they considered too voluminous.

In an introduction, Chao Hsüeh-min explains his motives. His most important thoughts are presented below:

1. Chao Hsüeh-min attempted to supplement those parts that had been mentioned in the *Pen-ts'ao kang mu* but had been insufficiently discussed.
2. He criticized the structure of the *Pen-ts'ao kang mu* which he felt was complicated by the division of the monographs (kang) into technical rubrics (mu) of drug description.
3. Chao wrote that in using drugs one is interested in those which can be obtained most easily. Therefore, he questioned the use of descriptions of expensive or rare drugs. Conversely, however, he noted that it is not advantageous to come upon the strange and peculiar things, which after all do exist between heaven and earth, without being able to do anything with them. For this reason, he finally decided to include such items anyway.
4. Chao differentiated from the subgroup "vines" (*man*)—which in the *Pen-ts'ao kang mu* was included among the herbs—a separate group of "climbing plants" (*teng*), which he discussed following the groups of tree drugs in his work. In this connection he expressed the assumption that the vines originally might have

Pen-ts'ao kang mu shih-i
"Additions to the Materia Medica Arranged according to Drug Descriptions and Technical Aspects"
10 + 1 chapters / 921 drug descriptions
Author: Chao Hsüeh-min (eighteenth century)
    tzu: Shu-hsüan
    from: Ch'ien-t'ang in Che-chiang
Written: ca. 1800
Published: 1871

been herbs and the climbing plants originally might have been trees. In addition, Chao established the new group "blossoms," since the blossoms had previously been discussed only in an appendix to the plant monographs and therefore had been neglected.

5. To make it easier for the user of his work to inform himself about innovations, Chao presented those drugs not previously described, in separate appendixes to the individual groups.

6. Chao eliminated the group of human drugs. This group, he wrote, was not suitable for helping humanity but, instead, constituted an obscenity. It is said: "If one kills living beings to save man, this causes the wrath of heaven!" How much more valid must this be when one uses men to cure men, Chao argued. He therefore abolished this group.

This introduction is followed by a preliminary chapter entitled "Correction of Mistakes," Here, Chao Hsüeh-min discussed in detail, for example, the false definition of some drugs, criticized the fact that Li Shih-chen had not recorded the complete prescription for the preparation of *she-wang*, an arrow poison containing aconite, and wrote a treatise claiming that the drug *ch'ien-fen*, alkaline carbonate of lead, is poisonous, whereas Li Shih-chen had maintained the opposite:

> *Fen-hsi* is the same as *ch'ien-fen*. [In order to produce this substance] one pounds lead into thin, small plates and steams these together in a pot with the contents of a bottle of vinegar. Through a process of transformation the [*ch'ien-fen*] powder is created. Today it is produced in large amounts in so-called powder factories in K'ang-ch'eng. Because the influences of lead and vinegar are poisonous, within three years [of employment there] the muscles and the bones of the workers there are dissolved and their nature turns wild. Once a month, the factory workers have to eat a goose to neutralize [the effect of the poison]. This shows how poisonous the substance [*fen-hsi*] is. Under the heading "Collected Explanations," P'in-hu quotes the *Yü-tung lu* by Ho Meng-ch'un. It also says: "The workers involved in the production of the powder have to eat fat pork or dog meat, drink wine, and partake of iron broth in order to suppress the toxic effects. If the poison gets into the empty stomach, the person immediately falls fatally ill. Old and young [workers] who are exposed to the poisonous fumes frequently suffer from paralysis and deformation, until they die." This description certainly shows that [*fen-hsi*] is poisonous! Elsewhere it is stated: "At the time of its production, the influences [generated by *fen-hsi*] contain poison. But once the powder is finished, it is not at all poisonous. If it contained poison, how could the people in former times, in their prescriptions, have put it into preparations that were to be eaten? And furthermore, there are no methods transmitted how to prepare an antidote." [P'in-hu] probably did not know that the nature of this substance is able to subdue sulfur and that it eliminates the acidity of wine. Auripigment, upon mere visual contact with it, will turn black. If it is added to crabs preserved in distiller's grains, [the crabs] will not turn brittle. Taken in drugs [this substance] can cause miscarriages. Rubbed on the face, it causes spots. Its destructive, cruel characteristics equal those of arsenic. Only the intake of small amounts is possible. Afterwards, the stool often turns black, but then [automatically] resumes its original appearance. Court records mention a case where a woman died from taking *ch'ien-fen*. Her hands and feet turned black. This, too, shows the toxicity [of

this substance]. However, in the section on [thermo-]influence and taste, P'in-hu writes the following about *fen-hsi:* "[Taste:] acrid; [thermo-influence:] cold; no toxicity *(wu-tu)*." All [subsequent] *pen-ts'ao* works have taken over this mistake. It is said universally: "No toxicity." But that constitutes a not-inconsiderable deception of people; for this reason, I have specifically pointed it out here."[207]

This criticism is a manifestation of the changed meaning of the term *tu.* In the classic traditional pharmaceutical literature, it had been used to designate the effect of the drug and had always indicated the strength of medicinal effectiveness. In contrast to the drugs with tu, that is, with distinct medicinal effectiveness, which were suited for the treatment of acute illnesses, stood the drugs without tu; these were the preventive drugs, which had to be taken over a long period of time in order to have an effect. Only after Li Shih-chen was the meaning "poison" or "poisonous" ascribed to the term *tu* in connection with the indication of drug effects, leading to the misunderstanding between Chao Hsüeh-min and Li Shih-chen.

Of the total of 921 drugs described by Chao, 205 belonged to the appended drugs mentioned under point five of the introduction. Many of the newly included drugs came from foreign countries. We encounter here *yen-ts'ao* [tobacco plant] and *chin-chi-lei* [cinchona bark], about which he wrote, among other things:

> In the *Jen-hai chi* by Ch'a Shen-hsing (1650–1727) it is said: "In Western countries exists a type of tree bark called *chin-chi-lei.* It is used to treat malaria fevers. The cure sets in after only one dose." In the fifth year of the period *chia-ch'ing* (1800), my relative Chin Chai returned from Canton. He brought this article back and showed it to me. It consisted of thin, hollow twigs. They resemble the drug *yüan-chih,* after one has removed from it the marrow [lit.: the bones]. The taste is slightly acrid. It is said "[this drug] is able to penetrate the construction and protection [influences of the body]. Its nature is fairly hot. It is particularly suited to penetrating the influences and the blood.
>
> Malaria therapy. This is being transmitted among the barbarians at Macao. Against any kind of malaria, one takes one *ch'ien* of *chin-chi-lei,* and five *fen* of *jou-kuei.* They are boiled together and then consumed. Strong and sturdy people may use two *ch'ien* of *chin-chi-lei.* Cure is achieved after one dose.
>
> Antidote against [the effects of] wine. A hot decoction [of *chin-chi-lei*] is brought down into the [patient's] throat. He will then become conscious again. This is also a tradition among the barbarians residing in Macao.[208]

Further, we find among the minerals, for example, a drug called "Protects-from-fright stone" *(pi-ching-shih)*[209] from Spain, and another called "wonderfully effective stone" *(ch'i-kung shih)*[210] whose origin is supposed to be in the Atlantic Ocean.

Various "drugs" that Chao Hsüeh-min categorized as "medicinally used utensils" are reminiscent of the old European *Dreckapotheke.* These include such things as worn-out children's shoes, old roof shingles, and tobacco wrapping paper, as well as latrine boards and "white autumn frost" (i.e., urinary sediments). They were, of course, subjected to a more or less complicated process of preparation—as, for example, incineration—before they were used medicinally.

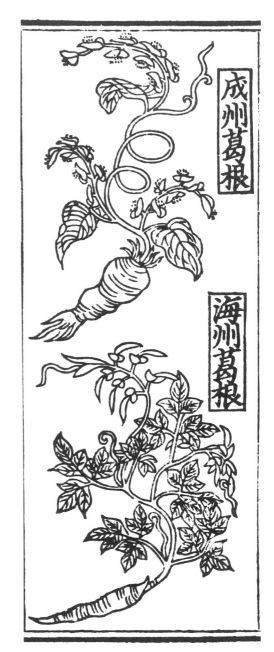

pachyrhizus root *(ko-ken)*—*Ch'ung-hsiu cheng-ho pen-ts'ao*

The individual monographs are of differing lengths. They are no longer subdivided according to various criteria. Frequently, the text is based on quotations from works of previous authors; particularly striking here are travel reports and local chronicles. The contents of the descriptions deal with the preparation, the origin, and the effects of the drugs; secondary names are mentioned as well. There are no explicit references to the Chin-Yüan doctrines; Chao did not argue in terms either of the yinyang theories or of the Five Phases theories. The work contains no illustrations.

The *Pen-ts'ao kang mu shih-i* is the first Chinese pharmaceutical work to convey to us a detailed description of opium smoking. The pertinent monograph is found as an appendix to the group "fire":

[It says in the] *T'ai-hai shih-ch'a lu:* for the preparation of opium tobacco, hemp or *ko* [plants] and opium cakes are cut into strips and heated together in a copper kettle. The resulting opium product is then mixed with tobacco. In addition, one fills a bamboo pipe with coconut fibers, and all these things are smoked together. The price asked for it is far greater than that of ordinary tobacco. [Shops] that deal specifically with the preparation of this product bear the name *k'ai ya-p'ien kuan.* After one has smoked opium tobacco once or twice, it is impossible to free oneself from it. The warm influences [of the opium smoke] flow directly into the *tan-t'ien* area.[211] Afterwards, one does not need to sleep all night. The natives also take [opium] as a medication that is supposed to procure a lascivious way of life for them. Their bodies and limbs become emaciated, their body's depots and palaces dry out. One cannot stop until the body has been destroyed. The police authorities issue strict prohibitions in every case. Frequently, the people are thrown into prison. They beg for reprieve and only a short while afterwards they smoke another pipe.

The opium cake comes from Java. [It says in the] *Hai-tung cha-chi:* Opium is a foreign product made in Java and Luzon. It is one of the goods that falls under the prohibition of importation from across the ocean. In Taiwan, many unstable people smoke opium mixed with tobacco. They say that it is useful for the mind and enables one to stay up all night, without having to sleep. Whenever it is smoked, several people must get together. In between, food is served repeatedly. Mats are spread out on the brick-bed, and everybody sits down there. In the center, a lamp is lit for the smoking. One inhales over a hundred up to several hundred times. The pipe consists of a bamboo cane, about eight to nine *fen* long. The inside is filled with coconut fibers and human hair. Both ends are fitted with silver caps. Into one side, a hole the size of the little finger has been drilled. One makes a gourd-shaped, hollow receptacle of yellow clay. It is baked in fire and is set on the hole between the two ends. The opium tobacco is placed on this gourd-shaped receptacle. Only a small amount of tobacco is needed. One fills one's entire mouth with smoke. That produces a strange sound. [The smokers] have drinks and food served several times; fatty and sweet dishes are demanded. Otherwise, their stomachs and intestines do not feel well. When one first smokes for a few months, it seems as if one were still able to give up [this habit]. But when one suddenly stops [smoking] after a longer period of time, one is very exhausted and feels ready to die. Finally, one's family and one's body are destroyed and ruined. All smokers can be recognized by their blackish faces and hunched shoulders. Their eyes water, their sensations are distracted and can no longer concentrate; finally, death occurs.

Main indications [for use as a drug]: miraculous effect in cases of pain in the stomach-bowel area.[212]

開鴉片館

丹田

poppy *(ying-tzu-su)—Chih-wu ming-shih-t'u k'ao*

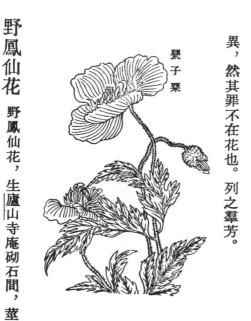

野鳳仙花

罌子粟

野鳳仙花，生廬山寺庵砌石間，莖葉

異，然其罪不在花也。列之羣芳。

Chao Hsüeh-min wrote the *Pen-ts'ao kang mu shih-i*, as well as eleven other works, which he combined as *Li-chi shih-erh-chung* ("Twelve Useful Works"). For many years, they were handed down only as manuscripts, and during the course of time, all but two were lost. In addition to the *Pen-ts'ao kang mu shih-i*, a work entitled *Ch'uan-ya* was preserved.[213] Of the other ten, we know only the titles. A man named Chang Ying-ch'ang finally acquired the *Pen-ts'ao kang mu shih-i* manuscript. With his own afterword, dated 1864, he published the work, three-quarters of a century after it had been written.[214] It was later published by the Commercial Press in Shanghai as a supplement in their edition of the *Pen-ts'ao kang mu*.

Because of the inclusion of numerous foreign drugs and of the quotations describing them, the work has a certain cultural-historical value. For the everyday practice of the physician, it scarcely constitutes an enrichment. Perhaps this fact has contributed to the minor interest shown in this work after its completion.

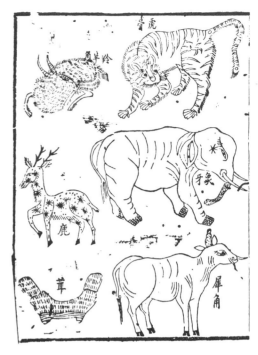

illustrations from the *Pen-ts'ao hui-yen*

The greatness of the *Pen-ts'ao kang mu* overshadowed the last centuries in the history of traditional Chinese pharmaceutical literature. There was scarcely a later pen-ts'ao author who did not refer, in some manner, to Li Shih-chen. Many viewed it as their responsibility to produce a handier work corresponding more closely to the requirements of the medical practitioner, a work that was often conceived as an outline of the *Pen-ts'ao kang mu*.

Thus developed a tradition whose authors had no individual intentions other than being of assistance to the medical practitioner. The contents of their works united, with no visible contradiction and, at most, with a changing emphasis, the conceptions of the Chin-Yüan doctrine and elements of the old main tradition. The model for this type of combination was, of course, the *Pen-ts'ao kang mu*; we have already found indications of such a tendency in the *Pen-ts'ao chi-yao* and in the subsequent works of the Chin-Yüan tradition.

Various authors of this direction termed themselves representatives of a Ch'i-Huang school. In so doing they made reference to the discussions recorded in the *Su-wen* between Huang-ti, the Yellow Emperor, and Ch'i Po, his minister, and expressed their conception of being representatives of the original doctrine. The pen-ts'ao works most frequently used today by traditional Chinese medical practitioners and pharmacists, at least on Taiwan, come from this tradition.[215]

1. The *Hui-t'u pen-ts'ao kang mu hui-yen*

Hui-t'u pen-ts'ao kang mu hui-yen
"Illustrated Materia Medica, Arranged by Drug Descriptions and according to Technical Aspects"
Short title: *Pen-ts'ao hui-yen*
20 chapters / 609 drug descriptions
Author: Ni Chu-mo (ca. 1600)
    tzu: Ch'un-yü
    from: Ch'ien-t'ang in Che-chiang
Written: ca. 1620
Published: 1624

In the "Annals of the Che-chiang Province," we find the following description of author and work and the comparison with the *Pen-ts'ao kang mu*:

> Ni Chu-mo—his *tzu* reads Ch'un-yü—penetrated secrets already in his youth and showed pleasure in old things. He studied the teachings of Mr. T'ung and Ch'i Po and gained access to their hidden meanings. He achieved outstanding successes in the treatment of illnesses. Many people traveled in great haste to consult him. If they could not receive [treatment from him], they became very annoyed. Chu-mo collected the pen-ts'ao works from all periods. He conducted exhaustive and extensive studies, made decisions in cases of doubt, and uncovered mistakes. Finally, he arranged and edited the results of his careful investigations, entitling [the work] *Pen-ts'ao hui-yen*. His son, [Ni] Chu-lung, arranged the publication and had the work distributed. In general, it is said: the subtleties [of pharmaceutics] are compiled in the *Pen-ts'ao kang mu* of Li; this work, however, combines the most important elements. I agree with this statement.[216]

We learn more about the intentions of the author from his introduction to the *Pen-ts'ao hui-yen*. There we can read that the author, beginning with the *Pen-ching* and continuing through the *Pen-ts'ao kang mu*, had thoroughly studied more than forty works on materia medica. From these works the author took over 609 frequently used drugs in order to create a "useful tool" for the medical practitioner.

Moreover, Ni Chu-mo expressed the view that, although very extensive pen-ts'ao works already existed, mankind had changed and that of necessity the pen-ts'ao literature had to be adjusted to these changes. He also claimed that although the *Pen-ts'ao kang mu* was indeed the best drug work, it had to be simplified.

In his work, Ni Chu-mo declined to include drugs used in Taoist prescriptions; there was too much "nonsense" involved, as he stated.[217]

The arrangement of the *Pen-ts'ao hui-yen* does not correspond completely to that of the *Pen-ts'ao kang mu*—herb and tree drugs are placed at the beginning—but the division into sections and subsections is reminiscent of that work.

The monographs are collected in chapters 1 through 9. They are very detailed and place a great value on the inclusion of the Chin-Yüan doctrines. For this reason, the name of a drug is followed by information on thermo-influence, taste, medicinal strength, rising, descending, floating, or diving properties, as well as the ability of the drug to penetrate certain conduits.

It is only after this information that commentaries of earlier authors are presented, beginning with T'ao Hung-ching, in which, among other things, details about origin, collection time, and the appearance of drugs, as well as on the original material (plants or animals, for example) are given.

Illustrations are combined on a total of forty-five pages, which are spread out in the text at the beginning of the respective chapters. Each individual page of sketches contains several quite lifelike illustrations of various drugs and also of the original sources for the drugs, that is, complete plants or animals.

The twentieth chapter contains general and theoretical treatises. Here we find numerous quotations, with which we are by now familiar, from both the works of the Chin-Yüan epoch as well as from the *Pen-ching* and from T'ao Hung-ching.

The work achieved a certain reputation. In 1645, a second edition was published; in 1699, this work reached Japan.[218]

Ku Yüan-chiao's conception scarcely differs from that of Ni Chu-mo. To compile a new work, he selected what he considered the most beneficial passages from a whole series of earlier works, adding his own commentaries. In choosing drugs, he limited himself to those most frequently used by physicians. The result was the relatively modest number of 397 monographs.

The emphasis in the drug descriptions was on references to connections with the Chin-Yüan doctrines and on information for prescriptions. Following the monographs, the author included fifteen sections, again devoted to the Chin-Yüan theories. The work is illustrated; all illustrations are grouped together.

Wang Ang (ca. 1700) later published a revised version of the *Pen-ts'ao hui-chien*.[219]

Wang Ang can probably be considered the most successful medical writer of the Ch'ing period. Even today, a large number of his works are widely circulated among practitioners of traditional Chinese medicine. In addition to the drug work *Pen-ts'ao pei-yao*, the *T'ang-t'ou ke-chüeh,* composed in verse, and the much more extensive *I-fang chi-*

2. The *Pen-ts'ao hui-yao chien-chu*

Pen-ts'ao hui-yao chien-chu
"Annotated Enumeration of the Important Elements of the Materia Medica"
Short title: *Pen-ts'ao hui-chien*
10 chapters / 397 drug descriptions
Author: Ku Yüan-chiao (seventeenth century)
    tzu: Yen-wen
    from: Pi-ling

3. The *Pen-ts'ao pei-yao*

Pen-ts'ao pei-yao
"Completion of the Important Elements of the Materia Medica"
8 chapters / 400 drug descriptions
Author: Wang Ang (ca. 1700)
    tzu: Jen-an
      from: Hsiu-ning in An-hui
Written: date unknown
Published: 1682

aconite tubers (*fu-tzu:* top) and aconite blossoms (*fu-tzu-hua:* bottom)—*Ch'ung-hsiu cheng-ho pen-ts'ao*

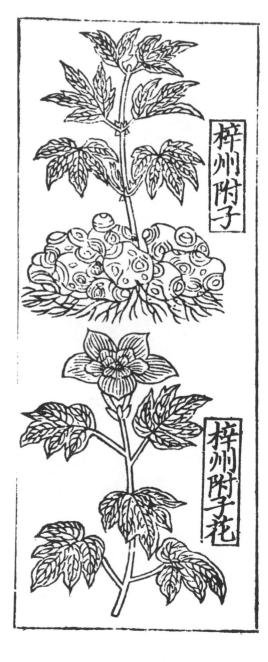

chieh could be mentioned here as two of his well-known prescription works.

Wang Ang's lasting success may have two explanations. First, he utilized an easily understood language. His works could be penetrated by those lacking a thorough education. Second, he apparently created the most advantageous combination of the two earlier traditions: the main pen-ts'ao and the Chin-Yüan traditions. Wang Ang repeatedly expressed his views on this matter; in the introduction to the above-mentioned *I-fang chi-chieh,* he emphasized the necessity of a theoretical foundation for the use of medications:

> The prescription literature, both old and new, is quite extensive, and yet always, the commentaries that precede the prescription state only: "cures this and/or that illness!" Explanations of the underlying causes of the illness are always lacking, as is information on which conduits are affected by the illnesses. In addition, within the individual prescriptions advice is given only to use this and/or that drug. However, information is always lacking on the effects of [thermo-]influence, taste, which of the various conduits are penetrated, and thus, on the causes of the drugs' abilities to cure certain illnesses. In fact, the works dealing with prescriptions were therefore written in a senseless manner, and the superficial capabilities of the common medical practitioners can be viewed as being characterized by ignorance. They limit themselves to treating living illnesses with dead prescriptions and not infrequently shower the world with their mistakes, thereby causing harm to mankind.
>
> Finally, during the Sung period, Ch'en [Wu-]che was the first to study the works of [Chang] Chung-ching. He placed the explanations of illnesses at the beginning and clarified the effective properties of drugs, so as to enable the reader to understand from beginning to end.[220]

That Wang Ang was not restricted to certain theories and kept an open eye for practical problems is indicated by the following excerpt from the introduction to the *Pen-ts'ao pei-yao:*

> In the descriptions of drug indications by [earlier] authors, general details are more frequent than differentiating ones. Thus, for example, among the drugs that cure mucous diseases are those suitable for the treatment of dry mucus and those suitable for moist mucus. But all works include only the information that mucous afflictions can be eliminated [with the drugs in question]. Drugs for headaches [as a further example] can be subdivided into those directed against headaches caused by internal sources and those caused by external sources. In all works, however, only the following can be read: "they cure headaches." But these are symptoms with opposite causes and cannot be approached in an undifferentiated manner. These are only two examples; the others can be deduced in a similar manner. In addition, [I would also like to mention] that it is only stated which drugs are suitable for use with specific illnesses. But references to which illnesses must not be treated with [these drugs] are lacking. For this reason, I have taken such incompleteness into account here, supplementing such material with detailed commentaries. In this manner, I have avoided deceptions.[221]

The thoughts that motivated the author during the compilation of the *Pen-ts'ao pei-yao,* as well as the models and the points of emphasis, are described in the preface:

The most important thing in medicine is the examination of the [movement in the] vessels. Only the person who can correctly recognize the [different movements in the] vessels and the manifestations [of illnesses] that appear in them is able to differentiate whether it is a question of depletion or repletion. Otherwise, the assaults [against illnesses] and the treatments for the replenishment [of conditions of depletion] are senseless, and instead of achieving a long life, the result is usually an early death. The second most important thing [in medicine] is the necessity of clearly understanding the properties of drugs. If, for example, an illness is present in a specific conduit, a very specific drug must be administered. It is also possible that [the illness] located in this conduit can spread to other conduits; a treatment of replenishment must then be carried out upon the associated mother [depot] or a treatment of drainage on the respective child [depot]—weakness must be supplemented and violence checked! The correct method of action is based upon many principles, and one cannot simply emphasize one alone as binding. If a person is incapable of uniting individual details, penetrating generalities, analyzing subtleties, and understanding the mysterious, he will not succeed in achieving brilliance, but he will approach evil and stray from the correct path. In earlier times, it was aptly said: "The use of drugs is similar to the employment of soldiers: one must really be careful!"

From antiquity to the present time, several hundred authors have written *pen-ts'ao* works. None of them, however, surpasses the [*Pen-ts'ao*] *kang mu* of Mr. Li in either spirit or accuracy. The examinations and studies [expressed in this work] are, at the same time, profound and extensive; information is comprehensive and clear. For this reason, I admire the attitude of this man and would like to speak praisingly of "extreme perfection." However, the chapters and volumes were written in such numbers that it is difficult to study [the work] completely during the course of a lifetime. Furthermore, it is rather cumbersome to bring along [the *Pen-ts'ao kang mu*] when traveling by boat or carriage. It is indeed an all-embracing work, but that which is essential cannot be [recognized immediately]. [Works] such as the *Chu-chih chih-chang* and the *Yao-hsing ko-fu* were written with the intention of facilitating for the student the learning and recitation [of pharmaceutics]. Although they concentrate on essential matters, comprehensiveness is lacking. In more recent times, the [*Pen-ts'ao*] *meng-ch'üan* and the [*Shen-nung pen-ts'ao*] *ching-shu* are generally considered good works. The newly added sections in the [*Pen-ts'ao*] *meng-ch'üan* are indeed of quite brilliant significance, but the language is limited to verse. As a result, the text is extremely gay and variegated, and there are numerous deficient and superficial passages. In the [*Shen-nung pen-ts'ao*] *ching-shu* the principles of the main curative effects and the meaning underlying the preparation of prescriptions and the mixture [of drugs] are explained. In addition [the author] has written an examination of mistakes [in earlier works] in order to explore their deficiencies. [His work] can be characterized as very good. Thus, there is no pause in his interpreting the way of earth, in his elucidating the preparation [of prescriptions] and the treatment [of illnesses], and in his differentiating genuine and false [products]. If [such extensive and manifold] commentaries accidently led to some forced conclusions, and very frequently used drugs were dismissed, this means only "a single mistake in thousands of plans."

I am not one of those who particularly follow the teachings of Ch'i and Huang, but I do like to read their work. For more than three years I collected the *pen-ts'ao* works of all authors—from comprehensive [reading] I returned to a concise [presentation]. I selected a total of 400 drugs suitable for use and arranged them in a small volume. [In this work I discussed] which drugs penetrate which specific conduits, and which afflictions they then relieve. For this one must be knowledgeable

aconite tubers resembling the heads of crows (*wu-t'ou*)—*Ch'ung-hsiu cheng-ho pen-ts'ao*

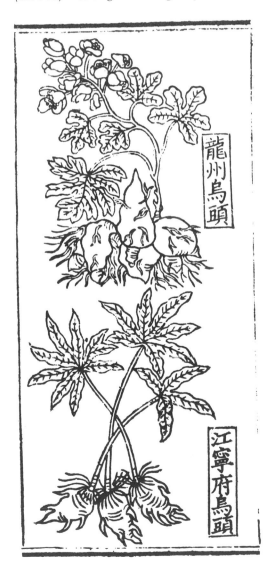

龍州烏頭

江寧府烏頭

about the [thermo-]influence, taste, appearance, and color [of drugs], since these properties are considered the foundations of the main curative effects. In between I have added the profound and broad meaning of the "extreme aversion and common action, of the formation of resistance, and of mutual aid," upon which the people of antiquity based the use of drugs. Following [the drug descriptions] I have added information concerning place of origin, method of preparation, and incompatibility. I have placed the ten types of prescription combinations and the [treatises on] diverting and penetrating properties and the depletion-restoring and repletion-relieving characteristics before [the drug descriptions]. In this manner, I have described the effectiveness [of the drugs] but have also elucidated their possible disadvantages, so that people will realize it while reading. As a result, the use [of this work and the drugs it describes] do not lead to mistakes. It can probably be said that, on the one hand, my work is comprehensive but that, on the other hand, the essential elements can be recognized. Intelligent scholars can use the work as a basis for their investigations, for the essence and subtleties of medicine can, for the most part, be taken from it. The title reads *Pen-ts'ao pei-yao*. By using this text, the correct way to the works of our ancestors is achieved.[222]

A chapter entitled "Summary of the Significance of Drug Properties" is placed before the main part of the *Pen-ts'ao pei-yao*. In this chapter, Wang Ang offered the reader nearly the entire spectrum of the most important theoretical foundations of pharmaceutics. He explained the sense and utilization of the doctrines of the five tastes and five colors, of the yin and yang correspondences, and of the mode of operation of drugs in the body.

The contents of the individual monographs in the main section were already indicated by the author himself in the preface reproduced above. They contain, like the preceding works of this tradition, a detailed consideration of the Chin-Yüan doctrines.

Originally the *Pen-ts'ao pei-yao* was not illustrated. Only in later editions were illustrations added for most of the drugs. Wang Ang himself, at the age of eighty, completed a revised edition of his work, expanded in comparison to the original by sixty drug descriptions.[223]

4. The *Pen-ts'ao ts'ung-hsin*

Pen-ts'ao ts'ung-hsin
"Restoration of Pharmaceutics"
18 chapters / 720 drug descriptions
Author: Wu I-lo (eighteenth century)
    tzu: Tsun-ch'eng
    from: Hai-yen
Written: date unknown
Published: 1757

With the *Pen-ts'ao ts'ung-hsin*, Wu I-lo picked up directly from the *Pen-ts'ao pei-yao*.[224] However, at least according to his statements, he was not quite as convinced by the Chin-Yüan theories as was his predecessor. In the preface to this work, Wu I-lo wrote:

Earlier generations of my family compiled an extensive library. Above all, they purchased books whose use was beneficial to the people. For this reason, there are also among these books many rare [editions] which contain teachings by those who are the followers of the Ch'i-Huang school. Since my youth, when I prepared for the [civil service] career, I have frequently chosen these books for extra reading. When I occasionally understood something in these works, I felt as if my spirit and my nature had been opened and purified. As a result, I have revealed [over time] the hidden [meaning of these works], and I have unraveled their innermost core. Forty years have now passed since that time.

The most important thing in medicine is the understanding of its principles. The second most important thing is the differentiation of symptoms; the third position is taken by the use of drugs. How can someone differentiate symptoms if the principles are not clear to him?

How are medications to be used if someone cannot differentiate symptoms? For this reason, I have composed ten medical works. One of them is entitled *I-yüan pi ch'e* ("The Entire Origin Must Be Understood"). A second [work] is called *Ssu chen hsü hsiang* ("The Four Diagnostic Methods Must Be Carefully Carried Out"). I carefully considered all teachings on the meaning of the classics and on the peculiar characteristics of illnesses and endeavored to find what was most appropriate for each case. In addition, it was my belief that heaven allowed medications to grow, so that the illnesses of man might be cured. Thus, it is quite certain that there is a drug for each illness; illnesses appear in a thousand variations—drugs also. If one can differentiate, in detail, [thermo-]influence and taste and selects one or two [substances] from the multitude of drugs, he will, in their application, be on one level with the spirits! If one is unable [to differentiate drug properties] he will have many doubts [about which ones to select] and his use of [the drugs selected will be] confused. All drugs can harm man. This is especially true if drugs with unbalanced, distinct effective properties are used contrary to their requirements.

Throughout the centuries, since the times of the old classics, the commentators of the *pen-ts'ao* have continuously introduced revisions and new regulations, and the *Pen-ts'ao kang mu* of Mr. Li is a magnificently complete collection. The evidence he has provided [concerning the effects of drugs] is correct and comprehensive and, therefore, quite apt to rectify the deficiencies of the *Erh-ya* and of the commentaries to the *Shih*[-*ching*] and to complete the art of practical medicine. Miu [Hsi-yung] deplored the great bulk [of the *Pen-ts'ao kang mu*] and, as a result, compiled the [*Shen nung pen-ts'ao*] *ching-shu*. [In this work] he not only described the effects of drug properties but also wrote treatises on their possible disadvantages. They contain much new information but were sharply criticized by Yü Chia-yen from Hsi-ch'ang. Finally, Mr. Wang from Hsin-an, on the basis of the above-mentioned two works, wrote the [*Pen-ts'ao*] *pei-yao*. It is not very extensive, but it is in accordance with current trends with its comprehensive selection of material. The only regrettable thing is that [his arguments] are not grounded in the Ch'i-Huang school and that, instead of orienting himself on symptoms, [Wang] gave special credence to earlier theories. Without differentiating, he took over the most diverse teachings and with them, unavoidably, mistakes. I have disregarded my own limitations and have subjected this work to another revision. In the process I have taken over half of the work, changing or writing the second half myself. In addition, I have plucked [some information from] older texts, and I have also taken into account my own experiences from the course of time. The completed work is entitled *Pen-ts'ao ts'ung-hsin*.[225]

After a short introduction, the illustrated monograph section of the *Pen-ts'ao ts'ung-hsin* begins immediately. A special treatise devoted to a detailed discussion of the theoretical foundation is lacking. Nevertheless, Wu I-lo does not totally dispense with this element. The individual monographs contain the usual information on thermo-influence, taste, appearance, color, conduit affiliation, and on the main effects of the drug. The annotations on theory are inserted in the form of commentaries between the individual statements on the various indications of drugs.

The arrangement of the work—sections and subsections—follows that of the *Pen-ts'ao kang mu*. The actual order, however, does not coincide with that of the great model; Wu I-lo also placed, as did his predecessors in this tradition, the description of herbs and trees at the beginning.

In addition to the *Pen-ts'ao pei-yao*, the *Pen-ts'ao ts'ung-hsin* is still one of the most widely disseminated pen-ts'ao works.

5. The *Pen-ts'ao ch'iu-chen*

Pen-ts'ao ch'iu-chen
"The search for truth in pharmaceutics"
11 chapters / 520 drug descriptions
Author: Huang Kung-hsiu (eighteenth century)
      tzu: Chin-fang
        from: I-huang hsien in Chiang-hsi
Written: ca. 1700
Published: 1778

In preliminary remarks to this work the author, Huang Kung-hsiu, strongly criticized what he considered unjustified admiration for the *Pen-ching* by his contemporaries:

The basic classic [*Pen-ching*] of pharmaceutical [literature] goes back to Shen-nung; its meaning is, of course, not simple. If the information it contains is examined, statements concerning the properties of drugs, such as the following, can frequently be found: they are able to soothe the five depots, strengthen spirit and mind, prolong life, relieve the body of its material weight, and blacken the hair, or, in the case of drugs such as *sang-pai-p'i* and *tzu-ts'ao,* fill one's center and benefit one's influences. This language is extensive but superficial and raises some doubts. If one examines further [the assertion] that Shen-nung tested the herbs and that [the knowledge he acquired in this manner] has been handed down to us, [it is clear] that there was no writing at that time. Thus, knowledge had to be transmitted orally. How else could anybody have received it? Where [in the *Pen-ching*] more specific information is given concerning the places of origin of the drugs, the names are frequently from the late Han period. K'ou Tsung-shih, T'ao T'ung-ming, and Chang Yü-hsi have all expressed the opinion that this book was completed during the Han period, but they had no way of determining in what century it had been written. It is indeed stated in the *Huai-nan tzu* that Shen-nung tested the herbs in order to assemble the medications, but the name *Pen-ts'ao* is not mentioned in this connection. Finally, the editions of [Mr.] T'ung and Lei[-kung] are said to have been written on bamboo panels and [with regard to contents] to have corresponded to the *Su-wen*. However, this would lead to the question of why they were changed so much in later times! The suspicion that someone other [than Shen-nung] probably wrote [the *Pen-ching*] is therefore justified. In later times [the text] was shortened and then expanded again, so that its authenticity was lost even further, and the information it contained became increasingly faulty. It is no wonder that Li P'in-hu, when he compiled his *Pen-ts'ao [kang mu]*, only arranged the main effects of the *Pen-ching* in the foreground and made no special effort to compose commentaries for them. Moreover, he doubted whether the statements of the *Pen-ching* were genuine at all and preserved them solely to retain what had not been completely lost. It was by no means his intention to value that which was contemporary and look down upon that which was old; in reality, he did not dare to equate the *Pen-ching*, which appears to be half questionable and half reliable and whose words are often so shallow, with the *Su-wen* and to consider both equally as precious works from ancient times. Chang Lu from Ch'ang-chou was the only one who displayed utmost efforts of veneration [when he prepared his version of the *Pen-ching*]. But he often [carried out] the intention of patching together individual portions [of the *Pen-ching*] with force, which is not the real sense of a veneration. For this reason, I myself concentrate on the properties of drugs and proceed solely from the facts. Thus, I do not cling to the old in order to despise the new, and I do not esteem what is new in order to reject that which is old! My sole effort is directed toward the harmony of theory and illnesses, so that drugs correspond to the illnesses, with the result that the sentiments of Yen-ti for the salvation of the world secretly coincide with my discussions, and that his venerable intentions will not be thwarted. My hope has always been directed towards this goal.[226]

These comments are only understandable if one keeps in mind a new direction in the development of the pen-ts'ao literature (to be discussed in the following chapter of the present study) that had gained some influence in the intervening period. Various authors, including the already-mentioned Chang Lu, had endeavored to reconstruct the *Pen-ching* and create works that would be free of all "Chin-Yüan ballast." In this light, Huang Kung-hsiu was one of the last significant representatives of the eclectic tradition and the Ch'i-Huang school.

His *Pen-ts'ao ch'iu-chen* differed significantly in form from the works of his predecessors in this tradition. What is most conspicuous is a general division into two parts. Chapters 1 through 7 contain the 520 drug monographs; chapters 8 through 10 discuss theoretical questions.

Huang Kung-hsiu completely reorganized the arrangement of monographs. He divided the first seven chapters according to the following seven types of drugs: (1) drugs that replenish conditions of depletion; (2) astringent drugs; (3) dispersing drugs; (4) drugs that relieve conditions of repletion; (5) drugs that control the blood and its afflictions; (6) various drug effects; and (7) food drugs. These seven sections are, where necessary, further subdivided. Each section or subsection is introduced by a defining treatise. As an example, the definition at the beginning of the subsection "poisonous things" in the group "various drug effects" is reproduced below:

> All drugs [that are] neutral and balanced [in their properties], whose [thermo-influence] is neither cold nor hot, are not poisons. Also not poisonous are those drugs that, although possessing a [one-sidedly] hot *yang* or cold *yin* [thermo-]influence, nevertheless have effective properties which are not excessively strong. All drugs that display an excessively marked *yin* coldness, engender a violent burning, and have lost the neutrality and harmony of their influences, are to be designated poisons. However, poisons can be used, with a suitable preparation, in the treatment of man. That means that some drugs are indeed poisons but do not have to be designated as such. When, for example, the [thermo-]influence and taste [of a drug] are developed one-sidedly hot and pressing, [when the drug] contains solely pure *yin*- but no *yang* [-influences], and it exerts such a strongly controlling effect that one does not dare to submit oneself to it, then this signifies extreme toxicity, and under no circumstances should its use be undertaken rashly. *P'i-shuang, nao-sha, pa-tou, feng-hsien tzu, ts'ao-wu, she-wang,* and *kou-wen* are hot poisons with the capability of killing people. *Shui-yin, ch'ien-fen, mu-pieh,* and *chü-jo* are cold poisons with the capability of killing people. *Pei-ma, shang-lu,* and *lang-ya* are neither cold nor hot—nevertheless, their effective properties are not neutral and balanced: they contain the influences of acrid poison and, thus, are also capable of killing people. Naturally, I am of the opinion that medical treatment using poisons cannot proceed carelessly; [but it should be kept in mind] that those drugs that originally, in terms of their effective properties, were not considered as such can also function as extremely strong poisons—with no way of rescuing anybody subjected to them. This occurs when the illness [against which they were used] was falsely diagnosed and the [movement in the] vessels was not differentiated according to the facts. Moreover, the drugs that are poisonous to man are generally known, and people are aware what they have to watch out for. However, when [drugs] do not belong to the group of poisons, they are then considered beneficial, and caution is neglected. I have

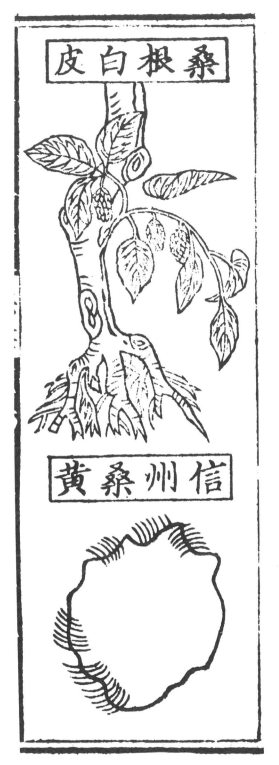

root epidermis of the mulberry tree (*sang-ken pai-p'i*)—*Ch'ung-hsiu cheng-ho pen-ts'ao*

often met patients who had taken nonpoisonous medications in the morning and had already died by evening. There are no other reasons [for such occurrences than the ones I mentioned]. To this end I have added these comments as a warning about the careless use of medications.[227]

Heading each individual monograph is the name of the drug. Beneath the heading is a number (in consecutive order) as well as information concerning the botanical, mineralogical, or zoological classification of the original material of the drug. This information usually corresponds to the designation of the individual subsections in the *Pen-ts'ao kang mu,* in which, for example, drugs had been defined as "swamp herbs," "high tree," and so forth, depending on the original plant or other matter.

The actual text of the monographs begins by repeating the name of the drug and referring to its capabilities of penetrating certain conduits. This is followed by a description of appearance, color, thermo-influence, taste, mode of operation, contraindications, combination in prescriptions, and pharmaceutical preparation.

The text has been compiled from the author's own statements and from comments by earlier authorities who are cited by name. There are almost no remarks in the text that refer to connections with Chin-Yüan doctrines.

The second part of the work begins with the treatise that constitutes the eighth chapter, "The Main Drugs for Illnesses in the Body's Depots and Palaces." Following a short introduction, there are twelve individual sections on the five depots, six palaces, and also on the *ming-men,* the "door of life."[228] These sections each begin with a theoretical observation, which is then followed by a table, in which a number of drugs are listed according to various effects. For example, the author divided the drugs for the liver into thirty possible effects.

命門

The ninth chapter carries the heading "The Main Drugs for Illnesses Caused by the Six Harmful Influences." The chapter also begins with a general introduction, followed by thirteen sections in the order: "Wind," "Cold," "Summer-Heat," "Moisture," "Dryness," "Fire," "Heat," "Mucus," "Influences," "Blood," "Obstructions," "Pain," and "Thirst Afflictions." Each section, in turn, is introduced by a short discussion, which is frequently based on the theories of the *Su-wen.* These introductions are followed by tables listing the suitable drugs, again subdivided according to individual effects.

The tenth chapter finally brings a summary. Quotations from Li Kao, Chang Yüan-su, Li Shih-chen, and Wang Ang, as well as from the *Su-wen* conclude the work.

There are no illustrations; with at least three Ch'ing period and two more newer editions, the work achieved a certain circulation. One of the Ch'ing editions was published in a small pocket format.

6. Concluding Remarks on the Eclectic Tradition of Pen-ts'ao Literature

In the present work, the least space has been devoted to the most successful individual tradition in all of the pen-ts'ao literature, from which came the drug works most popular with pharmacists and medical practitioners of the traditional curative system in China. The

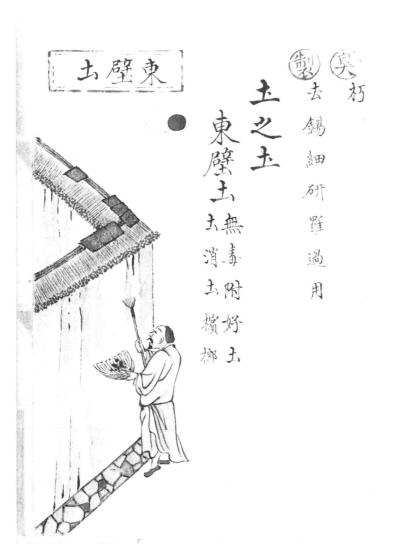

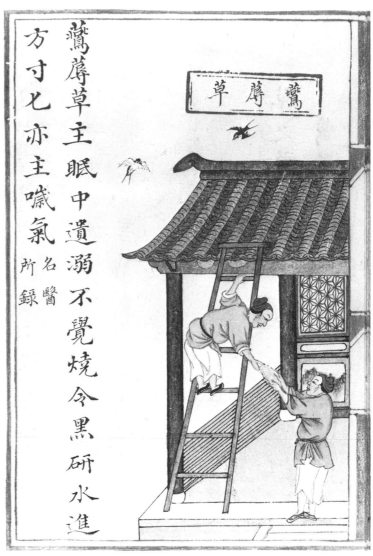

scraping soil from the east wall *(tung-pi t'u)*—
Pen-ts'ao p'in-hui ching-yao

removing swallows' nests for the drug "swallows' nest herb" *(yen-ju ts'ao)*—*Pen-ts'ao p'in-hui ching-yao*

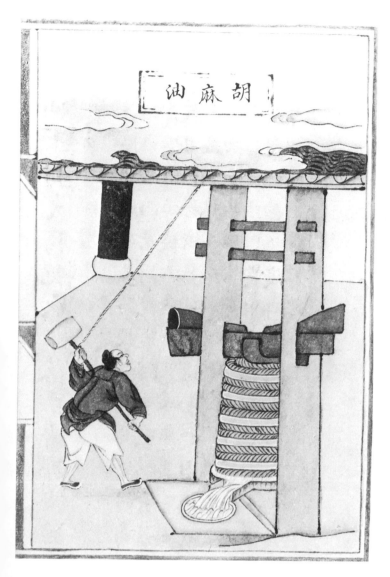

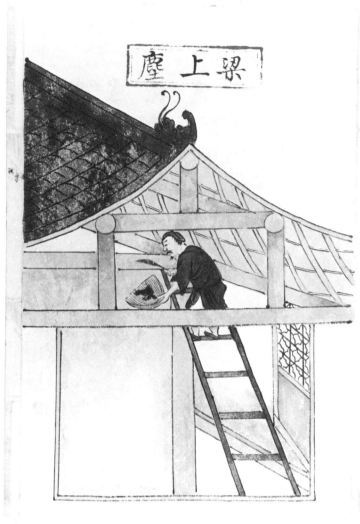

extracting sesame oil (*hu-ma-yu*) by means of
cold pressing—*Pen-ts'ao p'in-hui ching-yao*

sweeping up rafter dust (*liang-shang ch'en*)—
Pen-ts'ao p'in-hui ching-yao

explanation for this apparent contradiction can be found in the attribute "eclectic," which I have used to designate this tradition.

My presentation of this tradition is so brief because the elements from which the texts of the individual works were compiled have already been sufficiently discussed in connection with the two traditions from which they were taken. The works in the eclectic tradition contain no fundamentally new concepts. The authors were apparently thoroughly acquainted with the requirements of medical practitioners. The practitioners were offered a theoretical section for discussion and the description of drugs and prescriptions for actual practice. This system occasioned the success. It gave every practitioner the possibility to argue (and also, perhaps, to think) in the manner required by the profound theoretical claim, and to act in the manner that experience and the effectiveness of prescriptions called for.

1. The Intellectual Situation during the Ming and Ch'ing Period: The Return to the Sources

After early difficulties, Chu Hsi's (1130–1200) form of Neoconfucianism had been raised to the orthodox interpretation of Confucian doctrine. Even when influential philosophers and scholars had long since followed other traditions, the ruling circles of the Ming and Ch'ing period continued to adhere rigidly to it.

Chu Hsi's Neoconfucianism is designated "rationalistic" because he claimed that in order to investigate things, one had to approach them oneself. Li Shih-chen was probably one of the most prominent representatives to adopt this maxim for the investigation of nature. He placed himself, as we have seen, totally on the side of the official version of Confucianism.

良知 With Wang Shou-jen (1472–1528), an idealistic variant of Neoconfucianism had gained influence in the meantime. Wang believed that a given "intuitive understanding" (*liang-chih*) enabled every man to acquire a knowledge of the essence of things. Thus, one did not have to go to the things themselves to understand them, but had the capability within oneself; after all, he argued, things were only what we ourselves imagined them to be. That type of claim was bound to become an extremely fertile basis for a manifold individualism; Neoconfucianism disintegrated into numerous rival factions which were incapable of solving political and other problems.[229]

The reaction was not long in coming. Conservative forces, concerned about the welfare of the Chinese civilization, were aroused. They held Neoconfucianism and its consequences responsible for the empire's decline which had begun with the end of the Northern Sung dynasty. First the North was lost; then the entire empire became a victim of the Mongols. The subsequent Ming dynasty was indeed Chinese, but it brought with it no great reason for rejoicing—with its totalitarian form of rule, it seemed too much to resemble the preceding Mongolian period.

With the establishment of the Ch'ing dynasty, yet another triumph of northern barbarians over China occurred. Certain forces considered this sufficient proof that it was necessary to return from the heretical teachings of Neoconfucianism to the interpretations of Confucianism which had made China powerful and which, it was assumed, would be more suitable for dealing with the numerous problems than the introverted brooding of the Neoconfucians.[230] In this manner, the last crisis of Confucianism was ushered in. A solution was not found.

The opponents of Neoconfucianism, which by no means lost all of its advocates, advanced, in a nearly step-by-step dismantling, to earlier stages in time in the development of Confucianism, until they had finally returned again to Mencius and Confucius himself, placing even their concepts in question. The long journey back into the past ended, as Wolfgang Bauer emphasized, with no results; a suitable model for the solution of current and future problems was not found.[231]

The scholar Ku Yen-wu (1613–1682) was one of the first to attack publicly the "empty philosophizing of the Sung doctrine" and to hold it responsible for China's downfall. In his opinion, the officials trained under this doctrine had become incapable of assessing political realities and of preserving the country from internal and external harm. To overcome the "short-sightedness" of Neoconfucianism, especially in the version of Wang Shou-jen which resembled Ch'an Buddhism, he recommended the utilization of as many literary sources as possible. Ku Yen-wu took the view that the Han period commentaries of Confucian classics were closer to the true knowledge of antiquity than could be claimed for the initiators of the Sung doctrine. For this reason, he recommended strongly the study of Han period texts.[232]

The philosopher Yen Yüan (1635–1704) was also an advocate of looking to the past. After initial enthusiasm for the Sung teachings, he rejected all Buddhist and Taoist influences in the Confucianism of his time and carried out particularly sharp attacks on the "incessant theorization" of the Neoconfucians.[233] For him, such theorizing represented a blatant proof of Neoconfucianism's remoteness from reality.

The return to the sources of Confucianism, considered necessary by Ku Yen-wu, required that those texts containing the genuine and original doctrines and commentaries be clearly separated from imitators and falsifiers. The impulse for textual criticism, which yielded extremely valuable results, is attributed to Tai Chen (1724–1777). On the basis of their textual investigations, Tai Chen and his successors were able to expose the Sung teachings as a falsification of the original doctrine of Confucianism. To this end, numerous old classics and other texts were rescued from oblivion; others were freed from later emendations. Inevitably, these discussions were not restricted to the field of political philosophy alone, but also spread into adjoining areas, including medical thought.

Despite the appearance of a certain recognized professionalization (also recognized by the state) in the execution of medical skills, the connections between the learned Confucians and medicine had continued to be extremely close. Yen Yüan, for example, had studied medicine thoroughly and had utilized the resulting abilities in actual practice.[234]

When a reaction arose, the result was again, as had been observable during the course of Neoconfucianism, a parallel development in philosophical, political, and medical thought. It may have occurred subconsciously, but it seems plausible that something like a deliberately created symbolism was at work here. Thus, it is not surprising that in the development of pen-ts'ao literature, we very early come across the same elements that also characterized the "Han school" (Han-hsüeh) of Confucianism in other literary-philosophical fields. Demands emerged for the elimination of all Chin-Yüan "falsifications" of the works of Shen-nung and Chang Chi, and thus for all theorization. The original classic, the *Pen-ching*, was to be raised again as the guiding principle for all action.

As a result of these maxims, some authors attempted to reconstruct the *Pen-ching*. Later, some works were compiled that were supposed to correspond to the spirit of the *Pen-ching*, having been divested of as many Chin-Yüan reforms as possible. If these attempts at reconstruction only affected philological products, I could have discussed them at the beginning of this work with the *Pen-ching* itself. For the most part, however, they were written for actual medical-pharmaceutical practice; pharmacists and medical practitioners were supposed to orient themselves on these works. For this reason, it is justified to present them here as an integrated variant of the *Han-hsüeh* tradition of pen-ts'ao literature.

2. The Drug Works in the *Han-hsüeh* Tradition of Pen-ts'ao Literature

Shen-nung pen-ching (reconstruction by Lu Fu)
"Shen-nung's Original Classic"
3 chapters
Author: Lu Fu (ca. 1600)
    tzu: Pu-yüan
    from: Ch'ien-t'ang in Che-chiang
Written: 1602–1616
Published: 1624

2.1. The *Shen-nung pen-ching* (reconstruction by Lu Fu)

Lu Fu, who lived during the governmental period *wan-li* (1573–1619), initiated a series of attempts to reconstruct the Han period *Pen-ching*. He wrote the *Shen-nung pen-ching* as part of a collection of medical writings which he entitled "Seed-corns of Medicine" (*I-chung-tzu*). The work was divided into four sections: "Seed-corns from the Medical Classics" (*I-ching chung-tzu*), which included, among others, of the *Shen-nung pen-ching*, "Seed-corns of Medical Doctrine" (*I-lun chung-tzu*), "Seed-corns from Medical Prescriptions" (*I-fang chung-tzu*), and "Seed-corns from Medical Cases" (*I-an chung-tzu*).

Lu Fu's preface to the *Shen-nung pen-ching* was written in 1616. With this reconstruction, he anticipated the above-mentioned textual criticisms of Tai Chen and his successors by nearly one-and-a-half centuries in the area of pharmaceutics. For his task, Lu Fu was dependent on the white-on-black printed characters in the *Cheng-lei pen-ts'ao,* which indicated the share of the *Pen-ching* in that work. The division of his work and the arrangement of the drugs were probably made possible by the recently published *Pen-ts'ao kang mu,* in whose second chapter Li Shih-chen had included a table of contents of the *Pen-ching.* We do not know the source of this table of contents, or whether Lu Fu perhaps had access to it.

A Chinese edition of Lu Fu's work apparently no longer exists. Only two Japanese reprints dating from 1743 and 1799 are known.[235]

2.2. The *Shen-nung pen-ts'ao ching shu*

Shen-nung pen-ts'ao ching shu
"Commentary on Shen-nung's Classic of Pharmaceutics"
30 chapters / 490 drug descriptions
Author: Miu Hsi-yung (seventeenth century)
    tzu: Chung-ch'un
    hao: Mu-t'ai
    from: Ch'ang-shu in Chiang-su
Written: date unknown
Published: 1625

Miu Hsi-yung was harshly criticized for the first attempt to create a work that both revered the *Pen-ching* as a classic as well as utilized Chin-Yüan pharmacological theories to explain the activities and effects of drugs. In this manner Miu Hsi-yung created a compromise between the *Han-hsüeh* tradition and the Chin-Yüan teachings. Several later authors followed Miu Hsi-yung's example, among them Yao Ch'iu with his *Pen-ts'ao ching chieh-yao* (published under the name of the famous physician Yeh Kuei), Hsü Ta-ch'un with his *Shen-nung pen-ts'ao ching pai-chung lu* (see C, V, 2.6), Chang Chih-ts'ung with his *Pen-ts'ao ch'ung-yüan* (see C, V, 2.4), Chang Lu with his *Pen-ching feng-yüan* (see C, V, 2.5), Wu Shih-k'ai with his *Pen-ts'ao ching shu chi-yao,* Tsou Shu with his *Pen-ching shu-cheng* (see C, V, 2.8) and Chiang Kuo-i with his *Pen-ching ching-shih.*[236] These works and others like them constituted a subtradition within the *Han-hsüeh* tradition. Similar to the other works in the *Han-hsüeh* tradition, they were intended to explain the meaning of ancient pharmaceutics, but unlike the "pure" *Han-hsüeh* authors, Miu Hsi-yung and his successors did not believe they could dispense with later pharmacological insights.

Miu is described as a "Confucian scholar-physician."[237] The authors of the dynastic history of the Ming period considered him important enough to add a biography of his to that of Li Shih-chen. They emphasized the miraculous effects of many of his treatments and pointed out his special interest in elucidating the original meaning of the *Pen-ching*. Comparing the *Pen-ching* with the *I-ching*, Miu characterized the *Pen-ching* as the "classic" and later emendations as "appendixes," and he complained that the original textual differentiation by means of red and black characters had, during the course of numerous revisions and citations, become increasingly faulty. In addition, in the preface to the *Shen-nung pen-ts'ao ching shu*, Miu Hsi-yung expressed his dissatisfaction with the fact that the ancient works "had stated what is, but had not stated why it is."

For this reason, Miu set out to bring back to light the real meaning of the classic. Unlike Lu Fu, he did not intend to produce an exact reconstruction. This is shown, first of all, by the number of drugs described. Furthermore, Miu Hsi-yung devoted the first two chapters of his work to a discussion of theoretical and practical issues, which he dealt with in thirty paragraphs. While the first chapter focused on general, mostly theoretical information, the second chapter enumerated a large number of illnesses, surprisingly including demonological afflictions such as "demonic possession, possession by corpse[-spirits], and possession by flying corpse[-spirit]."

The monograph section begins with the third chapter. In the table of contents, a prefatory line points out for each section that, for instance, "of a total of seventy-three articles from the section of precious stones/minerals, now fourteen are commented upon here because they are important." Like Lu Fu, Miu Hsi-yung followed primarily the *Cheng-lei pen ts'ao*. He divided the drugs into ten sections which, with the exception of two changes, correspond to those in the *T'ang pen-ts'ao*. This fact may have prompted later criticism that Miu Hsi-yung probably mistook the *T'ang pen-ts'ao* for the *Pen-ching*.[238]

The monographs of the *Shen-nung pen-ts'ao ching-shu* begin with a quotation from the *Pen-ching* describing the particular drug, with the "Additional Notes of Renowned Medical Men" added. Then follows, under the heading, "Commentary," a discussion of the *Pen-ching* and *Pieh-lu* information in theoretical terms. For example, the "Commentary" following the quotation of the *Pen-ching/Pieh-lu* description of the drug *pa-tou* begins as follows:

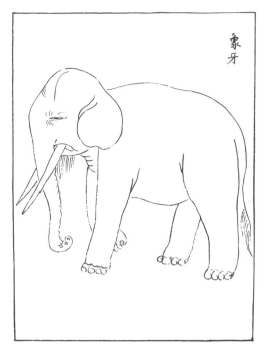

elephant tusks *(hsiang-ya)—Shao-hsing pen-ts'ao*

> *Pa-tou* grows in the season of flourishing summer and when the six *yang*[-influences are abundant]; it reaches maturity during the months of fall, [associated with the phase of] metal. As a consequence, its taste is acrid, its [thermo-]influence is warm, and it receives the influence of the wildness and ferocity of fire. As a consequence, its nature has a strongly developed medicinal effectiveness.[239]

A third section of the pa-tou monograph in the *Shen-nung pen-ts'ao ching-shu* is entitled "Main Therapeutic [Indications] and Combinations [with other Drugs]." It provides pragmatic information on formulas with pa-tou as an ingredient. The first line, for instance, reads as follows:

> [The effects of a combined use of pa-tou] with alum exceed those of pa-tou if used alone. The alum is ground to a fine [powder] which is blown into the throat. It washes out heat poison and, as a result, the throat is widened. It displays miraculous [effects] in treatments of acute throat closure.[240]

Finally, in a fourth section, Miu Hsi-yung pointed out inaccuracies and mistakes committed by previous authors in their descriptions of pa-tou.[241]

2.3. The *Pen-ts'ao ch'eng-ya pan-chieh*

Pen-ts'ao ch'eng-ya pan-chieh
"Four Beautiful Aspects of Materia Medica, Reduced by One-Half"
10 chapters/ 365 drug descriptions
Author: Lu Chih-i (seventeenth century)
    tzu: Yu-sheng
    hao: Chin-kung
    from: Ch'ien-t'ang in Che-chiang
Written: ca. 1625–1647
Published: ca. 1647

With this work, Lu Chih-i, a son of Lu Fu, tried a third method of revealing again the original sense of the *Pen-ching*. He himself declared: "The 365 drugs of the *Shen-nung pen-ching* corresponded to the number of days [in a solar year]. For this reason it is not permissible to reduce or increase [this number]. However, some drugs were used in antiquity that no longer exist."[242]

As a result of this insight, Lu Chih-i used only two-thirds of the drugs in the *Pen-ching*, (i.e., 222) for his own work. The remaining 143 monographs were compiled from drugs that appeared only in later works, beginning with the *Ming-i pieh-lu* and extending to the *Pen-ts'ao kang mu*.

Lu Chih-i had divided each drug description, in an original manuscript, into four sections, with the subtitles "Investigation," "Combination," "Interpretation," and "Decision." In an allusion to "a team of four horses" (*ch'eng*), he thus entitled his work "Four Beautiful Aspects of Pharmaceutics." During the political disorder at the end of the Ming dynasty, when roving troops burned and pillaged, Lu Chih-i's original manuscript was lost. The author compiled a new copy from memory; however, he was no longer able to achieve the completeness of the original. He therefore divided the monographs in the new version into only two sections—"Investigation" and "Combination," expanding the title of the work with the addition *pan-chieh* ("reduced by half").[243]

The first edition of the *Pen-ts'ao ch'eng-ya pan-chieh* is dated twice. The introduction carries a date from the year 1628; the preface was composed in 1647. Both were written by Lu Chih-i.

2.4. The *Pen-ts'ao ch'ung-yüan*

Pen-ts'ao ch'ung-yüan
"Reverence for the Origin of the Materia Medica"
3 chapters / 290 drugs
Author: Chang Chih-ts'ung (ca. 1650);
    tzu: Yin-an;
    from: Ch'ien-t'ang in Che-ch'iang
    Kao Shih-shih (seventeenth century);
    tzu: Shih-tsung;
    from: Ch'ien-t'ang in Che-chiang
Written: ca. 1662–1663
Published: 1767

Chang Chih-ts'ung considered himself to be a descendent of the famous Han period author Chang Chi. He was one of the best-known medical writers of the Ch'ing period, and he carried on the tradition of Lu Fu and his son. He founded the "Meeting Hall in the Mountains," in which for almost forty years he discussed textual investigations of the old medical classics with sympathetic minds. During the course of time he composed, among other works, commentaries to the *Su-wen, Ling-shu, Shang-han lun, Chin-kuei yao-lüeh,* as well as to the *Pen-ching.*

Chang Chih-ts'ung advocated absolute observance of the rules and regulations of all these old classics; undoubtedly he can be classified with the *Han-hsüeh* movement in medicine. Nevertheless, his *Pen-ts'ao ch'ung-yüan* stands out in a certain way from most other works in this tradition, since his commentaries express admiration for the *Su-wen* and the theories it contained on the Five Phases, as well as the five seasonal phases and six climatic influences (*wu yün liu ch'i*). He advocated very clearly, evident in the following excerpt from his preface to the *Pen-ts'ao ch'ung-yüan,* the necessity for drug use to be founded upon theory. However, the corresponding old classics, not the misleading later writings, were supposed to form the basis for theory and practice. To support his argument, Chang Chih-ts'ung quoted even a central slogan of Neoconfucianism, that is *ke-wu chih-chih* ("Expand knowledge through investigations of things"); he may 格物致知 have felt motivated to bridge the obviously widening gap between the Chin-Yüan principles of theoretically founded drug application on the one hand and the *Han-hsüeh* movement back to the real sources on the other hand:

The *Pen-ts'ao* of Shen-nung carries the designation "Original Classic." It contained 365 drug descriptions, corresponding exactly to the number of days in a solar year. One hundred twenty-five drugs constitute the ruler [drugs] of the upper class. They have no distinct medicinal effectiveness and exhibit their properties only after lengthy, continuous administration. They contribute to maintaining human existence and increasing life-expectancy. They benefit the influences and liberate the body from its material weight. [Whoever takes these drugs] is spared from old age, like the spirits and immortal ones. One hundred twenty drugs constitute the minister [drugs] of the middle class. Some possess a distinct medicinal effectiveness; others do not. Their main effect is the ability to penetrate the blood and the influences and bring them into harmony, to expel evil [influences] from the body, and to cure illnesses. The lower class is comprised of 120 assistant and aide [drugs]. Some [of the drugs in this group] are medicinally effective, others are not; some are extremely potent. They are especially suitable for expelling evil influences of a cold and hot nature and for destroying obstructions and constipations of all kinds. If they encounter an illness, it comes to a halt.

With the creation of heaven and earth began also the growth of herbs and trees. Emperor [Shen-]nung looked up to the six [climatic] influences in the heavens and observed the earth's Five Phases of Change. The six [climatic] influences are characterized by the three *yin* and the three *yang* [categories]: ceasing-*yin,* small-*yin, yin,* small-*yang, yang*-brilliance, and great-*yang.* As to the Five Phases of Change: the *shen-chi* [phase] moves the earth; the *i-keng* [phase] moves the metal; the *ping-hsin* [phase] moves the water; the *ting-jen* [phase] moves the wood; and the *wu-kuei* [phase] moves the fire. These five phases of [seasonal] movement constitute the Five Phases of Change. The characteristics of herbs, trees, metals, minerals, worms, fish, fowl, and quadrupeds can be differentiated on the basis of the theories of the five [seasonal] phases of movement and the six [climatic] influences; the treatments with cold

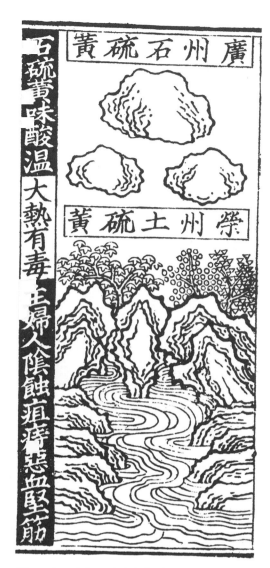

"Stone" sulphur (*shih-liu-huang:* top) and "earth" sulphur (*t'u-liu-huang:* bottom)— *Ch'ung-hsiu cheng-ho pen-ts'ao*

and hot drugs, drugs that rise or descend [in the body], and drugs that replenish depletions and drain repletions are connected with the body's five depots and six palaces, as well as with the twelve conduits in the human body. All things in heaven and on earth are covered by the Five Phases of Change. This is where they are brought forth first: in one of the five directions—east, west, south, north, and center; and this is when they are raised: in one of the five seasons—spring, summer, mid-summer, fall, and winter. The appearance of all things is composed of the five colors: green, yellow, red, white, and black. The influences are constituted by the five odors: penetrating, burnt, aromatic, strong, and putrid. In the substance [of all things] are found the five tastes: sour, bitter, sweet, acrid, and salty. All of these [characteristics] together form the nature of drugs. [In ancient times] one decided about the conduct of one's affairs through divination, and [pertinent texts] have been handed down to later times. Their language is old and their meaning is profound. It is difficult to read and fathom them. In later centuries, those who wrote treatises on the properties of drugs did not understand the *Pen-ching*. They spoke of specific drugs that cured specific illnesses and of specific illnesses that required specific drugs. They did not investigate the source [of affliction] but discussed only the treatment. That is [a concern with] drug usage but not [with] drug properties! If one understands these properties and applies [the drugs] in accordance with them, then this application has a basis and there is no obstacle to achieve miraculous changes. If, in administering drugs, one follows only examples of previous use, the [necessary theoretical] foundation is lacking; there will be barriers [on one's way toward success], which are difficult to overcome.

For this reason I have commented upon the *Pen-ching* and explained the properties of drugs. I have composed very detailed commentaries on the basis of the theories of the five [seasonal] phases of movement and the six climatic influences, so that the words of antiquity lie, as it were, before our eyes and the theory of [seasonal] movements and [climatic] influences can be recognized just as clearly as the sun and the stars. This is the way to expand knowledge through an investigation of things, and to unite the three powers [of heaven, earth, and man] into one.[244]

Chang Chih-ts'ung died before he could complete the *Pen-ts'ao ch'ung-yüan*. Among his students was a man named Kao Shih-shih. He came from a destitute family. He is said to have been interested in medicine already in his youth and to have read all accessible, popular works in which the medicinal concepts of his time were expressed. When he was twenty-three, Kao Shih-shih left his family to practice medicine, and he achieved a certain reputation. Later, he himself fell ill, and all attempts at treatment with the usual medicine of the time only worsened the affliction. Finally, after a long period of time, he regained his health without any medications. Ashamed, he wrote: "I have also treated my patients in such a manner; does that not mean 'dealing with human life as with a blade of grass'?"[245]

From that point on, Kao Shih-shih followed the school of Chang Chih-ts'ung. After the latter's death, he continued the work on the manuscript of the *Pen-ts'ao ch'ung-yüan* until it was ready for publication. He, too, died prematurely.

The position on medical theory held by Kao Shih-shih and his teacher—valuing the origin of theory but not later additions—is expressed in a statement attributed to Kao:

To a certain extent, medical principles resemble a banana that has to
be peeled. One peels until there is nothing left to peel—only then has
one advanced to the real principle. . . . In antiquity it was said "Whoever
does not understand the course of the conduits and their ramifications
will make mistakes as soon as he opens his mouth or raises his hand."
Whoever does not understand [the theories] of the five seasonal phases
and six [climatic] influences can read the entire literature on prescriptions and still will not benefit from it![246]

After Kao's death the manuscript of the *Pen-ts'ao ch'ung-yüan* came
into the possession of the family of a man named Hu Nien-an, whose
student, Kao Tuan-shih, received a copy of it, and who in turn passed
it on to Wang Ch'i (eighteenth century). In 1767 Wang Ch'i, finally,
published the *Pen-ts'ao ch'ung-yüan*—which had been revised in the
meantime and no longer corresponded exactly to the original work
of Chang Chih-ts'ung and Kao Shih-shih—in his medical collection,
I-lin chih-yüeh.[247]

醫林指月

2.5. The *Pen-ching feng-yüan*

Like all authors of the *Han-hsüeh* tradition of pen-ts'ao literature,
Chang Lu was an active Confucian. Especially in the areas of medicine
and pharmaceutics, he carried out years of study and compared all
opinions from the beginnings of the literature with those of his own
time.[248] During the disorder near the end of the Ming dynasty, Chang
Lu withdrew to the seclusion of a mountain for more than ten years
and was occupied only with the writing of books for the remainder
of his long life.

In the preface to his *Pen-ching feng-yüan*, Chang Lu explains the
position of the *Han-hsüeh* tradition in the total development of pen-
ts'ao literature. He despised the Chin-Yüan authors, who in his words
created "insignificant products which are certainly not worth discussing," but at the same time, he expressed his conviction that the
ancient theoretical classics are indispensable for therapeutic practice:

> The *Pen-ching* has the same importance for medical practitioners as
> does the marking-line for artisans. Once there is a marking-line, there
> are compass and square, and if there are compass and square, one may
> fall in with them. This falling in with [compass and square] produces
> skill, which then, in the last analysis, is grounded in the marking-line.
> Originally, the *Pen-ching* of Yen-ti represented the creation of a marking-
> line [for medicine]. The [*Ching-shih*] *cheng-lei ta-kuan* [*pen-ts'ao*] brought
> about compass and square. When the [*Pen-ts'ao*] *kang mu* was created,
> its collection [of information] constituted a magnificent creation, and
> yet it did not reach [the point of] falling in with [the compass and square
> as laid out by the *Ta-kuan pen-ts'ao*]. This can be compared with the
> fact that even great artisans are only capable of giving compass and
> square to men but not, however, their skills. Only the *Ling[-shu]* and
> the *Su[-wen]* of Huang-ti were able to give skills to men and allowed
> them to reach the path of falling in with [the compass and square]. And
> only one man, who [lived in] Ch'ang-sha during the Han period,[249] was
> capable of adopting, according to circumstances, the way of Yen[-ti]
> and Huang[-ti] without clinging to it like to a marking-line. The [man
> from] Ch'ang-sha was allowed by heaven to take over the way of

Pen-ching feng-yüan
"Elucidation of the Actual Meaning of the
Original Classic"
4 chapters / 831 drug descriptions
Author: Chang Lu (1627–?)
    tzu: Lu-yü
    hao: Shih-wan
    from: Wu-chiang in Chiang-su
Written: ?–1705
Published: 1715

Yen[-ti] and Huang[-ti] in a direct line. He could have complete faith in any movement of his hand; in each case it corresponded to the marking-line. I have not yet heard that a marking-line exists, except for the one [handed down] by Yen and Huang. I have often thought that in medicine there have always been famous men who have sought the origins and true source [of medicine]. The *Yü-han chin-kuei* [*yao-lüeh*] followed the information of the *Pen-ching* on the main effects [of drugs]. Beyond that, however, I cannot name another work. In the T'ang period, after [the man from] Ch'ang-sha, only the scholar living in seclusion [who wrote the] *Ch'ien-chin fang* comprehended the essential elements [of this tradition].[250] The boldness of his prescriptions surpassed even that of [the man from] Ch'ang-sha. In later times, people were no longer able to follow [these two men]: the authors of *pen-ts'ao* [works] disregarded the ancient methods of drug use according to what is in contrast and what is in accordance, what is opposed and what may stimulate. They were only concerned to conform, in a comfortable manner, to contemporary conditions. Only insignificant products, certainly not worthy of discussion, were created during this era. Even P'in-hu, who really did possess a comprehensive knowledge of old and new, pushed aside the fundamentals in the last analysis and preferred what was inessential. He emphasized the main effects [of drugs] listed in the *Pen-ching* [merely] to show that he wanted to preserve material not yet totally lost. Only Master Miu Chung-ch'un was able to penetrate the meaning of the classic. He brought forth all kinds of prescriptions which had been scattered and, in the case of difficult passages, cited additional information from the *Pieh-lu* and other works, thus creating classic statements. Now, who would not be bothered by the confusion of red and purple? In former times, Master Ch'iao San-yü wrote the one-volume *Pen-ching chu-shu*. I saw [the manuscript] thirty-five years ago in the library of Nien-o. Unfortunately, it was not published and can no longer be examined. Therefore, I have not concerned myself with the obsolete and superficial nature of my own views and have defined and commented upon the profound meaning of the *Pen-ching*. I have added the medical treatments published by various authors so that the student could reach the sources in every respect, without overstepping the marking-line of Yen and Huang. That should enable them to become great artisans. Yet even the most skillful artisan completely controls only six of ten cases [that he takes up]; even he lacks the skills of bringing a pale skeleton back to life. It is my wish that all medical practitioners of the world should act with caution and not rely frivolously on their abilities, in the hopes of achieving a short-term advantage. I would like to call people's attention to the rule that the outcome of an untreated illness is usually similar to the results achieved by mediocre physicians and [urge them] to overcome the circle of contemporary teachers. How could an [unjustified] limitation of the marking-line [then continue]?

Written in the year *i-yü* of the *k'ang-hsi* period (1705) during the first month of spring by Chang Lu, [with *hao*] Shih-wan in the Chün-yung Hall, at the age of seventy-nine.[251]

It was not Chang Lu's intention to allow the *Pen-ching* to rise again. He adopted 831 drugs from the *Pen-ts'ao kang mu* and described them in a rather pragmatical manner, without many theoretical embellishments, in the same arrangement as Li Shih-chen. The monograph of the drug *pa-tou* may again serve as a comparison with earlier drug descriptions:

Pa-tou [taste:] acrid, [thermo-influence:] hot; strongly pronounced medicinal effectiveness. [For medicinal use] the seed coat and heart [of the raw drug] should be removed and [the remaining portion] roasted

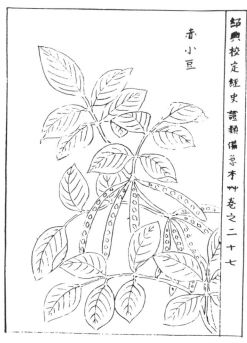

small red beans *(ch'ih-hsiao-tou)—Shao-hsing pen-ts'ao*

to a violet-black color; or [the drug] is burned with the retention of its nature, or one grinds it to a paste, wraps it in paper, presses the oil out, and uses the remaining material. In each case, the respective prescription is to be followed.

Pen-ching: [The drug *pa-tou*] masters harms caused by cold, moisture, malaria fevers, fits of cold and heat; breaks up bowel obstructions of different kinds, hardenings, stagnation of drinking liquids, mucous congestions, enlarged abdomen; cleanses the body's five depots and palaces; opens and penetrates obstructions; it clears the way for water and grains, removes spoiled meat, expels poisonings caused by demons, possessions by the *ku* and [other] evil things; kills worms and fish.

Explanation: *Pa-tou* possesses acrid [taste] and hot [thermo-influence]. [The drug] is capable of cleansing the body's five depots and six palaces. It penetrates not only indurations in the abdomen produced by various types of obstructions but can also be used for the treatment of afflictions caused by cold and malaria fevers occasioned by moisture that are connected with cold and hot fits. When, for example, [Chang] Chung-ching used the White Powder for the treatment of concentrations of cold in the upper abdomen, he understood fully the instructions of the *Pen-ching.* All editions [of the *Pen-ching*] say at this point "malaria fevers caused by warmth." That is, however, a misprint and should read "fevers caused by moisture." The effective properties of this [drug] can be quite harsh but can also offer milder benefits. [*Pa-tou*] has the power to break through [solidified] blood, drive out pus, attack mucus, and expel water. The amount used varies according to [the seriousness of] the symptoms. In a fresh state, [the drug] works abruptly and aggressively. In a prepared state, it develops a milder effect. The use of the material remaining after the oil has been pressed [has the effect of] pushing out the old and bringing in the new. The application must depend on the development of the symptoms. In treatments that return rectitude [in the organism], heroic usage has the effect of stabbing any disorder and destroying any illness. Even the use of small amounts shows admirable effects of soothing and harmonizing one's center. [The effect of the drug] is capable of penetrating the intestines and stopping diarrhea. In this are expressed the secrets of the oldest times. An old lady had already suffered from violent diarrhea for a long time. For her treatment she always took drugs that balanced the spleen, developed a rising effect in the body, and could stop and draw together. But the diarrhea worsened as a result of such treatment. The [movement in her] vessels became shallower and weaker. Chronic damage occurred in her spleen and stomach as a result of the accumulation of cold and obstructions. Here it was necessary to draw off [the accumulations of cold with drugs] of a hot [thermo-influence]. [After such treatment was carried out] the cold was removed and the diarrhea ended. Subsequently, cures could be achieved in numerous cases by the use [of *pa-tou*] for the treatment of diarrhea and for obstructions. It is important to understand the suitable manner of [*pa-tou*] use; otherwise, the *yin*[-influences] may be damaged. *Pa-tou* and *ta-huang* both serve as laxatives. [The difference is that] *ta-huang* possesses cold nature and is especially suitable for use against illnesses of the body's depots caused by too much heat. *Pa-tou,* conversely, possesses hot nature and is especially suited for illnesses of the body's depots caused by too much cold. If the shell of the drug is burned to ashes, maintaining its properties, it develops the power to end diarrhea and expel illnesses. Pregnant women should avoid the use [of *pa-tou*], since the power [of the drug] can trigger a miscarriage. [Chang] Yüan-su says: "*Pa-tou* resembles a general who breaks through barriers and opens gates. One must not use [this drug] carelessly. For a long time [*pa-tou*] has been used to treat alcohol afflictions and influences [pressing against the] diaphragm. With its acrid [taste] and hot [nature, this drug] is capable of opening and penetrating press-

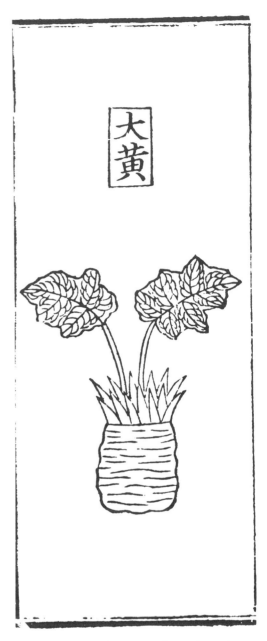

rhubarb root *(ta-huang)*—*Ch'ung-hsiu cheng-ho pen-ts'ao*

ing heat in the bowels and stomach. But while these pressing accumulations are penetrated, the blood and the fluids are lost as a
consequence. The yin-[influences] are damaged." The use [of pa-tou]
against afflictions caused by cold, against concentrations [of such evil
influences] in the upper abdomen, and against the afflictions in small
children produced by incorrect nutrition does not have to result in death
but is, nevertheless, dangerous. Why do the common people fear ta-
huang but not pa-tou? Because its nature is hot and because it is taken
in small doses only. If one undertakes the experiment of lightly rubbing
only a small amount [of the drug] on the skin, it will be completely
covered with blisters after a short time. When, however, the drug is
taken internally, is it not certain that the stomach and intestines will
suffer from burning and destruction [under the influence of this drug]?
If urgent symptoms cannot be eliminated otherwise, and one [has no
other choice but to] use it, the oil [of the raw drug] should be removed
by pressing it out, and a small portion from the remaining pulp should
be used for the medication. That is possible.[252]

Despite his detailed study of, if perhaps not the drug pa-tou itself,
at least the relevant older literature, Chang Lu made a statement here,
which I should like to look at more closely, since it may throw a
characteristic light on the research approach of this kind of author.

Right at the beginning of his pa-tou monograph Chang Lu writes:
"[For medicinal use] the seed coat [lit.: shell] and the seed [lit.: heart]
去殼及心 [of the raw drug] should be removed (ch'ü k'o chi hsin)." If this
directive were followed, not much would remain. The pa-tou seed
consists of a hard brown seed shell, a silvery-white membranelike
perisperm, and a neutral to yellow, oily endosperm.

The oldest pa-tou monograph containing such instructions was in
the Pen-ts'ao ching chi-chu by T'ao Hung-ching. The "Additional
Notes of Renowned Medical Men" (Ming-i pieh-lu), quoted here,
contained the following statement: "The seed coat [lit.: heart-peel] [of
the raw drug] must be removed for use (ch'ü hsin-p'i)." In his own
commentary, T'ao had taken over this same formulation when he
去心皮 wrote: "The seed coat should always be removed (ch'ü hsin-p'i)."

During the T'ang period, in place of the character p'i the author
of the Jih-hua tzu pen-ts'ao used the character mo, which is closer in
meaning to a skin or membrane. He wrote: "For [medicinal] usage . . .
去心膜 it is advantageous to remove the seed skin [lit.: heart-skin] (ch'ü hsin-
mo)." The expression hsin-mo may have meant either the same thing
as the older concept hsin-p'i, namely, the solid layer that surrounds
the pa-tou seed, that is, the brown seed shell, or it may have been used
to designate the membranelike perisperm. The latter alternative would
imply that the author took the removal of the outer shell for granted,
which is unlikely.

In the T'ang-yeh pen-ts'ao of Wang Hao-ku, dating from the thirteenth century, a new variant appeared as an ostensible citation from
Lei-kung. Hao-ku's formulation reads as follows: "In this case [the
drug] can be used in its fresh state following removal of the [seed]
去皮心膜 peel, seed skin (ch'ü p'i hsin-mo), and oil." It is not totally clear
whether the author joined these concepts together with the intention
of expressing the sense reproduced here in the translation—that is,
removal of the seed shell and of the membranelike perisperm—or

whether out of ignorance he meant to combine somehow the concepts *hsin-p'i* and *hsin-mo.*

In the sixteenth century, Li Shih-chen correctly cited the specific information of the *Ming-i pieh-lu* as *ch'ü hsin-p'i;* in the corresponding quotation of T'ao Hung-ching's commentary, however, a typographical or orthographical mistake perhaps crept in, for *ch'ü p'i hsin* is used with the literal meaning "remove peel and heart," which Li Shih-chen probably did not intend. In his own commentary, Li refrained, on the one hand, from referring to parts of the raw drug that should be rejected and instead expressed the problem in a positive manner with new terms: "[From the raw drug] *pa-tou,* the seed (*jen*), the seed coat (*k'o*), and the oil are used medicinally."

去 心 皮

去 皮 心

仁
殼

On the other hand, in the rubric "Thermo-influence and Taste," Li Shih-chen, surprisingly, states: "If one does not remove the seed skin (*mo*) [of the drug], it is harmful to the stomach. If the heart (*hsin*) is not removed, [the drug] induces vomiting."

Chang Lu, who had access to all these various expressions in his sources, may well not have completely grasped the development, and arrived, consequently, at the above-mentioned formulation *ch'ü k'o chi hsin.* Possibly, he believed that the character for *and* (*chi*) had been confused with the very similar character for *peel*—in one of his older sources.

及

Difficulties and misunderstandings of this kind are, of course, unavoidable when natural science is not carried out in nature itself but largely on the basis of literary evidence. This contributes substantially to the difficulties of a correct interpretation of the texts under consideration.

The first edition of the *Pen-ching feng-yüan* was brought to Japan, where a reprint was prepared in 1802. Copies of this Japanese edition, in turn, reached China and constituted the basis there for later editions.[253]

2.6. The *Shen-nung pen-ts'ao ching pai-chung lu*

One of the most striking personalities among the authors of the *Han-hsüeh* tradition was Hsü Ta-ch'un. His family was already known for generations because of its comprehensive education, and Hsü Ta-ch'un proved himself worthy of this reputation. Besides medicine, his interests included astrology, music, geography, and philosophy. He composed commentaries to Taoist classics, wrote a work on the regulation of rivers, and, above all, published numerous medical texts. His reputation as a physician reached the capital; he twice accepted invitations to Peking. However, he turned down an offer from the Imperial Medical Office.[254]

Shen-nung pen-ts'ao ching pai-chung lu
"One Hundred Drugs from Shen-nung's Classic of Pharmaceutics"
1 chapter / 100 drug descriptions
Author: Hsü Ta-ch'un (1693–1771)
    tzu: Ling-t'ai
    hao: Hui-hsi lao-jen
    from: Wu-chiang in Chiang-su
Written: ?–1736
Published: between 1736 and 1795

One of Hsü Ta-ch'un's works, "Treatises on the Origin and History of Medicine" *(I-hsüeh yüan-liu lun),* which interprets the development of Chinese medicine from the author's point of view, is very revealing of his position on the numerous medical currents that had arisen during the Ch'ing period. In the following "Treatise on the Old and Recent *Pen-ts'ao* [Works]," taken from this work, there are several sentences criticizing the post-Han changes in pharmaceutics and the demands raised during the Chin-Yüan period:

> [The tradition] of *pen-ts'ao* [drug works] begins with Shen-nung. [The number of] drugs [listed in his work] was limited to 360. [This shows] that the exemplary men [from the time] of the creation of the world acted in unity with heaven and earth. They were actually able to grasp the sense of the creation and fathom the principles of all things. Every single character [they wrote] was ingenious and true. Here lies a great difference to that knowledge deducted [hypothetically] by men of later times. When [exemplary men] treated symptoms of illness [in earlier times, symptoms and treatment] corresponded [like shout and] echo. All drugs in the prescriptions of [Chang] Chung-ching come from this [old] book [of Shen-nung]. The number of drugs in that work was limited, but they are capable of achieving miraculous transformations. Already at that time there were no longer any incurable illnesses. Later, the number of drugs increased daily until it had doubled by the time of T'ao Hung-ching to 720 specimens. Subsequently, new drugs were continually incorporated into the repertory of drugs. Exotic drugs and peculiar things, both from China itself and from foreign areas, which had shown their effectiveness in experiments, were adapted and utilized by medical practitioners. Each generation created [new] books. Finally, during the Ming period, Li Shih-chen expanded the *Cheng-lei pen-ts'ao* of T'ang Shen-wei and created the *[Pen-ts'ao] kang mu*. He analyzed differences and similarities; he distinguished genuine and false drugs and traced their origin. He gathered the opinions of all [earlier] authors, so that the *Pen-ts'ao* became even more complete. This is the reason for the increase in the number of drugs.

> Investigations of the effectiveness [of drugs] were also carried out later, and pertinent knowledge was accumulated. For this reason, the number of treated illnesses naturally expanded. However, by no means did all [these advances] match the genuine and true [knowledge] expressed in the *Pen-ts'ao* of Shen-nung. This is the reason why it was said during the Sung period: "When the drugs of Shen-nung are used, every treatment is successful; the drugs adapted by [T'ao] Hung-ching, however, are no longer particularly effective, and those drugs added in still later times are not at all trustworthy."

> In later centuries, interest in the commentaries [added to the drugs] was usually restricted to those drugs in old prescriptions which had been used to cure specific illnesses. Further comments were added. In some cases, this or that individual drug, erroneously claimed to be appropriate for the cure of a specific illness, was extracted from old prescriptions containing several drugs that had served as a cure for the same illness. Moreover [there were people] who deduced their knowledge from their own opinions. But it was also the case that someone cured an illness accidentally, a success that in reality had no connection with the drugs [used]. Although the [supposed] effectiveness [of the drug in question] was then emphasized in numerous words, such accounts are not to be trusted.

> Finally, Chang Chieh-ku and Li Tung-yüan [maintained] that certain drugs penetrate certain conduits. Now that is really far-fetched! Indeed, it is not at all necessary in the treatment of illnesses to make any sort of distinction among various conduits, depots, or palaces.

> Thus, when *pen-ts'ao* drug knowledge is discussed [the work of] Shen-nung must be used as a foundation. Other statements can be followed only after thorough examination. First of all, they should be tested clinically before being relied upon. In addition, one should investigate which drugs were already used in the prescriptions of antiquity. These [drugs] can be utilized [in prescriptions]. The [drugs introduced later]

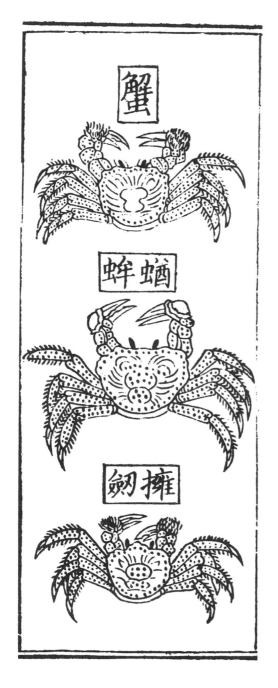

crabs (*hsieh*: top; *hsiu-mou*: middle; *yung-chien*: bottom)—*Ch'ung-hsiu cheng-ho pen-ts'ao*

are only suitable for application as individual drugs or for external use. There are, furthermore, strange drugs that were added [to the drug repertory] by people from later times. These drugs can come from the high mountains or deep valleys, from foreign countries or exotic areas. In earlier times, they had not yet been available. Only later were they adopted for use, and astonishing results were often achieved with them. [The discovery] of such [drugs] rests on the concurrence of one-sided geographical and extraordinary climatic conditions. Thus, the secrets of creation become more apparent with the passage of time. If [these strange drugs] are able to cure strange illnesses which the old prescriptions are not able to cure, the nobleman, with a comprehensive education in matters of nature, should also know them. These are [data] that lie outside [Shen-nung's] *Pen-ts'ao*.[255]

Hsü Ta-ch'un criticized the neglect of prescriptions found in the old works, thus contradicting, above all, Chang Yüan-su, who had expressed the view that each era required its own prescriptions. Hsü rejected the statements on guiding drugs and the theory concerning the penetration of specific conduits by drugs, thus clearly taking a stand against a doctrine from the Chin-Yüan period.

Nevertheless, he cannot be viewed as a dogmatic pragmatist who rejected theorization in its totality. Some elements from the Chin-Yüan influences on drug knowledge also found their way into his work.

For the *Shen-nung pen-ts'ao ching pai-chung lu* Hsü Ta-ch'un selected, from the ones described in the *Pen-ching*, 100 drugs that he believed were of special importance for the use of the two prescription works *Chin-kuei yao-lüeh* and *Shang-han lun*—both works, of course, by Chang Chi. In this selection he gave preference to drugs that had originally been classified in the "upper class" (63 specimens); drugs of the "middle" and "lower" classes, with 25 and 12 specimens, have been strikingly neglected in quantitative terms.

In each case, Hsü took over the original monograph of the *Pen-ching*, interspersing it with his own brief commentaries. He frequently appended another, detailed commentary to the monograph, because he was not content with—as the *Ssu-k'u ch'üan-shu* stated—the fact that the older commentaries had only described "that what is but not why it is."[256] Above all, Hsü Ta-ch'un discussed the main effects of the drugs and explained them with some theoretical indications, limited, however, to the Five Phases of Change and the yinyang theories. The monograph of the drug *tan-sha* (cinnabar) may serve as an example; the portions taken over from the *Pen-ching* are underlined:

Tan-sha; taste: sweet; [thermo-influence:] weak-cold.
"Sweet" indicates the taste, "cold" the nature. However, why are not color and odor also given? If [a drug] reaches the mouth, one can recognize its taste; if it reaches the stomach, one can feel its nature. Information on color and odor [of drugs] can be taken from the following statements about the main indications.

Masters the hundred illnesses in the body and five depots.
"The hundred illnesses" means here that [this drug] can be used against all illnesses, without any contraindications requiring consideration. By no means is it meant that [*tan-sha*] can heal all illnesses in the world. This is true for all drugs restoring harmony.

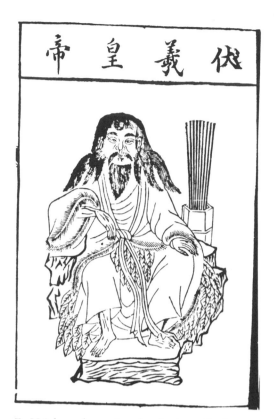

Fu Hsi, legendary ruler of antiquity—*T'u-hsiang pen-ts'ao meng-ch'üan*

Nourishes the spirit.
All substances that are accumulations of essential influences are appropriate to nourish the spirit. Man is equivalent to heaven and earth. Thus, because of corresponding similarities, the essential influences are of mutual benefit.

Pacifies the *hun* and *p'o* souls.
Deep red enters the heart and suppresses anxieties.

Supplements the influences.
If the influences sink, they are stored; storage means supplementation.

Clarifies the eyes.
All mineral drugs are able to clarify the eyes. Minerals are coagulations of the influences of metal. The fact that eyes are able to perceive things is also an achievement of the influences of metal. Furthermore, the essential [influences] of all the five depots flow upward toward the eyes. The size of the eyes as well as the corners of the eyes are associated with the heart. *Tan-sha* supplements the essential [influences] of the heart in the eyes.

Kills spiritual goblins; evil and malevolent demons.
Deep-red is the color of pure *yang* from heaven and earth, and it is therefore suitable for eliminating *yin*-evil.

After lengthy administration, one penetrates spirit-clarity, and one does not age. [The substance] is capable of being transformed into quicksilver.
Minerals are considered metals; quicksilver also contains the essence of metals. All drugs of the upper class receive, during the creation of their substance, the essential [influences] of the Five Phases of Change of heaven and earth. The body of man does not stand outside of *yin* and *yang* and of the Five Phases of Change. The essential influences [of all these categories] should be used in order to strengthen the true and original [influences of the body]. As a result, one's spiritual powers have transcending capabilities and one's appearance and substance remain firm. However, the nature of all items is one-sided. Too much and not enough of any thing may—contrary [to their beneficial potential]—cause harm. If one does not penetrate the mysteries of the creation, he will inevitably perish after one single test [of these drugs].

Thus, one follows here the color and substance [of the drug] in order to understand its effects. *Tan-sha* is genuine deep-red—the color of pure *yang*. The heart belongs to fire, whose color is also deep-red. For this reason [*tan-sha*] is capable of penetrating the heart and regulating the symptoms of illness in the corresponding conduits. With respect to its substance [*tan-sha*] is heavy. Therefore, [this drug] possesses the additional capability of suppressing influences and blood. Thus, when drugs are used, they should be selected according to odor, taste, color, appearance, nature, time of genesis, or place of origin, since all these one-sidedly manifest [variables] can be utilized in curing illnesses. Thus, one is able to fill up one-sided [conditions of the opposite nature] and to save from exhaustion, as well as to regulate and harmonize the body's depots and palaces. Whoever searches for the underlying principles will be able to understand [the meaning of this] himself.[257]

Elsewhere Hsü Ta-ch'un wrote very critical remarks concerning the possibility, advanced by practicing Taoists, of achieving a long, if not eternal, life by the use of certain drugs obtained through chemical processes. In a commentary on the monograph of the drug "quicksilver," which had already been ascribed such capabilities in the *Pen-ching*, Hsü Ta-ch'un gave free reign to his displeasure:

Quicksilver represents the essence of the five metals. It has received the essential influences of the five metals, but not their [actual metallic] substance. Through melting processes quicksilver can be transformed into such items as gold and silver. The [capabilities of quicksilver to] cure all skin afflictions, which should be considered a poisoning by [an unbalanced, preponderant influence of] heat, can be explained by the fact that the lung, which is also determinate for the skin and hair, is associated with the metal. Their influences affect each other.

In the oven and melting pot art of cinnabar experts, quicksilver and lead are considered dragon and tiger. [Alchemists] melt the two substances together and prepare an elixir from them. The administration of this substance [so they claim] can produce a long life. A lengthy administration is even supposed to enable [the consumer in question] to fly up into the air and become a feathered being. Since the [*Chou-i ts'an-t'ung-ch'i* ["Ideas of Taoist Self-Care Which Are in Agreement with the Book of Changes"] was written,[258] numerous such statements are found [in subsequent works]. Wise scholars have not refuted only one of them as false.

Quicksilver represents the essence of the five metals, but has, however, not yet received the body of metal. All metals fear fire, but quicksilver retains its original [quality], even after one hundred meltings. This is due to the fact that it has not yet achieved the substance of metals and contains the essence of water. Therefore, fire cannot harm [quicksilver]. That [quicksilver supposedly] can be transformed into yellow or white substances has its origin in the drugs that are added to the melting process. They change the external appearance [of quicksilver]; under no circumstances can gold or silver really be produced.

Since the composition [of quicksilver] is so constant, some people today would like to use the influences [of this substance] to strengthen their own appearance and body. However, there is virtually no link [between this drug and the desired effects], for man and the multiplicity of things have fundamentally different bodies. It makes sense to take advantage of the influences of things for attacking the six evils. But it makes no sense to take advantage of the substance of things in order to achieve eternal life. The proponents of such skills always claim to act intelligently; they speak of heaven and they speak of changes, and it almost appears as though they have something worth listening to. In reality, however, Fu Hsi sketched the oracle symbols, and a series of wise men wrote down the explanations of them. But where are the words "long life" [in these texts]? These are false claims, caused by ignorance and limited knowledge. It is fraudulently reported of some people, who have long since died, that they still exist. But when someone attempts this art, he ruins his family and destroys his body. If he has not yet died, he will not come to his senses; but whoever dies, of course, knows nothing about it.

[Such] blind men followed one another in close succession through all times. Their thoughts were filled with fear of death and a yearning for life, but they acted contrary to the mean, and thus only invited death, the opposite [of their goal], more rapidly. What a great pity![259]

2.7. The *Shen-nung pen-ts'ao ching* (reconstruction by Sun Hsing-yen)

Following Lu Fu, Sun Hsing-yen and his nephew, Sun P'ing-i, made the second attempt to reconstruct the Han period *Pen-ching* in its original form.

Sun Hsing-yen was a prestigious scholar. In 1786, he successfully completed the province exams and was awarded the rank of *chü-jen;*

Shen-nung pen-ts'ao ching (reconstruction by Sun Hsing-yen)
"Shen-nung's Classic of Pharmaceutics"
3 chapters / 360 drugs
Authors: Sun Hsing-yen (1753–1818);
    tzu: Yüan-ju, Po-yüan;
    hao: Chi-ch'iu, Wei-yin;
    from: Yang-hu in Chiang-su
    Sun P'ing-i (ca. 1800)
Written: 1781–1785
Published: ca. 1800

one year later he was already the second-best candidate to pass the central exams for the rank of *chin-shih*. His career as a civil servant brought him to numerous posts in various parts of the empire. In his private life he was particularly interested in the preparation and publication of old texts in their original form.

Besides the *Shen-nung pen-ts'ao ching*, Sun Hsing-yen devoted his time to the old work on the art of war, *Sun-tzu ping-fa*, the Taoist philosophical treatise *Pao-p'u tzu*, and the medical work *Ch'ien-chin pao-yao*, among other things. Other texts that he dealt with treated themes from the Han period administration, geography, topography, jurisdiction, and textual criticism. Most of his own works, and those that he reprinted, are assembled in two collections, containing more than sixty titles.[260]

For the reconstruction of the *Pen-ching*, Sun Hsing-yen and Sun P'ing-i followed the white-on-black printing of characters in the *Cheng-lei pen-ts'ao*. In three chapters they arranged 360 drugs into upper, middle, and lower classes. Each monograph began with the old, original text from the *Pen-ching*, to which they added commentaries from the *Pen-ts'ao* of Wu P'u, *Ming-i pieh-lu*, *Shuo-wen*, *Erh-ya*, *Kuang-ya*, *Huai-nan tzu*, *Pao-p'u tzu* and other texts.

Following the monograph section, the authors recorded the general prefatory paragraphs of the *Pen-ching*. However, they were of the opinion that these statements were to be considered the "Additional Notes of Renowned Medical Men." In addition, their work contains "lost sections of the *Pen-ching*," which they had taken from the *Pao-p'u tzu*, *T'ai-p'ing yü-lan*, and other works. In Okanishi's view, these fragments are quotations from drug compendia of the late Han period, which also carried a *Shen-nung pen-ts'ao* or similar title, but which were not identical with the texts used by T'ao Hung-ching.[261]

Most of the following "Twelve Sections from Mr. Wu's Materia Medica" (*Wu-shih pen-ts'ao*), which contain a list of drugs and a description of their effects when taken together, were also adopted from the *T'ai-p'ing yü-lan*.

At the end of their work, the authors placed the five-line quotation from the *Yao-tui* that had first appeared in the *Hsin-hsiu pen-ts'ao* and was later adopted by Li Shih-chen, and which was now included by Sun Hsing-yen, without one of the authors being able to interpret its meaning.

Sun Hsing-yen's preface to the *Shen-nung pen-ts'ao ching* is a philological treatise on the textual problems of *Pen-ching* reconstructions and contains no direct statement on whether Sun advocated a return to the therapeutic standards of the Han period. The medical relevance of the work is indicated, although only suggested, more by the two further prefaces of the first edition.[262]

2.8. The *Pen-ching shu-cheng*

Pen-ching shu-cheng
"Commentary on the Original Classic"
12 chapters / 173 drug descriptions
Author: Tsou Shu (1790–1844)
   tzu: Jun-an
   hao: Jun-an
   from: Wu-chin in Chiang-su
Written: ca. 1837
Published: 1849

Tsou Shu, whom we have already encountered as the author of a preface to the *Pen-ts'ao shu kou-yüan*, came from a destitute family. At the age of sixteen he lost his mother; only six years later, his stepmother also died. A lack of money hampered him, for his poverty eliminated the possibility of a tutor. All that remained to him was private study. With great diligence he read all the literature he could lay his hands on, achieving in this manner a reputation as a highly learned man. When, in 1821, an imperial decree requested that scholars living in seclusion be recommended to the court, the elders of the place where he was living decided to suggest Tsou Shu. Upon learning of this, Tsou Shu immediately prepared a petition and declined every call. He continued to live in seclusion with his books. He subsequently married, but the union remained childless. Following the death of his younger brother, Tsou Hsien, he adopted his brother's son, Tsou Meng-lung.[263] Tsou Shu's friends included Yang Shih-t'ai, who lived in the same district and is known to us as the author of the *Pen-ts'ao shu kou-yüan*.

Tsou studied medical questions thoroughly, but he expressed the regret that the works of Chang Chi, the *Shang-han lun* and *Chin-kuei yao-lüeh*, were in themselves not sufficient for medical activity. Yang Shih-t'ai suggested that he study the *Pen-ts'ao shu* of Liu Jo-chin, in which the theoretical background of pharmaceutics was also discussed. After reading this book, however, Tsou Shu felt that it contained too much of the Chin-Yüan theories while the prescriptions of Chang Chi and Sun Ssu-mo had been neglected.[264] As a consequence, Tsou Shu set out to compile a work on pharmaceutics himself which was to contain a blending of theoretical and practical information as he considered appropriate.

He first wrote the *Pen-ching shu-cheng*.[265] He regarded the *Pen-ching* and the *Ming-i pieh-lu* as the "classic" and the *Shang-han lun*, the *Chin-kuei yao-lüeh*, the *Ch'ien-chin yao-fang* as well as the *Wai-t'ai pi-yao* as "appendixes." In addition, he drew on a wide range of further sources, including historical, Buddhist, and Taoist works. Tsou Shu may well be considered to have been the most liberal of the *Han-hsüeh* authors. For the basic arrangement of the *Pen-ching shu-cheng*, Tsou adopted the three classes of the *Pen-ching*. Within these classes he described the drugs in sections ranging from minerals to vegetables. At the beginning of each of the 173 monographs he placed the original *Pen-ching/Ming-i pieh-lu* description of the respective drug and designated, when necessary, the sections from the *Pen-ching* and *Ming-i pieh-lu* by means of different type. These are followed by extensive commentaries compiled by Tsou himself and earlier authors.

The preface to the *Pen-ching shu-cheng* was written by Hung Shang-hsiang:

> The meaning of therapeutics can be learned from the [old] works. These include the *Ling-shu, Su-wen, Nan-ching,* and the even earlier *Shen-nung pen-ching,* the very first work. The first of the above-mentioned works emphasize the differentiation of illnesses; the *Pen-ching,* however, is devoted chiefly to [the problems of] treatment. Theory and reality complement each other, as internal and external. Unfortunately, the names of those who handed down this work can no longer be ascertained. Generally, it has been assumed that [the above-mentioned

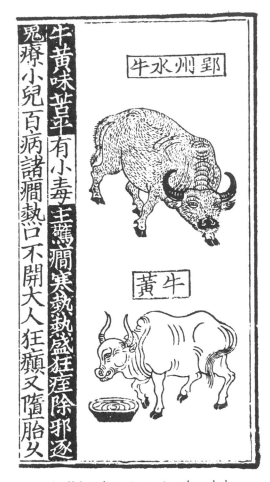

water buffalo (*shui-niu:* top) and cattle bezoar (stone) (*niu-huang:* bottom)—*Ch'ung-hsiu cheng-ho pen-ts'ao*

work] was written under pseudonyms during the Han period. But when the burning of books was carried out during the Ch'in period, medical texts were not affected, and it is therefore certain that this work was passed down from antiquity. Of the later authors who continued [the tradition of] this literature, T'ao Yin-chü and [his] "Additional Notes [of Renowned Medical Men]" are the most highly esteemed. Further on, during the Sung, Chin, and Yüan periods, more than ten scholars wrote *pen-ts'ao* works. Their explanations became more and more extensive; their theories became more and more diverse. Their language attempted again and again to surpass the newest things; the meaning of their words became more and more obscure. Thus, they all tried to outdo the *Pen-ching* and to expand the "Additional Notes"; all of these works, however, suffer from [the fact that their contents are both] disorderly and full of weeds. The physicians of all subsequent generations took over this material from one another and used it, without knowing that it was meaningless. Even so-called good medical practitioners discussed only books on how to prepare prescriptions if confronted by [specific] clinical symptoms; they considered the *Pen-ching* and the "Additional Notes" only ordinary herb books. They did not possess the abilities to work through these texts and study them in comparison with other works. They were unable to reach an understanding of these works and to relate their explanations to actual evidence. For this reason, the teachings on the intentions underlying the use of drugs by men in antiquity as well as the teachings on why drugs can cure illnesses remained hidden from them and were impenetrable. To this day they still do not know that a specific illness has a prescription that is specific for that illness, that a specific prescription has drugs that are specific for this prescription, and finally, that a specific drug has effects that are specific for this drug. If [medical practitioners] are unable to differentiate drugs, how should they be able to prepare prescriptions? If, however, they cannot prepare prescriptions, how should they cure illnesses? This was reason enough for Tsou Jun-an to write the *Pen-ching shu-cheng*.[266]

Tsou Shu's own introduction is dated 1827.

Shortly thereafter, Tsou prepared a continuation of the *Pen-ching shu-cheng*—the *Pen-ching hsü-shu* ("Continued Commentary to the Original Classic"). In six chapters arranged in the same manner as the first work, the author described 142 additional drugs, which had been chosen according to frequent usage. Some of them again came from the *Pen-ching* and the *Ming-i pieh-lu;* others were designated as having been taken from the *T'ang pen-ts'ao, Pen-ts'ao shih-i,* or the *Cheng-lei pen-ts'ao*. The type of commentary on the quotations from original monographs corresponds to that in the *Pen-ching shu-cheng*.

Finally, Tsou Shu compiled still a third work for his *Pen-ching* cycle—the *Pen-ching hsü shu-yao* ("Compilation of Commentaries on Important [Passages] in the Original Classic"). Containing eight chapters, the work lists several drugs under each of ninety-three illnesses and symptoms, with a very brief characterization of the drugs' properties. Tsou Shu wrote an introduction to this work in 1840.

A total of fourteen works by Tsou Shu are known. The great majority of them are devoted to medicine and pharmaceutics. In addition, Tsou Shu also published collections of prose and poetry. He was only fifty-five when he died.[267]

地漿主解中毒煩悶 名醫所錄

（地）

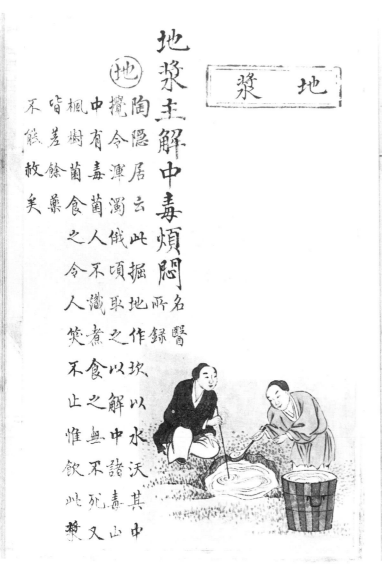

陶隱居云此掘地作坎以水沃其中
攪令渾濁俄頃取之以解中諸毒山
中有毒菌食人不識煮之
楓樹菌殺人
之令人笑不止惟飲此漿
皆差
不能救矣

地 漿

earth "soup" (ti-chiang)—Pen-ts'ao p'in-hui
ching-yao

井底沙主治湯火燒瘡用 名醫所錄

（地）

謹按井底沙即井中泥而具坤體
乃至陰之水也蓋井水靜而不流為陰
水也非江湖之
陽光為陽之水日夜浸
性愈冷故能祛大
熱湯火之毒也
浸漬成泥其

井底沙

sand from the bottom of the well (ching-ti
sha)—Pen-ts'ao p'in-hui ching-yao

200

石之金

鐵落 無毒

鐵落出神農本經

主風熱惡瘡瘍疽瘡痂疥氣除胸膈中熱氣食不

在皮膚中以上朱字神農本經

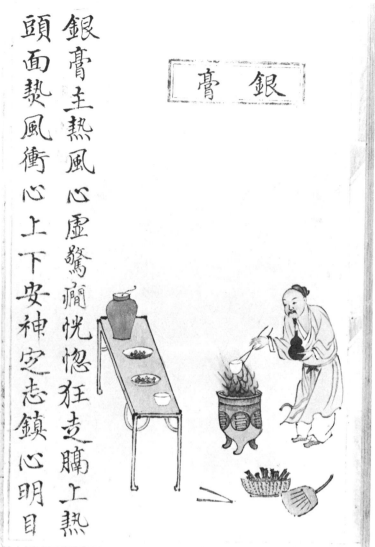

銀膏主熱風心虛驚癇恍惚狂走臟上熱

頭面熱風衝心上下安神定志鎮心明目

wrought iron chips (*t'ieh-lo*)—*Pen-ts'ao p'in-hui ching-yao*

the preparation of silver amalgam (*yin-kao*)—*Pen-ts'ao p'in-hui ching-yao*

201

2.9. The *Shen-nung pen-ts'ao ching* (reconstruction by Huang Shih)

After Lu Fu and Sun Hsing-yen, Huang Shih published the third "original version" of the *Pen-ching*. For this purpose he adopted almost unchanged the reconstruction of Sun Hsing-yen, adding only twenty-two monographs. Characteristically, the work appeared in the collection *Han-hsüeh t'ang ts'ung-shu*.[268]

Shen-nung pen-ts'ao ching (reconstruction by Huang-Shih)
"Shen-nung's Classic of Pharmaceutics"
3 chapters / 388 drug descriptions
Author: Huang-Shih (end of the nineteenth century)
Written: date unknown
Published: between 1875 and 1907

2.10. The *Shen-nung pen-ts'ao ching* (reconstruction by Ku Kuan-kuang)

Ku Kuan-kuang came from a family with a long medical tradition. He himself planned a civil service career. However, after three unsuccessful attempts to pass the necessary exams, he had no alternative but to follow the family tradition. A family named Ch'ien, living nearby, possessed an extensive library. It is said that Ku Kuan-kuang spent all available free time reading there. Besides medicine, he was especially interested in astronomy and the calculation of calendars. In both areas he achieved remarkable expertise.[269]

For his reconstruction of the *Shen-nung pen-ts'ao ching*, Ku Kuan-kuang followed the model of Lu Fu. New in his work were quotations from old pen-ts'ao writings that had been preserved in encyclopedias of the T'ang and Sung periods.[270]

Shen-nung pen-ts'ao ching (reconstruction by Ku Kuan-kuang)
"Shen-nung's Classic of Pharmaceutics"
4 chapters
Author: Ku Kuan-kuang (end of the nineteenth century)
Written: date unknown
Published: 1883

2.11. The *Shen-nung pen-ts'ao* (reconstruction by Wang K'ai-yün)

Since his youth, so report his chroniclers, Wang K'ai-yün had devoted himself most fervently to the study of literature. His erudition earned him a position as adviser to the influential statesman Su-shun (1815?–1861). Wang K'ai-yün was an advocate of the textual criticism tendencies of the Han school. He wrote numerous books dealing with the meaning of the old classics. Among others, he annotated the *I-ching, Shu-ching, Shih-ching*, and *Li-chi*. Although not possessing any special knowledge in the area of medicine, he also prepared an "original version" of the *Pen-ching*. It is considered extremely insignificant, however. Like the works described in 2.9 and 2.10 above, it received no appreciable circulation.[271]

Shen-nung pen-ts'ao (reconstruction by Wang K'ai-yün)
"Shen-nung's Original Classic"
3 chapters
Author: Wang K'ai-yün (1833–1916)
     tzu: Jen-ch'iu, Jen-fu
Written: date unknown
Published: 1885

2.12. The *Shen-nung pen-ching* (reconstruction by Chiang Kuo-i)

Chiang Kuo-i published under his name a version of Wang K'ai-yün's reconstruction, the contents and title of which had been changed only insignificantly. The work attained no importance at all and is mentioned here only for the sake of completeness.[272]

Shen-nung pen-ching (reconstruction by Chiang Kuo-i)
"Shen-nung's Original Classic"
1 chapter
Author: Chiang Kuo-i (end of the nineteenth century)
Written: date unknown
Published: 1892

VI. CONCLUDING REMARKS ON THE *HAN-HSÜEH* TRADITION AND ON *PEN-TS'AO* LITERATURE WITH COMPREHENSIVE CONTENTS

The presentation of the *Han-hsüeh* tradition of *pen-ts'ao* literature concludes the first part of the present work. This section has included the description of all recognizable traditions in Chinese pharmaceutical literature that were more or less closely connected with intellectual trends and that were based upon a unified medical conception.

I have chosen to present the individual traditions in the context of a chronological series of representative works, but at this point I should emphasize again that none of the individual traditions that came to be added to the main tradition of pen-ts'ao literature was able to eliminate a previously existing tradition. The continuous arising of individual traditions meant an ever-increasing fragmentation of the spectrum of therapeutic thinking. The main pen-ts'ao tradition was dominant until the Sung period, when the new Chin-Yüan tradition gained great influence. Proponents of both trends existed simultaneously. The *Ssu-k'u ch'üan-shu* contains the following apt remark: "The split of Confucians occurred during the Sung period; that of medical practitioners during the Chin-Yüan period."[273]

During the sixteenth century, the third trend developed—the eclectic tradition. Its adherents selected appropriate elements from all previous currents. Finally, the seventeenth century saw the emergence of the *Han-hsüeh* tradition.

This covers the four basic medical conceptions that were expressed in pharmaceutical works. The entire palette of medical tendencies during the Ch'ing period, however, was even more colorful. The diversity of philosophical and political opinions and conceptions during that period of the empire's dissolution was reflected exactly in the medical arena. Supporters of numerous trends competed with one another: modern doctrines, already influenced by the West, the teachings of the Ming period, of the Chin-Yüan period, of the T'ang and Sung period, of the Ch'in and Han period, and finally, many different independent ideas.[274]

It can be considered symbolic that the *Han-hsüeh* tradition of pen-ts'ao literature was discussed in the present work as the last predominant tradition. As in a great circular course, the adherents of this tradition returned to the point where recorded Chinese pharmaceutical knowledge had begun: to the originals of the Han period. With their restoration, of course, it soon became clear to some investigators that these works were scarcely capable of solving the contemporary medical problems.

In the same manner that Confucian ideology, despite a reconsideration of its sources, could not offer the appropriate conceptions for solving the internal difficulties and external threats in the political-philosophical sphere during the last centuries of the Empire, so too, traditional medical thought ended, temporarily at least, at a zero point. It is thus not astonishing that the same forces that sought a radical reorganization in China with respect to political structure and social ideology also demanded a complete overcoming of the old schemes of medical thinking and health care organization.[275] The correspondence of both spheres is obvious.

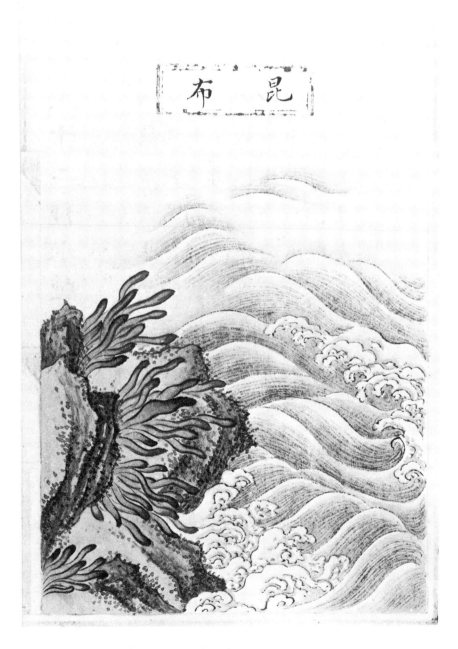

sea algae *(k'un-pu)—Pen-ts'ao p'in-hui ching-yao*

D. The Pen-ts'ao Literature with Specialized Contents

The Chinese pharmaceutical works presented in chapter C were distinguished by two characteristics. On the one hand, their contents were comprehensive, that is, each of these works discussed the total range of pharmaceutics, with animal (and human), mineral, and vegetable drug groups. On the other hand, the traditions to which these works belonged were closely connected with intellectual currents in Chinese culture. The genre of pharmaceutical literature defined in this manner can be contrasted with a second genre, one comprising those works that are technically specialized and that, with a few exceptions, could not be grouped in one of the traditions already described, even though they were influenced by one or another of the medical conceptions represented in these traditions.

In some works, specialization was expressed in the contents, in others in the form. The following works can be considered to have specialized contents: those devoted to preventive and curative dietetics; those whose contents were restricted to the description of a single drug; those that were particularly oriented to the presentation of pharmaceutical-technological methods; and those devoted specifically to the drugs originating in certain areas. In addition, I have included here the description of several pharmaceutical reference works that discuss the most suitable provenances, or synonyms for drug names. The group of pen-ts'ao works composed in verse should also be mentioned in connection with specialization of form. These were compiled with the special intention of enabling the beginning student to memorize pharmaceutical data more easily.

As will be shown, each of these individual genres can be traced back many centuries. The individual works, however, were directly connected with one another only in the rarest instances, so that the word *tradition* cannot be used in the same sense as in the first part of the present work.

I. PEN-TS'AO WORKS ON DIETETICS

The influence of a balanced diet on the well-being of the individual appears to have been observed in China very early. There is also early evidence for the conclusion that can be drawn from such observations—that is, that food can be helpful in eliminating some illnesses.

The *Chou-li*, the "Notes on the Rites of the Chou Empire," written no later than during the earlier Han period, describes among a total of four classes of physicians the institution of a *shih-i*, a medical specialist in dietetics:

食醫

> Dietetic Physicians. Their task is to care for the balance of the six foodstuffs, six drinks, six dishes, hundred provisions, hundred soups, and eight precious dainties of the king. When they prepare rice dishes, the [warmth of] springtime should be taken as an example. When soups are prepared, the [heat of] summer should serve as an example. When they prepare sauces, the [coolness of] fall should be taken as an example. When they prepare drinks, the [coldness of] winter should be taken as an example. All foods prepared in spring should be especially sour, those in summer especially bitter, those in fall especially pungent, and those in winter especially salty. In each case, the balance should be reestablished with sweetness. During the preparation of dishes [containing several ingredients, the dietetic physicians] must consider appropriate [combinations]. Beef should be combined with glutinous rice; lamb should be combined with glutinous millet; pork should be combined with panicled millet; canine should be combined with common millet; wild goose should be combined with wheat; fish should be combined with mustard. All foods for noble men must be prepared according to these principles.[1]

References to the curative power of foods were adopted by the *Shan-hai ching*, also recorded during the earlier Han period.[2] A quotation from the *Su-wen* may serve as an example of how dietetic treatment, as opposed to a therapy with drugs, was assessed. The more potent the latter, the smaller the range of illnesses against which they may be applied, whereas dietetic therapy may be applied against any affliction:

> Medicinally potent drugs can eliminate six out of ten illnesses. Medicinally normal drugs can eliminate seven out of ten illnesses. Medicinally weak drugs can eliminate eight out of ten illnesses. Drugs without marked medicinal effectiveness can eliminate nine out of ten illnesses. Grains, meat, fruits, and vegetables are suitable for dietetic nourishment against all illnesses. But even with these, certain limits should not be exceeded. Otherwise the proper [influences] of the [patient] might be harmed.[3]

The appreciation of dietetics was soon reflected in a special literature, whose titles, remarkably, appeared already in the bibliographical sections of the historical work on the Han dynasty—at a time, therefore, when there was not yet any mention of general pharmaceutical pen-ts'ao works.

For the discussion of several representative examples from dietetic literature, we must first distinguish three groups within this genre. The first group comprises those works that attempt to offer the reader all knowledge necessary for healthy daily eating and drinking. The writings of this group are thus limited in their monographs to the descriptions of common foodstuffs; some are conceived directly as cookbooks. In connection with this series of works, one should keep in mind the medical principle of a healthy life-style—a life-style pre-

"poisoning by means of foodstuffs"—*Yin-shan cheng-yao*

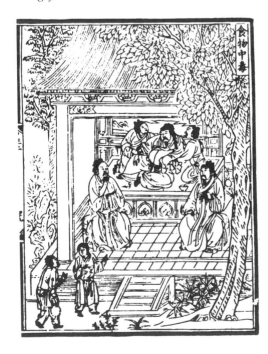

venting illness through nourishment, the realization of which is to be aided by these texts. A second group in this literary genre is devoted to the use of foodstuffs for treating illnesses that have already appeared, that is to say, a curative diet. Finally, a third group can be mentioned, comprising works offering the reader information on the simple foodstuffs found in nature that are necessary for survival in the wilderness or during times of need. The boundaries between the three groups are, of course, not totally rigid; various works deal with more than one of these subjects.

1. The *Shen-nung Huang-ti shih-chin*

Shen-nung's Huang-ti shih-chin
"Shen-nung's and Huang-ti's Nutritional Prohibitions"
7 chapters

2. The *Huang-ti tsa-yin shih-chi*

Huang-ti tsa-yin shih-chi
"Various Prescripts of Huang-ti Regarding Abstinence from Food and Drink"
2 chapters

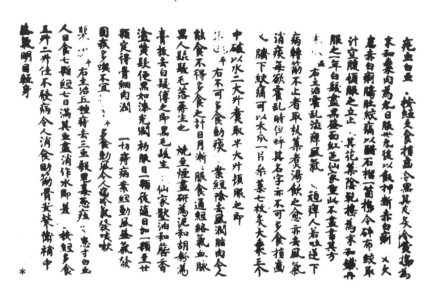

3. The *Lao-tzu chin-shih ching*

Lao-tzu chin-shih ching
"Lao-tzu's Classic on Dietetics"
1 chapter / number of drug descriptions: unknown
Author: unknown
Written: early Han period

All these works, the three earliest Chinese special texts on dietetics known by title, have long been lost. The first work was already mentioned in the *Han-shu*. The second and third were listed for the first time in the bibliography of the history of the Sui dynasty. The significance ascribed to the value of dietetic measures is also visible in the association of the contents of the above-mentioned works with the names of the early culture-heroes Huang-ti and Shen-nung, as well as with the Taoist philosopher Lao Tzu.[4]

4. The *Ts'ui Hao shih-ching*

Ts'ui Hao shih-ching
"Ts'ui Hao's Scripture on Nutrition"
9 chapters / number of drug descriptions: unknown
Author: Ts'ui Hao (?–450)
  tzu: Po-yüan
  from: Ch'ing-ho in Ho-pei
Written: ca. 430–450
Published: date unknown

Ts'ui Hao is known as a statesman and historiographer. He was interested in calendar science and astronomy, turning later to Taoism and dietetics.[5] In 436 he was commissioned to prepare the history of the Northern Wei dynasty, under which he lived. His outspoken language led to his premature death and the destruction of his entire family. All that remains of his dietetic work, which presented his mother's recollections of the preparation of good foods in times of surplus, is the preface:

> From the time of my youth until adult age, I have observed the domestic labors of my mothers and aunts with ears and eyes and have fully acquired [their knowledge in this area]. They themselves usually attended to the food and drink that was offered the mothers- and fathers-in-law in the morning and evening, and the sacrifices offered in all four seasons, although we had the necessary resources to entrust [such tasks] to employees. Once we were affected by destruction and

*10th century fragment of a manuscript of the *Shih-liao pen-ts'ao* found in Tun-huang. The names of food drugs recognizable here—*mu-kua*, *hu-t'ao*, and *fei-tzu*—were set in red, in contrast to the otherwise black script

unrest. Serious famines resulted, and we were no longer able to prepare all the necessary items to live on rich congee and vegetables. In the meantime, we had not prepared [such foods] for more than ten years. Only my mother, who has passed away in the meantime, expressed the fear that knowledge [of the methods of how to prepare good foods in times of surplus] could fall into oblivion with the passage of time, so that later generations would know nothing of such things. Since the time of her youth, she had been unpracticed in writing and now presented [this information] orally in nine sections. Her style was concise and beautiful. She was able to differentiate everything intelligently, and her memory was very distinct in every respect. Only after the death of my parents did our country experience another rise of the dragon. The rebels were pacified and disturbances were crushed; stability reigned in all directions. I myself obtained a position among the ministers in which I took part in important projects. As a result, I received great reward. My cows and sheep cover the land, and my fortune stretches into the ten thousands. However, when I think back about my life, I realize that the time when Chi Lu still carried rice will never return.[6] For this reason I am writing this preface to the work left [by my mother], so as to pass it on to posterity.[7]

The earliest Chinese work devoted specifically to dietetic therapy from which at least an extensive fragment has been preserved is the *Shih-liao pen-ts'ao*, dating from the T'ang period. From bibliographical entries of previous centuries it can be calculated that in the time from the Han to the T'ang period, nearly forty manuals and prescription works on dietetics had already been written.

The forerunner to the *Shih-liao pen-ts'ao* was a work entitled *Pu-yang fang* ("Prescriptions to Fill [Deficiencies] and Nourish"), written by a man named Meng Shen. An otherwise unknown author, Chang Ting, expanded the *Pu-yang fang* of Meng Shen some time between the years 721 and 739. His version expanded the original 89 sections to a total of 227 monographs; the new work was aptly entitled *Shih-liao pen-ts'ao*. When Ch'en Ts'ang-ch'i, in 739, published his *Pen-ts'ao shih-i*, he quoted both from the original version, the *Pu-yang fang*, and from the *Shih-liao pen-ts'ao*.[8]

Meng Shen appears to have been associated—at least conceptually—with Taoist circles of his time. In his work we encounter references to afflictions caused by various demonic entities, to longevity, as well as to the desired goal of "elimination of the body's material weight." In addition, Meng Shen alludes to specific technical terms used in Taoist circles for some of the substances he described. Emperor Jui-tsung (662–716), who was set up as titulary sovereign by the Empress Wu Hou in 684, and who ascended to the throne in 710, is known to have had a profound fondness for Taoism and alchemy. Meng Shen had served him as reader-in-waiting before his ascension to the throne and was asked to serve in an official position afterward. When Meng Shen excused himself on grounds of ill health and age, the emperor bestowed upon him valuable gifts. Further information on the background of this author is provided by his biography in the older T'ang history:

Meng Shen came from Liang in Jou-chou. He had passed the *chin-shih* exams and was given a position as an assistant in the Imperial

5. The *Shih-liao pen-ts'ao*

Shih-liao pen-ts'ao
"Materia Medica for Successful Cures through Nutrition"
3 chapters / 227 drug descriptions
Authors: Meng Shen (621–713);
from: Ju-chou in Ho-nan
Chang Ting (eighth century);
hao: Wu-hsüan tzu
Written: ca. 701–704
Enlarged: ca. 721–739
Published: between 721 and 739

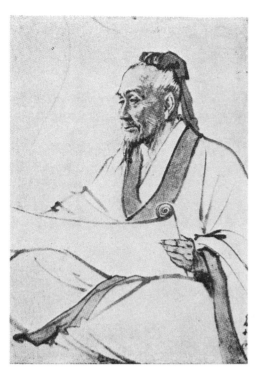

Sun Ssu-mo (581–682?), physician and author of well known prescription works

Grand Secretariat at the beginning of the governmental period *ch'ui-kung* (685–688). Already during his youth [Meng] Shen had studied prescription techniques [i.e., alchemy]. Once, when he saw gold in the house of the vice-president of the Imperial Grand Secretariat, Liu Wei-chih, which Liu had received as a gift from the throne, Meng Shen told him it was false gold. [This could be shown] by lighting a fire on the surface [of the gold] which would develop a five-color smoke. An experiment proved the [words of Meng Shen]. When the sovereign heard of this, she became angry and transferred [Meng Shen] on the basis of some matter to T'ai-chou as a subprefect. Later, [Meng Shen] rose to vice-president in the Department of Astronomy. . . . At the beginning of the *shen-lung* period (705–709), Meng Shen withdrew from the civil service and lived henceforth in a mountain hut in I-yang, where he studied drugs and dietetics. Despite his advanced age, he possessed the mental facilities of a man in the best years of life. He told those who were near to him: "Whoever is capable of protecting his body and nourishing his nature sees to it that good words and good drugs remain with him always!" . . . When Meng Shen finally died, he had reached the age of ninety-two.[9]

In his youth as a student, Meng Shen had followed the well-known medical practitioner and author Sun Ssu-mo (581–682?). Sun Ssu-mo, in chapter 26 of his comprehensive collection of prescriptions and relevant informations *Ch'ien-chin fang,* had published a treatise entitled "Dietetic Therapy" (*shih-chih*). In a preface he quoted earlier 食治 authorities and voiced his own opinions, on the advantages of a dietary treatment of illness:

(Chang) Chung-ching has said: For the human body to remain in a healthy and balanced state, nothing else is required but to care about its nourishment. By no means should drugs be consumed recklessly. The strength of drugs is one-sided, and there are occasions where they are of help. But they lead to an imbalance of the influences in man's depots and, consequently, an affliction will easily be acquired from outside [sources]. Living beings have always depended on food to maintain their life. But, at the same time, they are unaware of the fact that even food has positive and negative aspects. [Food] is in daily use with all the people, but one knows little about it. Water and fire are very near but difficult to comprehend! I regretted this and have, therefore—when I had spare time from my [other] writings—compiled a treatise on dietetic therapy [emphasizing] harms and benefits that can result from the five tastes, in order to inform our youth. . . . Now, those who practice medicine must first of all recognize the origin of an illness; they must know which violations [have caused the suffering]. Then they must treat it with dietary means. If dietary therapy does not cure the illness, only then can they employ drugs. The nature of drugs is violent, just like that of the imperial soldiers. Because the soldiers are so wild, how could anybody deploy them recklessly? If they are deployed inappropriately, harm and destruction will result everywhere. Similarly, excessive calamities are the consequence if drugs are thrown against illnesses (carelessly).[10]

As a second part of this introduction, Sun Ssu-mo quoted lengthy passages from the *Huang-ti nei-ching,* expounding the correspondences between the five tastes, the human organism, and possible illnesses. In the following four sections of chapter 26—devoted to substances from the realms of fruits, vegetables, grains, and animals (including man), respectively—the author presented a dietetic materia medica. In 149 short monographs resembling the style of contemporary pen-ts'ao works, Sun Ssu-mo described the curative properties of a large number of more or less common foodstuffs. Three examples may illustrate the kind of data he presented:

> *Areca* nut. Taste: acrid; [thermo-influence:] warm. Astringent. No marked medicinal effectiveness. Digests grains and drains water. Eliminates diarrhea [caused by] mucous [accumulations]. Kills the Three Worms. Drives out hidden corpse [spirits]. Cures tape worm.[11]

> Sow milk. Neutral. No marked medicinal effectiveness. Masters fright and cramps in infants. To drink it has miraculous [effects].[12]

> Wild horse penis. Taste: sour, salty; [thermo-influence:] warm. No marked medicinal effectiveness. Masters weakness of the male *yin* [i.e., sexual organ], lack of semen.[13]

In his compilation of the *Pu-yang fang,* Meng Shen appears to have been influenced by the knowledge of his teacher Sun Ssu-mo; the contents of numerous monographs in the *Pu-yang fang* correspond to those in chapter 26 of the *Ch'ien-ching fang.* Nakao Manzō believed that this proximity may have been one reason for the renaming of Meng's work as *Shih-liao pen-ts'ao* by Chang Ting a few years after Meng Shen's death.[14] A second reason may have been that a title like *Pu-yang fang* refers to a work focusing on prescriptions, a claim realized in Meng Shen's book only secondarily.

Of the three examples quoted above from Sun Ssu-mo's *Ch'ien-chin fang,* sow milk was not adopted by Meng Shen; neither was the *areca* nut, a monograph on which was only added by Chang Ting. The monograph on horse penis, though, coincides in the *Pu-yang fang* with that of the *Ch'ien-chin fang:*

> *Areca* nut. If one consumes much of it, heat develops. The people in the south eat it in a fresh state. In Fukien it is called *kan-lan-tzu* [i.e., olive seeds]. Those that come here are boiled, steamed, and dried for future use.[15]

> White horse penis. Supplements the *yin*-influences in males. [The drug] is dried in the shade and then pulverized. It is combined with *ts'ung-jung* for preparations of honey pills. They are swallowed on an empty stomach, with wine. Forty-nine pills are taken several times a day; after one hundred days the effect is manifest.[16]

In subsequent years the *Shih-liao pen-ts'ao* experienced the fate of so many pen-ts'ao works in the secondary tradition: the most important passages were adopted by a later work in the main pen-ts'ao tradition while the rest fell into oblivion and, sooner or later, were lost. Both versions, the original *Pu-yang fang* and the *Shih-liao pen-ts'ao,* appear to have been preserved until the eleventh century, for Chang Yü-hsi (992–1068), the author of the *Chia-yu pen-ts'ao,* cites statements from both Meng Shen and Chang Ting, presenting passages together that sometimes even agree nearly word for word.

From Japanese texts it can be observed that the *Shih-liao pen-ts'ao* was read in Japan as early as the ninth century.[17]

Until the beginning of this century, the most important sources for quotations from the *Shih-liao pen-ts'ao*, were the *Cheng-lei pen-ts'ao*, from China, and the *Ishinpō* (tenth century) and *Yenshu ruiyō* (eleventh century), both from Japan.[18] Fortunately, a fragment of the *Shih-liao pen-ts'ao* was also found among the materials discovered in the Tun-huang Caves of West China by Aurel Stein in 1907. A scroll glued to paper carrying the date 934, this fragment represents the oldest textual version known today and is probably the one most faithful to the original *Shih-liao pen-ts'ao*. The fragment contains twenty-five monographs. In each case, main indications, commentaries on them, and recipe guidelines are presented following the names of the food drugs. The main text of the fragment, which today is located in the British Museum, is written in black ink. The names of drugs and symbols separating sentences are designated by red ink. In 1930, Na-kao Manzō published a detailed analysis of the reconstructable portions of the *Shih-liao pen-ts'ao* in a scientific journal in Shanghai, comparing the contents of the twenty-five monographs of the Tun-huang fragment with statements ascribed, in the *Cheng-lei pen-ts'ao* and other sources, to Meng Shen and to the *Shih-liao pen-ts'ao*.[19] Apparently, in compiling his *Cheng-lei pen-ts'ao*, T'ang Shen-wei made thorough use of the *Shih-liao pen-ts'ao* but cited the original monographs in a significantly shortened or changed form. The quotations in the Japanese sources also did not reproduce the original. The monographs of the Tun-huang fragment on *fei*-seeds as well as the statement ascribed to the *Shih-liao pen-ts'ao* in the *Cheng-lei pen-ts'ao* on the same drug may demonstrate the differences:

1. Tun-huang fragment

榧子

> *Fei-tzu.* Neutral. This [drug] masters the treatment of the five kinds of hemorrhoids. Drives out the Three Worms. Kills demonic poisons and possessions by the malevolent. Furthermore, people suffering from tapeworm should eat seven seeds a day for seven days. Then all the worms are dispersed to water and are discharged. Commentary: It is good to consume large amounts of three or two *sheng;* no illness will result from this. [On the contrary,] it helps man to digest food and aides his muscles and bones; it pacifies one's defense, fills one's center, and supplements the influences; and it clears the eyes and eliminates the material weight of the body.[20]

2. *Cheng-lei pen-ts'ao* quotation

The *Shih-liao [pen-ts'ao]* states:

> for treating tapeworms, each day seven seeds should be eaten for seven days. All the worms will have been transformed to water [by then].[21]

6. The *Shih-hsing pen-ts'ao*

The *Shih-hsing pen-ts'ao* was written during the false T'ang period by Ch'en Shih-liang, vice-commander of the P'ei-jung army and assistant lecturer in medicine in Chien-chou. He proceeded from the assumption that there had already been dietary officials in antiquity who treated [patients] by means of [suitable] nourishment. For this reason, he went back to the *Shen-nung pen-ching* and compiled all drugs [from the works] of T'ao Yin-chü, Su Kung, Meng Shen, and Ch'en Ts'ang-ch'i that were related to food and drink. He then added his own comments. In addition, he wrote down all prescriptions of dietetic medicine and of the art of regulating the body's depots and nourishing the body's depots and palaces in accordance with the five seasons. The literary official and scholar Hsü Chieh wrote a preface to this work.[22]

Shih-hsing pen-ts'ao
"Dietetic Materia Medica"
10 chapters / number of drug descriptions: unknown
Author: Ch'en Shih-liang (ninth century)
            from: Ch'ien-t'ang in Che-chiang
Written: ca. 890–900
Published: date unknown

The *Shih-hsing pen-ts'ao* was described in these words in the *Chia-yu pen-ts'ao*'s list of sources. It has since been lost as an independent work. Only quotations from thirty-four monographs are preserved in the *Cheng-lei pen-ts'ao*.

The *Shih-chih t'ung-shuo* is a pharmaceutical work, whose author is described as an apothecary and apparently also a pediatrician. In the Sung bibliography *Chih-chai shu-lu chieh-t'i*, it is recorded that Lou Chü-chung was responsible for the pulverizing of metallic drugs in an apothecary in Lin-an; his son passed the state examinations and was supposedly promoted out of grace to a civil servant, first class.[23] Apparently, the family possessed a certain prestige and the necessary connections. Otherwise, it probably cannot be explained why the prime minister, Chao Ju-yü (died 1195) wrote an afterword to the *Shih-chih t'ung-shuo*, in which he left a lively portrayal of Lou Chü-chung:

7. The *Shih-chih t'ung-shuo*

Shih-chih t'ung-shuo
"Treatise on Dietetic Methods of Treatment"
1 chapter / number of drug descriptions: unknown
Author: Lou Chü-chung (twelfth century)
Written: date unknown
Published: date unknown

> [Lou] has practiced medicine since his youth; now he is already eighty-one years old. When Ch'ien-t'ang served as temporary capital, there were many men in high positions. [Lou] has not traveled even once to pay a visit to ministers or noblemen. The [latter] frequently attempted to meet him in person but without success. Each morning he proceeds to his drug shop in a sedan chair. Waiting for him at the shop are already many children, sobbing from afflictions, screaming, and filling the room with noise. [Lou] attends to all of them with unusual care. He sits down a good while, then rises slowly and observes each person in turn. He liked to say: "Children are not sick to begin with; those who love them, however, harm them. When, for example, children suffer from diarrhea, it is a symptom of deficiency in the spleen. Too much intake of milk causes this kind of affliction. Nothing else is required but to limit milk intake and to warm their stomach with a small dosage of [*jen-*]*shen* and *shu*. But those who love children [follow more frequently the following course of action]: a child suffers from persistent diarrhea and its body's influences are exhausted. It is not forced to eat and is thus unable to compensate the losses [of the body]. As a result, the stomach is empty and no longer capable of digestion, and the influences [emanating from it] suffer severe damage. At this point, [drugs like *jen-*]*shen* and *shu* are no longer effective and, therefore, must be strengthened by means [of the drugs] *chiang* and *fu*[*-tzu*]. But *chiang* and *fu*[*-tzu*] are also no longer sufficient and, finally, potent [drugs from the area of] metals and minerals are used. This is all the more dangerous for the child! Why, I ask myself, are not such prescriptions used with which the body is familiar? We [adults] consume two *sheng* of rice daily when we are healthy and strong, and that still is not quite sufficient to satisfy our need. If we do not feel particularly well one day, we ourselves do not want to take a single grain in our mouth. How much more does this apply to children?" Everytime I observed [Lou] holding medications

[I noticed] that he spoke so incessantly to the customer when handing it over that his mouth nearly burst. At the same time, he wrote his directions on the paper sack that serves as packing material for the medication, so that [the customers] could not forget anything after their return home.[24]

This work was also lost. The following observation about its contents was recorded in the already cited *Chih-chai shu-lu chieh-t'i:* "It expressed the view that 'when food is in order, the body is also in order.' This constitutes the art of the best practitioners to treat illnesses before they arise."[25]

8. The *Yin-shan cheng-yao*

Yin-shan cheng-yao
"Correct and Important Principles of Nutrition"
3 chapters / 228 drug descriptions
Author: Hu Ssu-hui (beginning of the fourteenth century)
Written: ?–1330
Published: 1456

The dietetic pen-ts'ao literature is quite manifold, and its authors frequently pursued differing goals. Hu Ssu-hui wrote a dietetic cookbook, in which he discussed the preparation and eating of food as a means of promoting health, a means against illnesses, and a means of achieving a long life. The author himself portrayed his opinions in an introduction to the *Yin-shan cheng-yao:*

Whatever is created by heaven and nourished by the earth has in it combined the influences of heaven and earth. Man arises provided with influences from heaven and earth. All three constitute the Three Parts. The Three Parts are heaven, earth, and man.

The most important thing for the life of man is his heart. The heart is the ruler of the body and the basis for all its action. If the body is in a condition of peace, the heart can respond to all changes and control all actions. If the body is neither protected nor nourished, how can it achieve a condition of peace? The best method of protecting and nourishing [the body] consists of "maintaining the middle." If the middle is maintained, there is no damage through too much or too little. If one adapts to the four seasons, if one is moderate and careful with food and drink, if one does not wake or rest unreasonably, if one brings the body's five depots into harmony by means of the five tastes, and if the five depots are in a state of harmony, then blood and influences will be amply present, the spirit will be healthy and cheerful, and the heart and the mind will be peaceful and stable. No evil [external influences] will penetrate easily; heat and cold cannot attack [the body]. In this manner, man finds himself in a state of quiet harmony. For this reason, the exemplary men of antiquity treated those who were not yet sick and did not [have to] treat the ones who had already fallen ill. Therefore, if one considers food important and is not concerned about the [financial] means [that must be spent for it], then this is [one method] to adopt. Therefore, it is said: "In eating, no effort should be spared in getting the best. For hashed fish, no effort should be spared to obtain the most finely cut. If a fish has spoiled or meat has deteriorated, if the color and odor are poor, if something is ill cooked and is not in time, one may not partake of any of it!" By no means did the exemplary men heed such regulations solely because of their craving for food and drinks, but rather because of [their intentions of] nourishing their influences and their body, and protecting them from harm. If one consumes items the influences of which affect one another negatively, one's essence is harmed. If the tastes of foods [consumed together] are not blended harmoniously, one's appearance is damaged. The appearance takes up the five tastes and constitutes the body with them. All this caused the exemplary men to make, first of all, use of dietetics in order to maintain their particular nature. Later [in the case of acute illness], they prepared medications to protect life itself. Now, there are drugs with potent

medicinal strength, and in therapy potent medicinal drugs will eliminate
six out of ten illnesses. Treatment with normal medicinal strength will
eliminate seven out of ten illnesses. Treatment with drugs of little medicinal strength will eliminate eight out of ten illnesses. Treatment with
drugs of no marked medicinal strength will eliminate nine out of ten
illnesses. Finally, if one nourishes with grains, meats, fruits, and vegetables, one will achieve a complete cure in all cases. One should not
exceed the limits [even with foods, though] so as not to harm the proper
[influences].[26]

Although there are many types of food and drink, one should always
see to it that one gets them unadulterated. One must find out whether
they are suitable for filling, supplementing, assisting, or nourishing. The
difference between fresh and aged [foods must be considered]. The
warm, cool, cold, or hot nature [of the food must be taken into account],
as well as the damage that can result from one-sided effects of the five
tastes. If one prefers to eat in an unbalanced manner, does not distinguish
fresh or aged foods, if one neglects the established standards in the
preparation [of food and drink]—these all lead to illnesses. "That which
is allowed should be carried out; one should avoid what is not allowed."
If, for example, a pregnant woman does not pay careful attention to
her conduct, and a nursing mother does not check her craving for food,
the child will suffer harm. If one pays homage to the joys of the palate
and overlooks the dietetic prohibitions, illnesses will arise, and a person
is afflicted before he is aware of it. There are one hundred years of life
available; if, however, a person forgets himself only one time during
eating, it is a pity [for life is thus shortened]. Sun Ssu-mo says: "Those
who practice medicine must first of all recognize the origin of an illness;
they must know which violations [have caused the suffering]. Then, at
the very beginning, they must treat it with dietetic means. If this remains
unsuccessful, they can employ drugs." Thus, they eliminate nine out of
ten [illnesses]. Whoever understands how to nourish life will first of all
attentively pursue this approach. With this method of sustaining life,
how could anyone not be in good circumstances?[27]

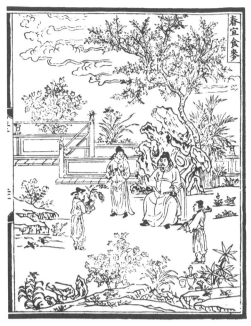

"Wheat should be consumed in spring"—illustration to the section "Correspondences to
the four seasons" in the *Yin-shan cheng-yao*

"Beans should be consumed in summer"—illustration to the section "Correspondences to
the four seasons" in the *Yin-shan cheng-yao*

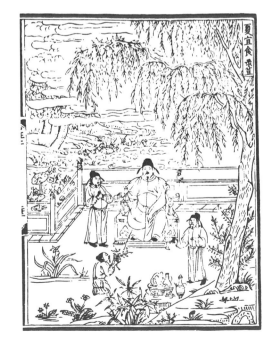

The theoretical foundation of the necessity for a dietetically con-
scious life-style corresponded completely to the demands of Confucian
ideology. In particular, the maxim to maintain the middle had been
filled with new life by the Neoconfucian Chu Hsi (1130–1200), not
very long before. He had annotated and published, as an independent
work, the relevant chapter *Chung-yung* from the old classic *Li-chi*.
For Chu, the middle way meant a fixed standard amid all imaginable
contrasts.[28] The concept of the middle way was transposed by Hu Ssu-
hui from the moral-social sphere, in which the Confucian was assigned
an unshakeable place in the variety of contradictory world views and
behavioral patterns, to a natural-cosmic sphere. In this sphere the
human organism must find its solid reference point between such
opposites as hot and cold, waking and sleeping, and sour and sweet,
in order to assert a middle way of mind and body—that, in the final
analysis, is "good health."

The quotation from the *Su-wen* and the reference to taste and
thermo-influence also indicate, in addition to the proximity of Chu
Hsi's Neoconfucianism, a slight influence of Hu Ssu-hui by the Chin-
Yüan reforms in medical thought. Seen as a whole, however, the author's pharmaceutical statements were on the level of the main pen-
ts'ao tradition.

The creation of the *Yin-shan cheng-yao* and the background of its compilation become visible in the following excerpt from the accompanying letter for the delivery of the work to the emperor:

In my humble view, the present dynasty grandly embraces the four seas. From all areas, near and far, valuable food items and rare goods are submitted as tribute and stored in the treasure vault. The local conditions here are unsuitable for some of the foods. For others, the appropriate degree of moisture, for example, cannot be found. If those responsible in the kitchen do not know how to differentiate the nature and taste [of these substances] but use them carelessly [in foods] for the emperor, it is to be feared that their consumption will unavoidably lead to illness.

Emperor Shih-tsu [i.e., Kublai Khan, 1214–1294] possessed sagelike wisdom. Based on the fact that in the "Rites of the Chou" *(Chou-li)*, section "Heavenly Officers," medical professors, physicians of dietetics, physicians for acute illnesses, and physicians for ulcerous afflictions had been listed, [Emperor Shih-tsu] proceeded along the lines of this old code and employed four imperial medical practitioners for dietetics. Their assignment was to select from the *pen-ts'ao* works medicinally ineffective, mutually nonopposing, nutritious drugs that can be taken over long periods of time, and to regulate and harmonize their five tastes in order to adapt them to drinks and food. In addition, they were to instruct, in detail, who had to be in charge and which items had to be used in the daily preparation of precious articles and imperial provisions. When wine was offered to the emperor, cups made from deeply aromatic wood, from gold [washed out of] sand, or from crystal had to be used. It had to be considered what was best suited to avoid extremes [so that the emperor was always able] to manage governmental affairs and to fulfill his responsibilities. In addition, daily entries had to be made in the calendar concerning [items] used, in order to verify later effects. As for decoctions, pastes prepared from precious jade, *huang-ching, t'ien-men-tung,* and *ts'ang-shu,* or the boiling of bone marrow from rind and of *kou-ch'i,* as well as all precious and unusual delicacies—they all were to receive suitable treatment. Because of this, Emperor Shih-tsu enjoyed sagelike longevity, extended to eternity, without any illness. Since the present revered emperor has assumed his treasured position, he has—in his spare time from his occupation with the manifold and important matters of the state—followed the rules established by his ancestors as, for instance, in the art of nourishment and protection [of one's life]. [Thus], the most suitable of all items [to be used] as drinks or food are offered [to the emperor] each day anew and, consequently, his sagelike body has achieved perfect peace. This official [Hu] Ssu-hui has been appointed—during the *yen-yu* years [1314–1320]—to be responsible for [the emperor's] drinks and dishes. In this position I have enjoyed heavenly favors for years. When I retire and ponder about this, it appears that I have nothing to repay [these favors]. Could I dare not to exhaust all my loyalty and sincerity in order to recompense at least one out of ten thousands of all-encompassing graces [extended to me]?! Therefore, in my daily spare time, together with the official P'u-lan-hsi of the Duke of Ch'ao, I set out to select from the exotic valuables and unusual delicacies, prepared as decoctions, pastes, and boilings, which I had offered [to the emperor] for his perusal as his waiter-in-person every morning and, furthermore, from the *pen-ts'ao* works of all authors and from the prescription techniques of famous physicians, as well as from grains, meat, fruits, and vegetables, all those [items] whose nature and taste fill [depletions] and supplement [the influences], and to compile a book in three chapters which I entitled

"The Proper and the Important in Drinks and Dishes." We have collected and added information that had not been adopted by [earlier] *pen-ts'ao* authors. We humbly hope that the emperor will forgive us our arrogance, and that he will consider our naive loyalty. In the confines of the capital, the protection and care of former sages is reflected, and [life proceeds] in accordance with the climatic conditions. Deficiencies are warded off and abundance was brought here. We hope that with the achievement of peace [the emperor's] sagelike longevity will be extended beyond all limits and that his virtue will be of benefit everywhere.

With due respect we present this collection of "The Proper and Important in Drinks and Dishes," and we humbly beg that his Majesty perceives the feelings of those below who are overcome with utmost awe, excitement, and agitation.[29]

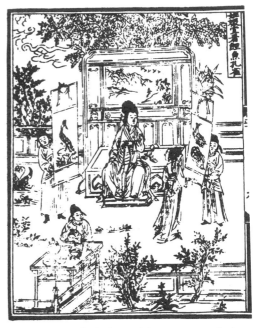

A pregnant lady-in-waiting contemplating paintings of carp and peacocks—*Yin-shan cheng-yao*

The *Yin-shan cheng-yao* contains three chapters, each of which forms an independent unit. Following the table of contents, the first chapter devotes a separate treatise to the life and achievements of each of the three legendary rulers and culture heroes—Fu Hsi, Shen-nung, and Huang-ti. Four sections follow, dealing with dietetic regulations and prohibitions:

"What To Avoid for the Nourishment of Life"
"Food To Be Avoided During Pregnancy"[30]
"Food To Be Avoided by Nursing Mothers"
"What To Avoid When Drinking Wine"

The argumentation and contents of these sections, which were largely based on concepts of magic correspondence, can be seen in the section on "Food To Be Avoided During Pregnancy":

The sages of antiquity were acquainted with a process of teaching the embryo while it was still in the womb. When a woman in antiquity was carrying a child, she did not lie on the edge of the bed and always sat in the middle of chairs. She did not lean toward one side when she stood and did not consume evil foods. If foods were not properly cut up small, she did not eat them; when the mat was not straightened out, she did not sit down. She did not look at any evil colors and did not listen to any frivolous noises. At night, she had blind musicians sing songs and tell unobjectionable incidents. Such behavior produced a child with a handsome appearance and above-average talents. Thus, when T'ai Jen [who lived in this manner] gave birth to Wen Wang, the latter was distinguished by outstanding intelligence and sagelike wisdom: if he became acquainted with only one [aspect of some matter], he knew it entirely! These are the possibilities of educating a child in the womb.

The sages [of antiquity] also frequently had emotions rise in pregnant women. Accordingly, [pregnant women] were to avoid observing persons occupied with mourning rites, those with mutilated bodies or bodies destroyed by illness, or people in poverty. Instead, [pregnant women] were supposed to view things that were outstanding and virtuous, happy and joyful, as well as beautiful. If [a mother-to-be] wished her child to possess great knowledge, she was supposed to observe carp and peacocks. If she wished a pretty child, she was supposed to look at pearls and precious stones. If [the future mother] expected a strong and powerful child, she was to observe flying falcons and runnings dogs. Thus, a good or fateful [development of the child] depends on the correspond-

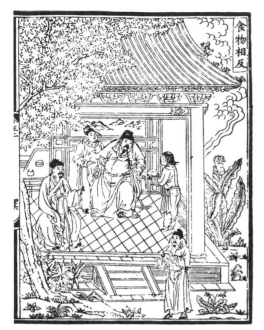

Emperor vomiting after consuming foods in the wrong sequence—*Yin-shan cheng-yao*

ing sensations [of the mother during the pregnancy]. And how much more important yet are the rules and prohibitions in connection with the consumption of food and drink!

Dietetic Prohibitions for the Period of Pregnancy:
[If a pregnant woman]
—eats hare meat, the child will be mute and lack an upper lip;
—eats the [meat of] mountain lamb, the child will be frequently ill;
—eats young chickens and dried fish, the child will often be afflicted with skin disorders;
—eats mulberries and duck, the child will enter the world as a breech baby;
—eats peacock and drinks wine, the child will have an obscene attitude, not control his passions, and disregard any sense of shame;
—eats chicken and glutinous rice, the child will bring forth a tapeworm;
—eats peacock and bean curds, the face of the child will be spotted and streaked;
—eats tortoise flesh, the child will have a short neck;
—eats donkey meat, the embryo will be carried beyond the normal term of pregnancy;
—eats icy soups, a miscarriage will result;
—eats mule meat, a difficult birth will result.[31]

Several illustrations accompanied the text. The illustrations, executed in great detail, portray not only, for example, pregnant ladies of the court observing paintings of carp but also such surprising motifs as an emperor vomiting because of stomach irritation.

The second half of the first chapter of the *Yin-shan cheng-yao,* entitled "Precious and Unusual Foods," consists of a list of ninety-one exotic foods, including detailed prescriptions and the respective medical indications.

The second chapter begins with the heading "All Kinds of Decoctions," followed by information on the preparation of a total of fifty-six foods in liquid form, from paste to tea. Additional sections carry the following headings:

"All [prepared] Waters [i.e., waters meant for human consumption]"
"Foods Consumed by the Immortal Ones"
"The Correspondences of the Four Seasons"
"One-Sidedness with Respect to the Five Tastes"
"The Cure of Illnesses with Food" (a list of 61 foods, with recipes and information on preparation and indications)
"Dietetic Prohibitions during a Period of Taking Drugs" (missing in the table of contents)
"General Prohibitions during an Extended Intake of Drugs" (missing in the table of contents)
"Harmful Foods"
"Foods Incompatible with One Another"
"Poisonings with Foods"
"Strange Changes [of Appearance] in Fowl and Quadrupeds"

Partial translations of two sections chosen from these titles may again serve as examples:

Dietetic Regulations During a Period of Taking Drugs.

During a period when medications are being taken, the following foods should not be consumed in large amounts: fresh coriander, garlic, and various other fresh vegetables, all smooth things, fatty pork, dog meat, oily and fatty things, fish, and chopped meat with a strong, biting odor. In addition, the sight of corpses and mothers in labor, as well as bloated and impure things should be avoided; aged and stinking foods should not be eaten. . . . During the taking of *pa-tou*, reed and bamboo shoots, as well as wild boar meat, should not be eaten.[32]

Harmful Foods.

It is possible to know which foods are harmful and to avoid them. Meat that does not change color during cooking must not be eaten. Meat that has not been slaughtered must not be eaten. Meat that smells and is spoiled must not be eaten. Meat that was offered in sacrifices and moves by itself must not be eaten. Horse and cow liver must not be eaten. During the second month no hare meat must be eaten. Lamb liver with holes must not be eaten. All livers of greenish color must not be eaten. Peaches and apricots with two pits must not be eaten. That which is out of time must not be eaten. Garlic must not be eaten in the third month; otherwise, the eyes become clouded.[33]

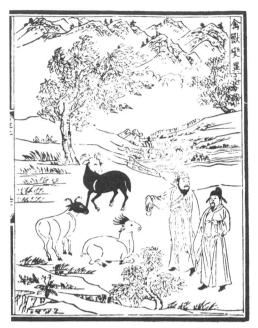

"Strange transformations in animals"—*Yin-shan cheng-yao*

Finally, the third chapter contains 204 monographs on food drugs from the areas rice/grains (these also include honey, vinegar, salt, and thirteen kinds of wine), quadrupeds, fowl, fish, fruits, vegetables, and seasonings/spices. Most monographs contain one illustration. The drug descriptions are very brief, consisting in most cases of only one line, which contains information on thermo-influence, taste, degree of medicinal potency, as well as brief details concerning indications.

The medical value of the *Yin-shan cheng-yao* is less important to us than its cultural-historical value.[34] The ingredients of meals, their preparations, and the spices reflect traces of an East-West cultural exchange. From the study of details in the *Yin-shan cheng-yao*, the size of the Mongolian Empire, which flourished when the book was written, can be estimated.

The composition of the committee responsible for the textual revision of the *Yin-shan cheng-yao*, and the person of the author himself, show a symbolic diversity. Hu Ssu-hui, whose name is given as Ho Ssu-hui in the *Ssu-k'u ch'üan-shu tsung-mu t'i-yao* because of a taboo, appears to have been a Moslem from the West.[35] Ishida Mikinosuke believed to have recognized in his name a sinicized form of Khosuki. This would explain the fact that, except for the monograph "pork," the *Yin-shan cheng-yao* mentions only one meal containing pork, although the Mongolian emperors themselves were not adherents of the Islam religion. The names of the editorial committee are given as Keng Chiu-ch'ien (perhaps a Chinese), Ch'ang-p'u-lan-hsi (a foreigner from the West?), Pai Chu (a Mongol?), and Chang-chin-chieh-nu (a Juchen?).[36]

chickens *(chi)*—*Yin-shan cheng-yao*

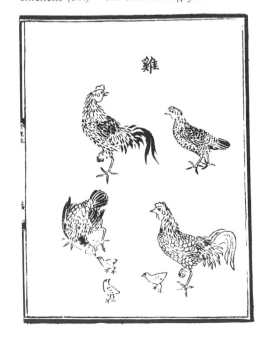

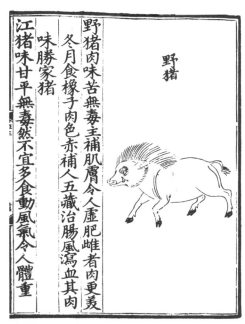

野豬肉味苦無毒主補肌膚令人虛肥雌者肉更美
冬月食橡子肉色赤補人五藏治腸風瀉血其肉
味勝家豬
江豬味甘平無毒然不宜多食動風氣令人體重

野猪

wild boar (yeh-chu)—Yin-shan cheng-yao

domesticated goose (o)—Yin-shan cheng-yao

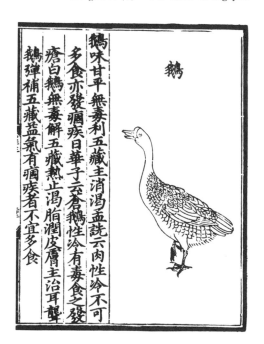

鵝味甘平無毒利五藏主消渴孟詵云肉性冷有毒食之發
多食亦發痼疾日華子云蒼鵝性冷有毒食之發
瘡白鵝無毒解五藏熱止渴脂潤皮膚主治耳聾
鵝卵補五藏益氣有痼疾者不宜多食

鵝

The foods and seasonings in the *Yin-shan cheng-yao* are as manifold as the nations that comprised the Mongolian Empire and with which it traded. The meat of sheep dominates. In the first chapter it appears in seventy-six of the ninety-one recipes under the heading "Precious and Unusual Foods." The emphasis clearly lies on northern dishes. Fish is mentioned in this list only four times. Some items, used in Southern China only for medications, belonged to daily meals in the North and are described in detail. Conversely, those items known as foods in Southern China are discussed much more briefly in the *Yin-shan cheng-yao* than in the Sung period pen-ts'ao works of the main tradition, in which the practices of the South were more frequently recorded.[37]

Numerous terms for dishes and their ingredients are foreign words, with Mongolian, Persian, Turkish, and Arabian origins. Let me give several examples.

A-la-chi designates an alcoholic beverage. This transcription stands for the Arabian word *araqi* ("strong liqueur"), known to us as *arrack*.

Pi-ssu-ta is derived from the Persian *pista* and Turkish *pistä* and corresponds to our usage of *pistachio*.

The term *hu-lu-pa* has its origin in the Arabian *hulba* and Persian *hulbat* and signifies the *fenugreek*.

A substance known in our pharmacies as *mastic* carries, in the *Yin-shan cheng-yao*, the name *ma-ssu-ta-chi;* the original Arabian-Persian word in this case was *mastaki*.[38]

Finally, *syrup* should be mentioned, which became known in China during the Mongol period but later fell into oblivion again. The Chinese term in the *Yin-shan cheng-yao* was *she-erh-pieh,* and apparently goes back to the Arabian *särbat*. It corresponds to the English term *sherbet*. The transcription *she-li-pieh* was used by a contemporary of Hu Ssu-hui, Chu Chen-heng (1281–1358), in his prescription work *Chü-fang fa-hui*. In a third work from the Yüan period, the "Complete Collection of All Things Necessary for the Household" (*Chü chia pi-yung shih-lei chüan-chi*), the similar term *she-li-pai* can be found.[39]

In thorough studies devoted to the identification of all forty-five foreign words in the *Yin-shan cheng-yao*, H. Franke and Y. S. Lao were able to clear up, with a few exceptions, the questions of origin. It is interesting that Franke was able to establish that the terms used for noodles and noodle dishes were all borrowed from Turkish, which suggests that such preparations were perhaps introduced in China during the Mongol period. This would include the *chiao-tzu* products, so admired and widely known in China today.[40]

Plants, animals, and animal parts are designated in the *Yin-shan cheng-yao* by Mongolian loanwords; Arabian-Persian names are usually found for spices, beverages, and vegetables.

The author of the *Yin-shen cheng-yao* doubtlessly compiled his work for the "requirements" of life at the court, not for the general public. Outside of the court there was scarcely anyone who could afford such choice and extravagant foods, or who could carry out the totally independent life-style that Hu Ssu-hui advocated. From the strikingly frequent references to certain illnesses in the indication information of the prescriptions, conclusions can be drawn about the values placed upon alcoholic and sexual pleasures at the court of the Mongolian emperor.[41]

In 1330, the completed manuscript of the *Yin-shan cheng-yao* was handed over to the throne. Yü Chi, a Han-lin official, wrote the preface. However, the book did not appear until 1456, when it was published at the command of Emperor Tai-tsung (1428–1457) by the Court Chancellery. The emperor is said to have contributed a preface to the work. The *Yin-shan cheng-yao* was later included, without the Ming preface, in the large collection *Ssu-pu tsung-k'an*. This edition was the basis for all later versions.[42]

At nearly the same time Hu Ssu-hui wrote his dietetic work for the emperor and his court, another servant of the court, the imperial physician Wu Jui, completed a dietetic manual which, unlike the *Yin-shan cheng-yao*, may have benefited larger segments of the population. Wu Jui's goal consisted in selecting and describing from those foods in everyday use the ones that were particularly suitable for preventing possible afflictions and curing various illnesses. In addition, he also adapted for his work numerous prescriptions containing medications.

Wu Jui arranged the monographs in the following order: rice/grains, melons/vegetables, fruits, flying fowl, quadrupeds, scaly animals/crustaceans, spices. The contents of the individual monographs comprised, in addition to the names of the drugs, information on the thermo-influence and taste, as well as various indications.

It is probable that the *Jih-yung pen-ts'ao* remained unpublished for a long time, with the manuscript being handed down through several generations of Wu Jui's family. As a result, a portion of the text was lost. Finally, a descendant in the sixth generation, Ching-su, decided to publish the work. However, he died prematurely, and it was left to his son to realize the plan. This occurred during the governmental period *chia-ching* (1522–1566); the work included the preface of one Li Fan:

> [Jui] chose drugs among those [described] in the *pen-ts'ao* works as suitable for daily use those that could also function as foods. Foods serve to nourish man, and one must not stop taking them for even one day only. But [among foods] are those that harm man. Knowledgeable men consider that fact, but most people know nothing about it. Therefore, it is not at all rare that their bodies, which are a thousand times more valuable than gold, are harmed unwittingly in the short time needed to use chopsticks. Jui deeply regretted [this possibility] and thus organized a total of more than 540 food [drugs] into eight chapters. He entitled [his work] "Materia Medica for Daily Use" and then published it. In taking to heart the basic principle—"What is past cannot be pursued; one should offer a helping hand to the future of mankind!"—[Jui proved] that he understood how to realize his moral sentiment and the attitude of humaneness![43]

The first edition of the *Jih-yung pen-ts'ao* was subsequently lost. A second and final edition from 1620, undertaken by Ch'ien Yün-chih, has been preserved. Ch'ien prepared a revised version, publishing it

9. The *Jih-yung pen-ts'ao*

Jih-yung pen-ts'ao
"Materia Medica for Daily Use"
3 chapters
Author: Wu Jui (ca. 1330)
    tzu: Jui-ch'ing
      from: Hai-ning in Che-chiang
Written: ca. 1330
Published: between 1522 and 1566

in three chapters in a double edition along with a *Shih-wu pen-ts'ao* in seven chapters (see D, I, 11).[44]

10. The *Chiu-huang pen-ts'ao*

Chiu-huang pen-ts'ao
"Materia Medica for Survival during Famines"
2 chapters / 414 drug descriptions
Author: Chu Hsiao, Chou Ting wang (? –1425)
Written: ca. 1403–1406
Published: 1406

Several authors of dietetic pen-ts'ao works attempted to write manuals for survival in difficult times, during famines, or also in the seclusion of the wilderness. Chu Hsiao's work, the *Chiu-huang pen-ts'ao*, belongs in this group.

Chu Hsiao was the fifth child of the Emperor T'ai-tsu (1328–1399), the founder of the Ming dynasty. In 1370, Chu received the title of Wu-wang, and in 1378, that of a Chou-wang. He is usually cited, under the name Chou Ting-wang, as the author of the *Chiu-huang pen-ts'ao*. Li Shih-chen mistakenly wrote that Hsien-wang, a son of Chu Hsiao, was the author of this work.[45]

Chu Hsiao had selected more than 400 herbs and trees, 138 of them from the *Cheng-lei pen-ts'ao,* which could function both as foods and drugs. Supposedly, he had all of them planted in his garden in order to test them himself. He commissioned a committee to observe and describe these plants in all stages of development. He had illustrations prepared for the individual monographs which portrayed the respective original plants. They have been sketched extremely true to life.

The entire work is divided into four parts by two double chapters. The Chinese original did not contain a preface or afterword. The first edition appeared in 1406, with numerous new editions following at the beginning of the sixteenth century. These new editions were frequently revised texts, and the number of drugs, chapters, and the contents no longer corresponded exactly with the original. The oldest edition preserved in China dates from 1586. It is unknown whether copies of the subsequent edition from 1593, containing a preface by the writer Hu Wen-huan from the same year, have been preserved.

In 1716, an edition appeared in Japan which combined Chu Hsiao's *Chiu-huang pen-ts'ao* with the *Yeh-ts'ai p'u* ("Book of Vegetables in the Wilderness") by Wang P'an (ca. 1506–1566) and the *Chiu-huang-yeh p'u* ("The Book of Survival in the Wilderness and During Famine") by Yao K'o-ch'eng, two works with similar objectives.[46] The last edition to date was published in the People's Republic of China in 1959.

The *Chiu-huang pen-ts'ao* was not the only medical work Chu Hsiao felt compelled to write, perhaps owing to the misery of the population during the disorders caused by the downfall of Mongolian rule and the rise of the Ming dynasty. In addition, he compiled the *P'u-chi fang,* an extensive collection of prescriptions published in 168 chapters. Li Shih-chen adopted numerous prescriptions from this work for his *Pen-ts'ao kang mu.*[47]

11. The *Shih-wu pen-ts'ao* (Lü Ho)

Shih-wu pen-ts'ao (Lü Ho)
"Materia Medica of Nutrition"
4 chapters / 391 drug descriptions
Author: Lü Ho (sixteenth century)
Written: mid-sixteenth century
Published: 1571

Various dietetic pen-ts'ao works were given the general title *Shih-wu pen-ts'ao* ("Materia Medica based on Food"). Lü Ho was the first to publish a work under this title. In arranging the 391 monographs, he oriented himself on the *Jih-yung pen-ts'ao* by Wu Jui, whose arrangement he changed slightly by adding the section "waters" to the beginning. Lü Ho divided the contents of his work as follows (the figures indicate the number of monographs in each section): waters (35), grains (35), vegetables (87), fruits (57), fowl (56), quadrupeds (38), fish (and other aquatic animals) (60), spices (23).

The individual monographs vary greatly in length. In many cases, one line is sufficient; in others, the author required two or three pages for the drug description. Lü Ho was influenced by the Chin-Yüan theories, but they do not shape the entire work. A large number of monographs contain purely pragmatic information, without any hint of theoretical additions. The description of the drug *ping-lang,* known to us as areca, or betel nut, may serve as an example:

> *Ping-lang.* Taste: acrid; [thermo-influence:] warm; no distinct medicinal strength. [The drug promotes] the digestion of grains and eliminates water. It removes mucous congestions. It relieves sensations of repletion, breaks through [obstructions in the flow of] the body's influences and drains obstructions in the body's depots and palaces. It is added to all medications meant to descend [in the body]. It kills the Three Worms and the tapeworm. If [this drug] is consumed in large amounts, it damages one's original influences. The people in Fukien and Kanton wrap the *ping-lang* in the leaves of the *chü-chiang* [plant]. The resulting taste is acrid-aromatic, and a pleasant feeling in the area of the diaphragm is produced. If lime prepared from shells is added, the effect should be even better. However, [after the use of this preparation], a red substance must be spit out, which is not particularly aesthetic. Another name [for *chü-chiang*] is *fu-liu;* thus the saying "the effect of *ping-lang* is based upon the addition of *fu-liu.*"[48]

In many other monographs the initial description by Lü Ho himself is followed by further commentaries, usually quoted from the works of the Chin-Yüan authors Wang Hao-ku and Chu Chen-heng. Occasionally, there are also sections from the *Su-wen,* and from nonmedical sources, such as the *Lü-shih ch'un-ch'iu.* For a number of drugs, Lü Ho made reference to their inclusion in the yin or yang categories and gave brief details on the conduits they were capable of penetrating. An example of this is the following passage from the beginning of the monograph on peach pits (*t'ao-jen*), which otherwise contains no theoretical statements:

betel nut *(ping-lang)—Shao-hsing pen-ts'ao*

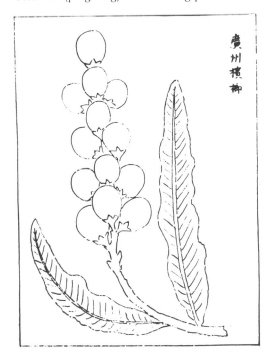

> *T'ao-jen.* Taste: bitter-sweet; [thermo-]influence: neutral. If the bitter taste is stronger than the sweet, it is a matter of the *yang*-in-*yin* constellation. No distinct medicinal strength. Penetrates into the hand- and foot-ceasing-*yin* conduits. Masters blood effusions, stagnations of blood, coagulations of blood, blood dryness, constipation, and evil influences. [The drug] kills small worms and functions as a laxative.[49]

At the conclusion of each of the eight sections, Lü Ho added a general treatise on all waters, grains, and so forth. Concerning fruits he wrote:

> All above-mentioned fruits are products of the earth, and [therefore] *yin* [items]. They are all subdivided again into *yin* and *yang,* hot and cold but, on the whole, belong to the *yin* [category] and are, therefore, suitable for nourishing *yin* [influences]. The illnesses of man are fre-

quently due to a depletion of *yin* [influences]. In such cases, it is advisable to eat [fruits]. The consumption of fruits produces cold [in the body]. Some [fruits], however, produce [the sensation] of moist heat. Dry [fruits] produce indurations and dryness. They are difficult to digest and create constipation. In particular, small children must be prevented from eating them. This is the origin of the proverb: "With well-cooked food the nobleman is served first; with mature fruit the nobleman is served last." The reason for this is that the people of antiquity were extremely careful [only to select what is] good.

But there are so many types of fruit in the world. Each region produces those appropriate for it; all the names and colors vary greatly, and all the [thermo-]influences and tastes have some [affliction] they can be used against. It is no longer possible to state everything in detail.[50]

The oldest preserved version of Lü Ho's *Shih-wu pen-ts'ao* is also most likely the first edition. It is a version from the year 1571, revised by Wang Kuei, to which Kuo Ch'un-chen contributed a preface.

At approximately the same time, or a little later, Hsüeh Chi adopted Lü's text and published it unchanged as the third and fourth chapters of the *Pen-ts'ao yüeh-yen*, discussed below.[51]

12. The *Pen-ts'ao yüeh-yen*

Pen-ts'ao yüeh-yen
"Survey of Pharmaceutics"
2 chapters / 676 drug descriptions
Author: Hsüeh Chi (sixteenth century)
    tzu: Hsin-fu
    hao: Li-chai
    from: Wu in Chiang-su
Written: mid-sixteenth century
Published: between 1550 and 1643

During his lifetime, Hsüeh Chi was a renowned physician. His reputation was based particularly on successes in the treatment of skin and ulcer afflictions and of organically caused illnesses. Hsüeh Chi's father, Hsüeh K'ai, had already made a name for himself with his medical knowledge, and during the governmental period *hung-chih* (1488–1505) was active as a medical scholar in the Imperial Department of Medicine. His son advanced even further. The emperor appointed Hsüeh Chi as personal physician during the *cheng-te* period (1506–1521).[52]

Hsüeh Chi proved to be an industrious author of medical works. He himself wrote numerous works in the most varied fields and reedited others. A compilation of his writings appeared in the collection *Hsüeh-shih i-an*. This work contains seventy-eight chapters, sixty of which come from Hsüeh Chi's own pen.[53]

The *Pen-ts'ao yüeh-yen* is composed of two parts. The first part carries the detailed title *Yao-hsing pen-ts'ao yüeh-yen* ("Outline of Medicinal Pharmaceutics"). In two chapters, containing 285 monographs, the author described what he felt to be the most important drugs for daily use. The monographs were arranged as follows: herbs (134 monographs), trees (56), fruits (18), vegetables (12), rice/grains (8), metals/minerals (26), man (5), fowl/quadrupeds (12), worms/fish (14).

The second part is entitled *Shih-wu pen-ts'ao yüeh-yen* ("Outline of Dietetic Pharmaceutics"). Its text coincides exactly with that of the *Shih-wu pen-ts'ao* by Lü Ho—whose name is nowhere mentioned—and thus needs not be discussed once more.

The style of the first part is quite similar to that of the *Shih-wu pen-ts'ao*. A slight suggestion of Chin-Yüan theories is indicated in the monographs themselves and by means of quotations from the authors of that period. There are often references to the yinyang categorizations of drugs and their capabilities of penetrating specific conduits. More far-reaching theoretical explanations are seldom included.

Several drugs are represented by a monograph both in the first part of the *Pen-ts'ao yüeh-yen,* probably written by Hsüeh Chi himself, as well as in the second part, composed by Lü Ho. To some extent, the contents of such monographs are contradictory, so that the entire work does not impress one as an organic whole. Compare, for instance, the monograph of the drug *ping-lang* in Lü Ho's *Shih-wu pen-ts'ao* (*yüeh-yen*) (see p. 222), with an excerpt from the description of the same drug in the *Yao-hsing pen-ts'ao yüeh-yen:*

> *Ping-lang.* Taste: acrid-bitter; [thermo-]influence: warm; no distinct medicinal strength. [The drug belongs to the] *yin*-in-*yang.* It descends [in the body]. It penetrates the chest and abdomen and breaks through obstructions in the flow of the body's influences; it cannot be stopped. It penetrates the intestines and the stomach, removes mucous congestions and moves directly downward. In all medications that are supposed to fall through [in the body, this drug] shows itself to possess the properties of a piece of iron or of a stone. After treatment, a powerful success occurs. As quickly as a running horse [this drug] penetrates the hand- and foot-*yang*-brilliance conduits. Its taste is bitter, and therefore the drug is able to draw together; but [the drug] also carries a slight acrid [taste] and thus has the sinking properties of iron and stone. As a result, it can be used in conjunction with all medications that are supposed to descend [in the body]. . . . In another work, the following is recorded: "[*Ping-lang*] kills tapeworms." The drug, however, cannot kill worms at all. Because of its descending property, it is able to force worms downward out of the body. This drug is frequently taken in Kanton and Fukien. There it is steamed in the moisture of the warm earth. The population of these areas suffers frequently from an [abnormally] rising flow of influences; thus, they take [*ping-lang*] to depress [this flow]. If the drug is taken over long periods of time, it injures one's original influences. If it is taken in large doses, it even drains the influences in the uppermost areas of the body. This [drug] is even better than green-peel *chih-shih.*[54]

The *Pen-ts'ao yüeh-yen* has survived in only two editions; it is also probable that no more were printed. There is a Chinese edition of the Ming period and a Japanese edition from 1660.[55]

If Hsüeh Chi had copied the text of the *Shih-wu pen-ts'ao* completely unchanged from Lü Ho, Wang Ying made the effort to change the order of the drugs somewhat and to undertake some improvements of the text when he wrote and published "his" *Shih-wu pen-ts'ao*— under the name of Li Kao, however. Lü Ho's work once again formed the basis. This work was revised once more by Ch'ien Yün-chih and was published in seven chapters, again under the name of Li Kao, in the already mentioned double edition with Wu Jui's *Jih-yung pen-ts'ao* (see p. 220). In addition to the changed text of Lü Ho, the *Shih-wu pen-ts'ao* part of this edition includes the following three new sections:

"Commands and Prohibitions Concerning Food"
"Poison Antidotes"

13. The *Shih-wu pen-ts'ao* (Wang Ying)

Shih-wu pen-ts'ao (Wang Ying)
"Materia Medica of Nutrition"
7 chapters
Authors: Wang Ying (ca. 1600)
       Ch'ien Yün-chih (beginning of the
       seventeenth century)
Written: ca. 1600–1620
Published: 1620

"The Conditions for a Harmonious Preservation [of Life] in Accordance with the Course of the Months, According to Sun Chen-jen"

These sections were probably added by Wang Ying.[56]

14. The *Pei-k'ao shih-wu pen-ts'ao kang mu*

Pei-k'ao shih-wu pen-ts'ao kang mu
"Materia Medica of Nutrition, Organized according to Drug Descriptions and Technical Aspects and Arranged for Reference Purposes"
Short title: *Shih-wu pen-ts'ao*
22 chapters / 1699 drug descriptions
Author: Yao K'o-ch'eng (seventeenth century)
    hao: Hao-lai yeh-jen, Lin-an tao-jen
    from: Wu (?)
Written: 1600–1638
Published: 1638

Under the name of Li Shih-chen, and with a title that refers to Li's *Pen-ts'ao kang mu*, an otherwise little-known author named Yao K'o-ch'eng published the most extensive work in the dietetic pen-ts'ao literature. It is highly probable that the details concerning the authors of the prefaces, like those of the author of the work himself, are falsified; one of the prefaces was attributed to Li Shen-chen, the other carries the name of Ch'en Chi-ju (1558–1639), a scholar and author living in seclusion during the Ming period.[57]

In a preliminary chapter, Yao K'o-ch'eng combined four treatises on dietetics:

"Foods" by Li Shih-chen
"Recipes for Rapid Aid against Starvation" by Sun Ssu-mo
"Simple Recipes without Grains for Rescue from Starvation" by Liu Ching-hsien (3rd–4th century)
"Guidelines for Cooking Beans" by Huang T'ing-chien (eleventh century)

In each case, the authorship is questionable.

The first chapter of the actual monograph section contains a work entitled *Chiu-huang-yeh p'u* ("The Book of Survival in the Wilderness and during Famine"), separate from the subsequent main part of the *Shih-wu pen-ts'ao*. It is reminiscent of the *Chiu-huang pen-ts'ao* and other works with similar titles, which had been conceived as manuals for times of famine and for survival with the aid of common plants in the wilderness.

A total of 120 drugs are described in the *Chiu-huang-yeh p'u*. Sixty monographs were taken from Wang P'an's *Yeh-ts'ai p'u;* the remaining sixty were written by Yao K'o-ch'eng himself. This small work is divided into two sections, herbs and trees, which in turn are further subdivided:

Herbs: edible stalk-leaves, edible leaves, edible moss, edible roots, edible sprout-leaves, edible fruits, edible root-sprouts.
Trees: edible roots, edible fruits, edible radical leaves, edible leaves, edible blossoms, edible bark, edible sprouts.

Each monograph contains an illustration of the plant. The text is divided into two sections. A prose commentary briefly characterizes the plant; such information may be lacking for very well-known herbs, being replaced with a short story. The second part of the text is always in verse. Two examples are given below:

Ho-shou-wu; the root is edible. In earlier times, Mr. Ho ate this [plant]. His hair, which had already turned white, became black again;

both eyes became clear again. Later, the people gathered and consumed the roots. It can also be used against hunger.

Ho-shou-wu both of my eyes still were jade-green.

> I was not very old, my hair was already white.
> Hunger and anxious thoughts often distressed me.
> *Shou-wu* stilled the hunger and cured the pain.
> Returned my youth and banished old age.
> Its effect to provide relief in times of pressing need
> seems to be especially good.[58]

Ch'e-ch'ien-ts'ao;[59] the leaves are edible. Other names are *tang-tao* and *ch'e-lun;*[60] it carries such names because it grows primarily alongside paths. The sprouts appear at the beginning of spring; the leaves cover the earth. They are round and slightly pointed. On their upper side are thread-like edges, like the leaves of *pai-o-hua.* The plant should be gathered as long as it is tender and eaten with water.

Ch'e-ch'ien-ts'ao grows alongside of paths.

> Horse's hoof, wagon wheel hub.
> Powerful spring wind.
> Just now, no traces of man for a thousand miles.
> The herbs of the wilderness grow abundantly,
> even at desolate places.[61]

Only at the conclusion of the *Chiu-huang-yeh p'u* do the twenty-two chapters of the *Shih-wu pen-ts'ao* begin. They are arranged as follows: Waters (with 5 subdivisions), grains (7), vegetables (5), fruits (6), scaly animals (2), crustaceans (2), snakes/worms (2), fowl (4), quadrupeds (4), spices (4), herbs (8), trees (5), fire (1), metals (1), precious stones/minerals (1), soils (1). This total of sixteen sections corresponds to the number, but not the order, in the *Pen-ts'ao kang mu.* The total number of subdivisions—58—is four fewer than in the *Pen-ts'ao kang mu.*

The first section, devoted to "waters," is particularly interesting. This description alone comprises four chapters of the entire work. The first chapter is divided into the four categories: "Waters of Heaven," "Waters of Earth," "Famous Waters," and "Poisonous Waters." Chapters 2 through 4 constitute what could be termed a first detailed guide to Chinese mineral springs and spas. They contain the fifth subdivision of the section "waters," carrying the heading "Famous Springs," with descriptions of the curative effects of mineral waters from 656 places in the empire. Following the name, the individual monographs contain a brief reference to place, and then a more or less detailed commentary on the curative effects of the spring and, if known, peculiar occurrences connected with it. This is illustrated by two examples:

> The water of the Runs-Like-A-Tiger spring.
>   [The spring is] located seventy miles south of Lu-chiang hsien, beside the *kuang-ming* temple.
> The water of the Runs-Like-A-Tiger spring. Taste: sweet. Masters clarification of the heart, enrichment of the lung, expulsion of heat. It stills thirst, cures from adversely rising breath, and generates bodily fluids.[62]

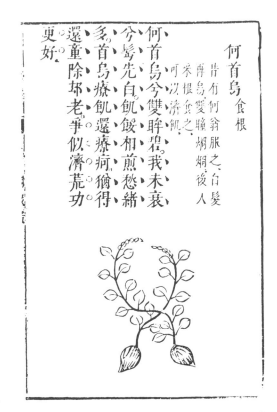

knotgrass root *(ho-shou-wu)—Chiu-huang-yeh p'u*

The water of the Life-Generation spring.

    [The spring is] located in the city of Kuang-hsin fu, to the west of the Inspection Office.

Weng Ta-li, from Yü-yao, wrote the following report during the Ming dynasty: In the year *ping-wu* of the governmental period *chia-ching* [1546], I undertook a tour of inspection through Kiangsi as senior secretary in the Ministry for Punishment. In the fifth month of the following year I reached Kuang-hsin and was given accommodations in the residence of the local censor. When I wanted to leave, in order to report on my mission, all of my attendants fell ill with an epidemic. Strange creatures resembling large dogs appeared in the censorate. Although everything had been hermetically sealed, these creatures entered daily at midnight and left only after consuming everything in the kitchen. At this time, a great epidemic had spread through Hsin-ch'eng. The people beat gongs and struck drums, in order to exorcise the demons of the illness. The noise continued night and day. When my attendants heard this, they were all very frightened and thought they had to die. They wept and informed me about the occurrences. Thereupon, I adjusted clothing and cap and, with a concealed light, waited secretly in the kitchen [for the questionable creatures]. Indeed, they appeared at midnight. I gave the order for a servant to intercept and attack them. He struck several hundred blows to the creatures before succumbing himself. The fears of the patients were a little relieved after this occurrence. An immortal then appeared to me suddenly in a dream and spoke: "The illness of your assistants can only be cured by T'ien-i sheng![63] He will arrive tomorrow; tomorrow is the day of the new moon in the sixth month!" I arose early and warned the gatekeepers: "If someone named T'ien-i sheng comes, don't let him wait at the door!" However, by afternoon, they still had not announced a new arrival. Filled with doubts and speculations, I strolled down the steps to take a short walk. [I] suddenly [noticed] a moist spot on the west side of the building. With a tool of some sort, I uncovered the cause: a clear spring bubbled forth from the depth of more than a foot. It emerged like a spout of water through a hole in an otherwise dry location. I drank from the spring and ascertained a cold and sweet taste. Delighted I cried out: "This is the water of T'ien-i, of which the immortal spoke!" I immediately ordered each of the patients to drink several ladles full; they were soon cured. As a result, all of those afflicted in the city drank from the [spring], and no one remained ill. I then gave the order for workers to bring stones and build a well. It was given the name "Life-Generation."

    The water of the Life-Generation spring has a sweet taste. It masters illnesses caused by cold, cold and heat in the body, headaches and pain in the eyes, pains in bones and joints, as well as indisposition combined with thirst and a strong sensation of heat. [It is advisable to drink this water] during epidemics, when the climate does not correspond to the four seasons and, as a result, all men fall ill; finally, the water is advisable for feverish diarrhea, cholera, as well as for mental confusion and depression resulting from rising influences caused by mucus.[64]

The remaining monographs comprise chapters 5 through 21. Like the text in the first four chapters, they contain no illustrations. Following the example of the *Pen-ts'ao yüeh-yen*, Yao K'o-ch'eng adopted the practice of adding another general, summarizing treatise at the end of the individual monographs. The contents of these treatises are similar to the corresponding texts in the *Pen-ts'ao yüeh-yen*, as the following information shows, which Yao K'o-ch'eng added at the conclusion of the description of fruits:

All poisonous fruits.
All fruits that have not yet developed stones produce ulcerous afflictions, as well as [sensations of] cold and heat [in the body] when consumed.
All fruits that have fallen on the ground and, as a result, have been infested by harmful worms produce, when consumed, the nine leaks [i.e., ulcers in the arms and on the neck].
All fruits with two stones are poisonous and fatal.
All melons with two stalks are poisonous and fatal. The melons that sink in water are also fatal.
All fruits that suddenly show changes from their normal appearance conceal with certainty a poisonous snake beneath the root [of the mother plant]. Consumption would be fatal.
All fruits listed above are products of the earth and are [therefore] yin-items. Although one may further differentiate them according to yin and yang, cold and hot [subdivisions], generally spoken, they are yin items and are, therefore, suitable to nourish yin [influences]. The illnesses of man are frequently caused by a depletion of yin [-influences]. . . .[65]

Chapter 22, under the heading "Everything Important for the Preservation of Life," included twenty sections dealing with dietetic injunctions and prohibitions, details on the toxicity of certain animals, and much more.

But this extensive work does not end here. Yao K'o-ch'eng also devoted a detailed treatise to the notorious ku poison. Under the title "Prescriptions for the Treatment of Ku [Poisonings]" (Chih-ku lun fang), Yao K'o-ch'eng wrote what is probably the most comprehensive presentation in the pen-ts'ao literature of all information concerning the causes, symptoms, and methods of treatment of ku poisonings. The four chapters of this appendix indicate the scope of his presentation:

"Symptoms of Ku Poisoning"
"Methods for Determining the Presence of a Ku Poisoning"
"Preventive Measures against Ku Poisonings"
"Prescriptions for the Treatment of Ku Poisonings"

Yao K'o-ch'eng's ambitions of connecting his work with Li Shih-chen in order to secure for it a certain admiration and circulation with the public, apparently remained largely unfulfilled; the first edition of the Shih-wu pen-ts'ao also remained the last. Today, only a few copies are preserved in libraries.

The Shih-wu pen-ts'ao is the last work of the dietetic pen-ts'ao literature to be discussed here. It is true that numerous additional works of this type were written up to the beginning of this century; however, they were unable to establish new trends.

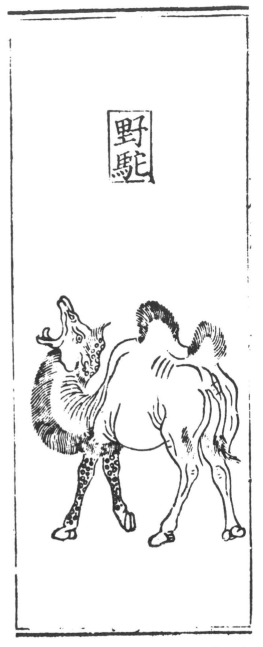

wild camel (yeh-t'o)—Ch'ung-hsiu cheng-ho pen-ts'ao

II. MONOGRAPHIC PEN-TS'AO WORKS

It does not require very much space to describe that genre of the pen-ts'ao literature whose works are devoted to the detailed presentation of one single drug. Only a few drugs were so highly valued. As we shall see, the examples selected for the present work (as well as the rest) are often those drugs to which an ability to prolong life was ascribed.

1. The *Chih-ts'ao t'u*

Chih-ts'ao t'u
"Illustrated (treatise) on the *chih* herb"
1 chapter / 1 drug description
Author: unknown
Written: before 500
Published: date unknown

In the bibliographical section *Ching-chi chih* of the history of the Sui dynasty, in the section "Medical and Prescription[-Literature]" (*I-fang*), we find a reference to what may have been the first Chinese *pen-ts'ao* work devoted to one drug.[66]

The plant *chih* was already mentioned in the *Pen-ching*. It is possible that the reference was to certain fungi. In the *Pen-ching*, the description of the chih drugs held a prominent position among the herbs, similar to that held by cinnabar, most highly coveted by the Taoists, among the precious stones and minerals. The first six monographs in the upper class of drugs were devoted to the green, red, yellow, white, black, and purple variants of chih. With the exception of the purple variant, the other five corresponded to the colors associated with the Five Phases of Change. It is also striking that their sequence in the *Pen-ching* corresponds to the mutual production order of the Five Phases. When one compares the references to tastes and indications of the first five chih monographs, the result is another parallel to the theories of the Five Phases:

chih-variant	taste	affected depot	secondary name
green	sour	liver	dragon-chih
red	bitter	heart	cinnabar-chih
yellow	sweet	spleen	gold-chih
white	acrid	lung	jade-chih
black	salty	kidneys	dark-chih

In the *Pen-ching*, all of the different chih drugs are ascribed the effect, after they have been taken for many years, of relieving the body of its material weight, of prolonging life, and—with the exception, however, of the purple variant—of transforming the consumer into a supranatural being.[67]

Consequently, the entire complex of chih drugs must have been given an enormous significance, at least in Taoist circles. Five variants reflected the five phases of the whole process of nature; combined, they had to appear to be the ideal drug for a uniform strengthening of all five depots of the body and of the functions connected with them.

This symbolic power may explain why it is the drug chih that constitutes the subject of the first known monographic pen-ts'ao work. Well-known thinkers and naturalists such as Wang Ch'ung (27–97), Chang Hua (232–300), Ko Hung (282–341), and Sun Ssu-mo (581–682?) studied this drug.[68] In the bibliography of the Sung history, the

229

authorship of the *Chih-ts'ao t'u* is even associated with Sun Ssu-mo; the work lists a *Sun Ssu-mo chih-ts'ao t'u*—containing, however, thirty chapters.[69]

In the *Cheng-lei pen-ts'ao*, we find in the list of source works a *Shen-hsien chih-ts'ao t'u* ("Illustrated [Treatise on the] Chih-herb of the Immortals"). The title again points out the promise associated with this drug.[70]

Even the *Pen-ts'ao kang mu* still devotes a very detailed monograph to the chih-drug. Li Shih-chen discusses its effects in a long commentary. He quotes various authors from the past, including Ko Hung, and lists in detail all the effects associated with a large number of different chih species. He cites the magic techniques developed in ancient times to obtain this drug in the mountains, referring to the white dog, the white chicken, and the salt that have to be taken along, to the steps of Yü that have to be performed, to suitable times of the day and year, as well as to the chastity of the person trying to discover this precious drug. Li Shih-chen believed that this substance resembles a human tumor in that it constitutes an outgrowth of rotten influences from the matter on which it develops, and he rejected as erroneous any belief in the drug's ability to transform a person into an immortal.[71]

The contents of the *Chih-ts'ao t'u* have not been preserved. This is rather strange, because the briefness of the work would have made possible its complete reproduction in an encyclopedia or another suitable work. Therefore, all we can learn about this work comes from the title: the monograph was illustrated.

The *Ho-shou-wu lu*, also called *Ho-shou-wu chuan* in some quotations and bibliographies,[72] is the oldest monographic pen-ts'ao work preserved in its entirety. The text which comprises a total of only 609 characters, has been transmitted to us in the collected works of Li Ao. More or less abridged versions can be found in various other works, from the *T'u-ching pen-ts'ao*, whose version was included in the *Cheng-lei pen-ts'ao*, to the *Pen-ts'ao kang mu*. The complete version from the *Shuo-fu* is given in the following:

2. The *Ho-shou-wu lu*

Ho-shou-wu lu
"Notes on [the drug] *Ho-shou-wu*"
1 chapter / 1 drug description
Author: Li Ao (?–844)
       tzu: Hsi-chih
       shih-hao: Wen
       from: Chao-chün
Written: 813
Published: date unknown

Notes on [the Drug] *ho-shou-wu*.
    The Buddhist priest Wen-hsiang was devoted to the art of nourishing life. On the eighteenth day of the third month in the seventh year of the governmental period *yüan ho* [812], he was on the Mao-shan [Mountain] early in the morning, and there, in the vicinity of the Hua yang cave, he met an old man who said to him: "You have the appearance of an immortal. I will reveal to you a secret formula. An ancestor of Ho Shou-wu, who lived in the district of Nan-ho in Shunchou, was originally named T'ien-erh and was later called Neng-ssu. He was born impotent and had turned to drinking wine. At the age of fifty-eight, he returned home drunk one night and was overcome by sleep while still outside. When he awoke again, he noticed on the field two shoots of climbing plants, which stood about three feet apart. The sprouts of these shoots were twisted around each other and then separated, three or four times. T'ien-erh considered this to be strange and, therefore, dug out the root of the plant and asked all the people in the village and in the wilderness, but no one was able to tell him its name. Thereupon he dried the plant in the sun. A man living nearby was an

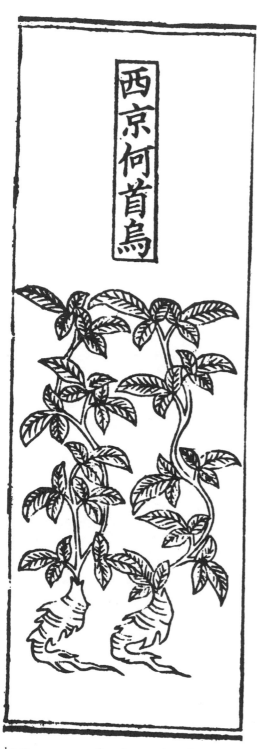

西京何首烏

knotgrass root (ho-shou-wu)—Ch'ung-hsiu cheng-ho pen-ts'ao

excellent jester and said to T'ien-erh: 'You are impotent, you are old and childless. This climbing plant struck you as peculiar, now surely it is supposed to serve you as a divine drug. Why don't you take it?' Thereupon T'ien-erh sifted out a fine powder of the drug and took it with wine. After seven days, he suddenly recognized clearly the principles of human life. After several tens of days had passed, he felt unburdened and strong, and he could barely control his sexual desire. He married a widow named Tsen and continued to take the drug regularly after that. He increased the individual dose to two ch'ien. After over 700 days, all of his previous complaints had disappeared, he regained his youthful appearance and begot a son. The people in the neighborhood were very astonished at this. During the following ten years, T'ien-erh became the father of several sons. He ascribed all this to the drug and said: 'This was caused by the climbing plant. When one takes it, one can live to be 160 years old, and yet it is neither listed in the old prescriptions nor in the pen-ts'ao literature!' I," continued the old man, "have received this [secret prescription] from my teacher, who was told about it in Nan-ho. Taking it helped me, also, to father children. Originally, I preferred peace of mind, and under no circumstances did I want to take this drug, because it is harmful to peace of mind. My spouse took it accidentally and we attained the greatest happiness. Subsequently, I recorded all the effects of the [drug] for T'ien-erh, and I changed his name to Neng-ssu ['capable of begetting']. He died at the age of 160 and left nineteen sons and daughters. His son Yen, who also took the drug, reached the age of 160 as well, and left thirty sons and daughters. Yen's son Shou-wu lived to the age of 130 by means of this drug, and fathered twenty-one children. An Ch'i[73] reports the following about this climbing plant: 'It has a sweet taste, warm [thermo-influence], and belongs to the drugs without markedly curative power. It masters the five hemorrhoidal complaints as well as all hidden illnesses and emaciating influences in the loins and abdomen. It expands the muscles and helps people to have many children because it increases one's semen. Taken as a food, this substance supplements the body's influences and strength, nourishes the skin, and prolongs life. Other names [of the plant] are: yeh-miao ["wild sprout"], chiao-ching ["joining stalks"], yeh-ho ["meeting at night"], ti-ching ["earth-semen"], and t'ao-liu ["peach and willow," i.e., sexual joy]. This climbing plant grows on the fields of Shun-chou, in the district of Nan-ho. It is also frequently found in all regions of Ling-nan. The sprouts [of the plant] are of the same size as those of mu-kao and have a moist shimmer. They resemble the shape of peach and willow trees. The leaves are bent, grow individually with their backs facing, and are not opposite. There are male and female types [of the plant]. The sprouts of the male plant are yellow-white, those of the female yellow-red. They grow at a distance from each other and unite at night. Some then become invisible. The female and the male specimens should be gathered on cloudless days at the end of spring, in midsummer, or at the beginning of fall, and they should be dried in the hot sun. The drug is taken pulverized, together with wine. When gathering, one ought to make sure that the whole root is obtained. The root must not be washed, must be protected from moisture, and is rubbed clean of sand and soil by means of a piece of cloth; the rind must not be damaged. It is stored in a tightly closed container. Every month [the drug] should again be dried in the sun. It must be taken only on even days, that is, on the second, fourth, sixth, eighth [etc.] day; and its use must be discontinued as soon as the clothes are soaked with perspiration, [indicating that one's influences] were brought into motion. [While taking the drug] the consumption of meat and blood from pork and lamb are to be avoided.'" Here, the old man ended and left. His walk resembled a swift wind. Censor Meng from the Provision Distribution Office in East Chekiang, was acquainted with

Mr. Ho Shou-wu. After he had tasted his drug, he said: "Its effects correspond to the tradition. It comes from the Niu-t'ou Mountain in Ping-chou. The sprouts grow in a crawling fashion similar to that of *pei-hsieh*. The root resembles a threatening fist. [The drug] is taken fresh, after removal of the black rind. Because of (the story related above,) the people in the South call [the drug] *ho-shou-wu*." Recorded in the eighth month of the eighth year of the governmental period *yüan-ho* [813].[74]

One might ask why Li Ao recorded this monograph. Li Ao is known as a philosopher and author of various works; along with Han Yü (768–824), he is considered an early pioneer of the Neoconfucianism of later centuries. If we recall that the Neoconfucians sought to prevent the death of the Confucian idea through the inclusion of certain Taoist and Buddhist elements into the doctrine of Confucius, a doctrine which had originally been restricted solely to the worldly-social sphere, the *Ho-shou-wu lu* of Li Ao might acquire the value of an excellent parable.

T'ien-erh, impotent, might embody the Confucianism of the time. In the wilderness, that is, outside of Chinese civilization, he encounters two plants which are combining, symbols of Taoism and Buddhism. Only by taking a carefully "sifted fine powder" of these two "drug"-parts can T'ien-erh become a "Neng-ssu," a man once again fruitful over many generations. Only Neng-ssu is able to recognize the "principles of human life"; T'ien-erh had given himself to wine, symbol of the superficial diversion through worldly things.

The narrator Li Ao himself suggested such an interpretation, as he quite openly moved the story into the triangle by bringing together the Buddhist priest, an old man who appears suddenly and rushes off like the wind (Taoist), and Confucian officials.

The medical value of the drug *ho-shou-wu* received no attention from medical-pharmaceutical circles until the Sung period. The *K'ai-pao pen-ts'ao* and the *Jih-hua tzu pen-ts'ao*, both from the tenth century, are the first drug works in which a ho-shou-wu monograph was included. The drug is still well known to practitioners of traditional Chinese medicine; it was described to the present author as an excellent remedy for regaining black hair.[75]

Under the term *shih-chung-ju*, stalactites had already been described in the *Pen-ching*, where they were eleventh among the precious stones/mineral drugs of the upper class. Their strange "growth," their age, and their permanence were particularly attractive, at an early time, to those specialists concerned about the prolongation of life without aging. In the *Ming-i pieh-lu* section of the *Pen-ts'ao ching chi-chu* of T'ao Hung-ching, the drug is ascribed the usual capabilities of the preventive drugs so highly valued by the Taoists. Among its numerous powers, it is supposed to clear the eyesight, bring peace to the five depots of the body, strengthen weakened legs, prolong the life span, bring back a youthful complexion, and aid in the production of numerous offspring.

The contents of the *Chung-ju lun* have not been preserved as a whole; nor can a quotation of its author be found in any of the known pen-ts'ao or similar works. Only the title is mentioned in a bibliog-

3. The *Chung-ju lun*

Chung-ju lun
"On Stalactites"
1 chapter / 1 drug description
Author: Ch'u Chih-ts'ai (Sung period)
Written: date unknown
Published: date unknown

stalactites (*shih-chung-ju*)—*Ch'ung-hsiu cheng-ho pen-ts'ao*

raphy of the Sung period, and in the section *I-wen chih* of the Sung history. The latter gives the author's name as Ch'u Chih-i. Further bibliographical information on a man of this or of the above-mentioned name could not be found.[76]

4. The *Jen-shen chuan*

Jen-shen chuan
"Notes on Ginseng"
1 chapter / 1 drug description
Author: Li Yen-wen (ca. 1500)
    tzu: Tzu-yü
    hao: Yüeh-ch'ih
Written: date unknown
Published: date unknown

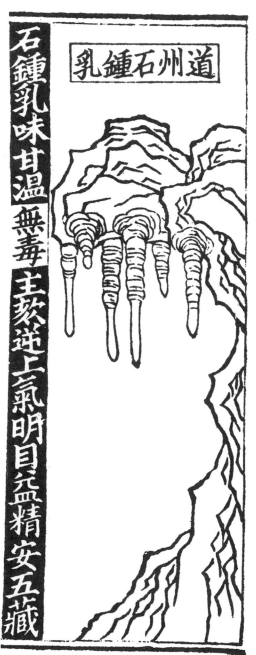

Although ginseng had been described in the *Pen-ching*, in the upper class of drugs, and had already been recommended at that time with all the characteristics that still guarantee its high esteem in Asia today, monographic pen-ts'ao works devoted specifically to this drug did not appear until the sixteenth century.

Li Yen-wen wrote the first ginseng treatise whose title is known to us. His son, Li Shih-chen, repeatedly quoted extensive excerpts from his father's work in the ginseng monograph of the *Pen-ts'ao kang mu;* but the extent to which these correspond to the complete original cannot be determined.

I have already pointed out that Li Shih-chen frequently argued on the basis of Chin-Yüan theories in his medical statements. In this he seems to have followed his father who, as is evident in the quotations from the *Jen-shen chuan,* had been strongly influenced by Chang Yüan-su, Li Kao, and others. In the section "Explanations" of the ginseng monograph of the *Pen-ts'ao kang mu,* for example, one can read the following excerpt from Li Yen-wen's treatise:

[Li] Yen-wen wrote: Used fresh, ginseng displays a cool [thermo-]influence. When [the drug] is used after preparation, its [thermo-]influence is warm. The slight sweet taste [of the drug] strengthens the *yang* [influences of the body]; the somewhat bitter taste [of the drug] strengthens the *yin* [influences]. Influences control the genesis of things; their origin is in heaven. The tastes control the completion of things; their origin is in the earth. [Thermo-]influence and taste, genesis and completion are realizations of *yin* and *yang* [influences]. The cool [thermo influence of fresh ginseng] expresses the *yang* influence of spring, of genesis and development. This is the *yang* [influence] of heaven. It has the nature of rising. Sweet is a taste that has been formed through transformation of moisture and earth. These are the *yang* influences of the earth. They have the nature of floating. The somewhat bitter taste has been formed through reciprocal interaction of fire and earth. These are the *yin* [influences] of the earth. They have the nature of submerging [in the body].

Taste and [thermo-]influence are both equally weak in ginseng. Whatever has a weak [thermo-]influence descends [in the body] when fresh, and rises when prepared. Whatever has a weak taste rises [in the body] when fresh and descends when prepared. In case of illnesses in which [the depot of the body associated with] soil [i.e., the spleen] shows a depletion and [the depot of the body associated with] fire [i.e., the heart] shows vigor, the weak cool [thermo-]influence of fresh ginseng is suited to diminish the blazing of the fire and to replenish the soil. This could be called a pure use of [thermo-]influence.

In the case of illnesses characterized by a depletion in the spleen and weakness in the lung, the sweet, warm taste of prepared ginseng is suited to replenish the soil and to generate metal. This would constitute a pure use of the taste [of ginseng].

[Li] Tung-yüan recommends the application of [the drug] *huang-po* with ginseng as an assistant drug in cases where a minister fire[77] takes hold of the spleen, with heat and confusion [resulting], when the influences rise in the body and [the patient] begins to pant, when he suffers

from headache and feels severe thirst, [the movement in] his vessels is
very strong and quick.

In cases of damage to the original influences through the heat of the
summer months, when a person perspires and suffers from severe diarrhea, and when paralyses and convulsions occur, Sun Chen-jen recommends the use of the *sheng-mai* powder to diminish the heat and   生脈
fire and supplement metal and water. As the ruler drug [in this pre-
scription] he uses the sweet coolness of ginseng; it diminishes the fire
and strengthens the original influences. As the minister drug [Sun Chen-
jen uses] *mai-men-tung* with its bitter-sweet [taste] and cold [thermo-
influence]. It purifies the metal and nourishes the source of the water.
He also added [the drug] *wu-wei tzu* as an assistant drug. Its sour [taste]
and warm [thermo-influence] are able to stimulate the formation of
essence in the kidneys and to reaccumulate lost influences. All this
constitutes a strengthening of the original influence which is founded
in heaven. By no means is this a replenishing of heat or fire. Pai Fei-
hsia wrote: "When one takes ginseng as a paste after an alchemical
preparation, [this drug] is able to restore the original influences into a
utopian condition." Whenever one suffers—after an illness—from influence depletion and from a depletion in the lung, combined with cough,
[ginseng] is appropriate [for the treatment]. When an influence depletion
exists together with fire, one should take [ginseng] together with [the
drug] *t'ien-men-tung*.[78]

The second monograph written by Li Yen-wen was devoted to the
leaves of the mugwort (*ai-yeh*). These leaves, pulverized, are formed
into the balls and bars that are burned on the skin, or above the skin
in suitable containers, during moxabustion treatments. All that is known
of Li Yen-wen's monograph, however, is its title; even the *Pen-ts'ao
kang mu* does not include a quotation from its text.[79]

5. The *Ai-yeh chuan*

Ai-yeh chuan
"Notes on Mugwort Leaves"
1 chapter / 1 drug description
Author: Li Yen-wen (ca. 1500)
 tzu: Tzu-yü
 hao: Yüeh-ch'ih
Written: date unknown
Published: date unknown

Following Li Yen-wen's initiative, several more studies devoted solely
to the ginseng appeared in subsequent centuries. In 1808, Huang Shu-
ts'an published a work entitled *Shen-p'u,* consisting of one chapter,
in which he attempted in a space of eighteen double-pages to distinguish and define the various ginseng types. This brief work has been
preserved.[80]

6. The *Shen-p'u*

Shen-p'u
"The Book of Ginseng"
1 chapter / 1 drug description
Author: Huang Shu-ts'an (1722–1806)
 tzu: Chin-t'ai
 hao: Mu-ts'un
Written: date unknown
Published: 1808

Somewhat less space, that is, ten double-pages, was used for the
Jen-shen k'ao, a study T'ang Ping-chün published in his literary collection *Wen fang ssu-k'ao.* An individual edition of the *Jen-shen k'ao*
appeared only in Japan. In China, the study was included in the collections *Ling-chien ko ts'ung-shu* and *I-yao ts'ung-shu.* It is not illustrated. The following table of contents indicates the problems that
concerned the author:

7. The *Jen-shen k'ao*

Jen-shen k'ao
"Investigations of the Ginseng Drug"
1 chapter / 1 drug description
Author: T'ang Ping-chün (Ch'ing period)
 tzu: Heng-ch'üan
 from: Chiang-ning
Written: date unknown
Published: date unknown

> How to distinguish the ginseng, and what one has to know about it in
> order to prevent disaster
> Differences between the present and previous places of origin
> [Ginseng from] Feng-huang ch'eng
> [Ginseng from] Ch'uan-ch'ang
> Products from [Ning-ku] t'ai
> Differentiation of [ginseng] ware by Soochow traders
> The weighing [of ginseng ware] by the Soochow traders
> Evaluation of the product in pharmacies according to color and name

Large ginseng specimens have been rare in the past years; stored spec-
  imens have not been destroyed by worms in the past years
Methods of storing ginseng
The time for preventive measures against infestations by mildew
[Drugs] bearing the name of ginseng [without having the same effects]
[Drugs that] resemble ginseng externally [without being ginseng]
Various tricks [to mix] genuine and false [specimens]
General comparison of all ginseng types[81]

The longest text section by far is found under the heading "Evaluation of the product in pharmacies according to color and name."
The evaluation of the quality of ginseng products, however, is discussed
here not only according to criteria of color and of name, which indicates the origin, but by other empirical criteria, such as the age,
as well.

Little is known about the life of the author, T'ang Ping-chün. We
may assume that he lived toward the end of the nineteenth century.

8. The *Kuei-k'ao*

Kuei-k'ao
"Investigations of Cinnamon"
1 chapter / 1 drug description
Author: Chang Kuang-yü (nineteenth century)
Written: date unknown
Published: 1891

To round out the picture of the drugs described in the monographic
pen-ts'ao works, a study entitled *Kuei-k'ao* should be mentioned here.
The work has been preserved, but I have not seen its contents.[82]

The earliest information in Chinese literature on the preparation of drugs is just as old as the sources on Chinese pharmaceutics. Pharmaceutical preparation is a process whereby certain original materials of a vegetable, animal and mineral nature are transformed to raw drugs and, finally, to the completed medicinal form.

The earliest Chinese pharmaceutical sources suggest a dual origin of the therapeutic use of substances found in nature or prepared by man. It appears that attempts to treat wounds, sores, or aching locations by covering them with leaves, pastes, juices, or other liquids led to an external pharmacy. We may assume, by contrast, that the intake of medicines, like dietetics, may have been considered in early times only a special form of food intake. Therefore, it is not surprising that some parallels can be discovered between the preparation of foods and the traditional preparation of drugs. In China, the latter measures fall under the concept *p'ao-chih,* which originally meant the thorough cooking of foods.

Obviously, in times predating medical and pharmaceutical literature, a rather subtle system of processing raw drugs was developed in China. It may have been based primarily on information gained through experience; it also included—at the latest by the T'ang dynasty—theoretical insights. Two areas can be differentiated. One comprises the pharmaceutical preparation of drugs. This includes the processes by which the original plant (or animal, etc.), through the removal, cleaning, and drying of the medicinally usable portions, is first processed into a raw drug and then into a refined drug. The second area comprises the preparation of certain medicinal forms from raw or refined drugs.

The processing of raw drugs into refined drugs was of special importance—and assumed even greater importance as a consequence of Sung-Chin-Yüan theorization. The purpose of this operation is, by means of a reagent added during the course of the preparation, either to guide the drug's original effect to a specific depot or palace in the patient, or to weaken the original effect of the drug, completely change it, or perhaps only support it. To achieve these effects, two different methods of preparation were developed—moist and dry. Examples of agents added during a moist preparation include, among others, honey, wine, brine, vinegar, ginger decoction, water used for washing rice, and urine of boys. The most widespread dry method of preparation is the "charring" of drugs. Since one and the same drug can usually be subjected to several different methods of preparation, thereby developing different effects, the result is an enormous multiplicity of uses for the Chinese materia medica.[83]

The taking of drugs prepared in this manner (the complexity of which could be only hinted at here) usually occurs individually or in combinations as decoctions, which the patient makes at home. In addition, raw, and even refined drugs, can be processed into a multitude of further medicinal forms. Various types of pills, powders for internal and external application, drops, plasters, ointments, pastes,

1. On the Preparation of Drugs in Traditional Chinese Pharmacy

炮灸

Lei-kung, demigod and legendary minister of the Yellow Emperor knowledgeable in medicine—*T'u-hsiang pen-ts'ao meng-ch'üan*

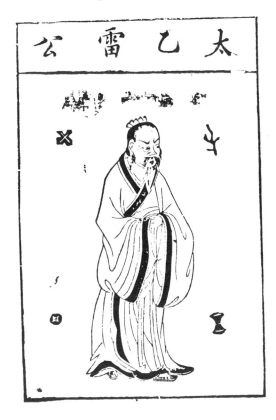

medicinal wines, distilled preparations, and others indicate a spectrum corresponding to that which was typical for the traditional European pharmacy.

For the most part, the methods of preparation described in Chinese medical-pharmaceutical literature were simple enough to be carried out in private homes, a fact corresponding to the low level of professionalization in health care that has characterized imperial China. In the comprehensive, encyclopedic materia medica literature of the Sung period and in the *Pen-ts'ao kang mu,* however, the reader also encounters the presentation of elaborate techniques hinting at the large-scale production of some substances used for medicinal purposes.

It would exceed the limits of the present work if I were to discuss here all the accomplishments, many centuries ago, of pharmaceutical technology in China. Many of the early Chinese efforts in "chemistry" and "physics" were devoted to the manufacture of medications, and would therefore fall into the field of pharmaceutical technology.

As an outstanding example, I will mention here only the processing of urine, practiced since the eleventh century. This process was meant to isolate, by means of distillation, precipitation, and sublimation, products of various kinds that may have contained a high concentration of sexual hormones.[84] We should, of course, not overlook the fact that the theoretical frame of reference that led some Chinese Taoists or "pharmaceutical chemists" to attempt a purification of sediments found on the bottom of urine collectors, as well as the scope of therapeutic usage of the substances so produced are hardly comparable to the origins and significance of steroid sex-hormones in Western medicine. While the discovery of androgens and estrogens revolutionized certain aspects of Western therapeutics, and while the ability to produce these substances and standardize their dosage had a remarkable effect on Western culture, the preparation of sublimation products from urine in China remained, in contrast, an insignificant, temporary aspect of traditional Chinese pharmaceutics, which was noticed and described, like some other achievements that impress the modern scientist, by only a few authors, and even that lost its limited attraction at some time between the sixteenth and eighteenth centuries.

The earliest records known today of the remarkable tradition of Chinese pharmaceutical technology can be found in the medical manuscripts unearthed from the Ma-wang-tui tombs in 1973. The *Wu-shih-erh ping fang,* one of these scripts, compiled, like the others, probably around 200 B.C., is characterized by an astonishing level of pharmaceutical technology. Besides a total of 224 drugs, numerous items were named that served as carrier-substances. These include various fats, named *chih* if they originated from horned animals such as ox and goat, and named *kao* if they originated from animals without horns such as the pig—lard being the most frequently recommended carrier-substance of the *Wu-shih-erh ping fang.* Such substances also include children's urine, gall liquid, human semen, animal blood, the contents of eggs, water used for washing rice, turtle-brain, cart-grease, and grease scratched from the human head. These items were used, for example, as binder for external medications, as binder for pills, as solvent for external medications, and as a medium for medical baths.

脂
膏

Different ways of drug application are specified in the *Wu-shih-erh ping fang* by eighteen different technical terms, most of them indicating external treatment. References to the collection of the original materials from which raw drugs or refined drugs were to be produced recommended suitable seasons of the year; they distinguished between drying under the sun and in the shade, and they advised the removal of those parts of an original plant, or material, that were deemed useless in therapy.

A small number of prescriptions in the *Wu-shih-erh ping fang* refers to the use of raw drugs (including those that have been merely chewed or pounded). Most prescriptions include an application of refined drugs or medicinal forms. Instruments recommended for their preparation include mortar and pestle, made from cedar wood, for pulverization; cauldron, pot, and pan for treating the drugs with heat; bowl, cup, jar, and tube for various other purposes. Nine technical terms designate different methods to grind, pound, scrape, scratch, break, split up, chew, knock, or melt original materials. Two technical terms distinguish different kinds of mixing substances. Five terms denote different methods to extract medicinal effects from a raw drug; twelve different terms indicate a broad range of techniques to treat raw drugs with heat before they are used medicinally.

Medicinal forms named in the *Wu-shih-erh ping fang* include:

1. Medicinal powders. These could be ordinary powders prepared from one or more substances after they had been dried and ground either individually or together. Other powders were prepared from so-called ashes, that is, from charred raw drugs.

2. Pills. The *Wu-shih-erh ping fang* names wine, vinegar, and fats as binders for pills. Other medical scripts discovered at Ma-wang-tui recommend honey, date pulp, the contents of birds' eggs, animal blood, pine resin, and "grain-juice" (the last possibly referring to water that has been used for washing rice).

3. Aqueous preparations. These include ordinary aqueous solutions, turbid suspensions, decoctions, and liquids produced by steaming a substance.

4. Medicinal wines. These were either ordinary wines recommended for therapeutic usage, or cold or hot solutions of drugs in wine. Other medical Ma-wang-tui scripts refer to the preparation of true medicinal wines from drugs.

5. Vinegar preparations. These were prepared by methods similar to those used to produce aqueous preparations and medicinal wines.

6. Pastes and ointments. These were medicinal forms for external applications only, prepared—with or without heat—from raw drugs and any of the carrier-substances mentioned above that appeared suitable for a particular therapeutic purpose.

Approximately four centuries later, Chang Chi (142–220?) mentioned, in his prescription works *Chin-kuei yao-lüeh* and *Shang-han lun*, eight methods of preparing the drugs he had recommended, namely *ao* (decocting), *hsi-chiu* (washing in wine), *ch'u-han* (removing the drug's inner dampness), *ch'u-hsien* (removing the salty elements), *ch'u-hsing* (removing the odor), *shui-chi* (watering), *t'ang-chi* (soaking in some decoction), and *shao* (charring).

Probably only another two or three centuries later, Yen Feng completed a work entitled "How to Make Herbs and Minerals Subservient" (*Chih-fu ts'ao shih lun*). The contents of this text are no longer known. It appears to have been the first pen-ts'ao work devoted especially to the preparation of drugs. Li Shih-chen mentioned it as a possible alchemical model for the *Lei-kung p'ao-chih lun*, the oldest manual for the preparation of drugs that has been at least partially preserved.[85]

2. The *Lei-kung p'ao-chih lun*

Lei-kung p'ao-chih lun
"On Lei-kung's [Methods] of [Drug] Preparation"
Short title: *P'ao-chih lun*
3 + 1 chapters / 300 drug descriptions
Authors: Lei Hsü (?) (fifth century); *tzu-hao: nei-chiu shou-kuo an-cheng kung*
Hu Hsia (?) (fifth century)
Written: date unknown
Published: date unknown

To this day we have been unable to learn very much more about the author and origin of the *Lei-kung p'ao-chih lun* than what Li Shih-chen said in a preliminary chapter of the *Pen-ts'ao kang mu*:

The author [of the *Lei-kung p'ao-chih lun*] is Lei Hsü from the Liu-Sung period, not the Lei-kung from the time of the Yellow Emperor. [Lei Hsü] called himself *nei-chiu shou-kuo an-cheng kung*. Perhaps this is a civil service title. Hu Hsia, a scholar living in seclusion, expanded the text, thereby establishing the final version. A total of 300 drugs [are described] in three chapters. The [information in the *Lei-kung p'ao-chih lun* concerning] the nature and taste [of drugs] as well as concerning differing processing procedures, is very old and obscure. The literary style is also ancient and belongs to someone other than Lei Hsü. Large portions of it go back to Mr. Yen from Ch'ien-ning. The preface at the beginning [of the work] describes the basic principles of things; it is also very obscure and mysterious. The actual writings then follow. The man from Ch'ien-ning was named Yen Feng. He wrote the *Chih-fu ts'ao shih lun* in six chapters; it was probably written by an expert on elixirs and minerals.[86]

However, only if we proceed from the assumption that Lei Hsü was indeed the author and lived before or during the same time as Hu Hsia, as Li Shih-chen has written, can the *Lei-kung p'ao-chih lun* be dated from the fifth century. While there are no exact reference points for the life of Lei Hsü, Hu Hsia is mentioned in the *I-yüan*, a literary collection by Liu Ching-shu, who died in approximately 468. It is peculiar that Su Sung (1020–1101), the author of the *T'u-ching pen-ts'ao*, is the first to speak of Lei Hsü. Su wrote: "It is said that Lei Hsü lived during the Sui period, but one also discovers drug names from the T'ang period in his work."[87]

As far as is known, the alleged work of Lei Hsü was not mentioned earlier by any pen-ts'ao author. Even the first bibliographical references date from the Sung period.

T'ang Shen-wei, a contemporary of Su Sung, was apparently the first to make extensive use of the contents of the *Lei-kung p'ao-chih lun*.[88] He adopted the preface of Lei Hsü and a total of 252 monographs from the work. In the process, however, it is uncertain whether the originals were perhaps shortened—as in other cases—or quoted in their entirety. As a result, these portions of the *Lei-kung p'ao-chih lun* were saved for posterity.

In 1932, in Szechwan, a man named Chang Chi published a *Lei-kung p'ao-chih lun*. In this work he had collected all Lei-kung quotations from the *Cheng-lei pen-ts'ao* and added further methods of preparation that he had taken from other pen-ts'ao works, from the *Ming-i pieh-lu* to the *Pen-ts'ao kang mu.*[89]

Nothing can be said with certainty about when the original *Lei-kung p'ao-chih lun* was prepared or completed. Okanishi also finally came to the conclusion that the archaic style of the text could not possibly have come from a Sung period author.[90]

Several details in the *Lei-kung p'ao-chih lun* can give us an idea of the contents of this work:

[On the preparation of *pai-shao yao:*]
[Immediately] after collection, [the drug] should be dried in the sun. The coarse bark should be removed with a bamboo knife and [the drug] steamed from 9 A.M. until 3 P.M. with hydromel. It should then [again] be dried in the sun and used.[91]

[On the preparation of *p'i-p'a yeh:*]
After collection the leaves are weighed. Moist leaves should each weigh one *liang;* when dried, three leaves should weigh one *liang.* In this way, they indicate that they contain the influences required for [medicinal] application. With a coarse cloth the fuzz should be removed from [the leaves], which are then washed with *kan-ts'ao* decoction. Then, a soft cloth is used to dry the [leaves] and, over a fire, each *liang* [of leaves] should be combined with one *fen* of cheese. In the process, the cheese should be completely absorbed.[92]

[On the preparation of *shou ti-huang:*]
Following the collection of *sheng ti-huang* [i.e., fresh *ti-huang*], re-move the white fuzz [of the plant]. Then, steam the plant on a willow-wood boiler above a porcelain pot; after a certain time, open [the cover] to allow the steam to escape. Now mix the drug with wine, steam it once more, and again allow the steam to escape after a while. The drug should then be dried. It must not be damaged by coming into contact with copper or iron. That would diminish one's kidneys [if it were later consumed] and turn hair white prematurely. In addition, [such a faulty treatment] damages the construction [influences] of males and the pro-tection [influences] of women.[93]

[On the preparation of *p'u-huang:*]
In preparing [this drug] for application, be careful not to use mis-takenly *sung-huang* or *huang-hao.* Both resemble [*p'u-huang,*] only the tastes are different. If one wishes to prepare *p'u-huang,* [the drug] must be wrapped in three layers of paper and dried [in a pot] above a fire until it has turned yellow. It is then steamed for half a day and then dried again in the same manner. As a result, application [of the drug] will produce outstanding [effects].[94]

[On the preparation of *t'ing-li:*]
In preparing this drug, be careful not to use [mistakenly] *ch'ih-hsü-tzu.* [This drug] is very similar to *t'ing-li*—its taste, however, is some-what sweet-bitter. In contrast, the bitter taste of *t'ing-li* is quite strongly pronounced. During preparation for medicinal use, [the drug] is com-bined with glutinous rice and heated carefully on a stove until the rice is cooked. The rice is then discarded, and the *t'ing-li* alone is pulverized and utilized as medicine.[95]

The *Chih-yao fa lun,* the *Hsiu-chih yao fa,* and the *Chin-shih chih-yao fa* are examples of Sung works devoted especially to the prepa-

3. The *Chih-yao fa lun*

Chih-yao fa lun
"On Methods of Drug Preparation"
1 chapter
Author: unknown
Written: Sung period (?)
Published: date unknown

4. The *Hsiu-chih yao fa*

Hsiu-chih yao fa
"Methods of Drug Preparation"
1 chapter
Author: P'ang An-shih (1042–1099)
    tzu: An-ch'ang
    from: Ch'i-shui in Ch'i-chou, Hu-pei
Written: date unknown
Published: date unknown

5. The *Chin-shih chih-yao fa*

Chin-shih chih-yao fa
"Methods of Preparing Drugs from Metals and Stones"
1 chapter
Author: Chang Chi
Written: date unknown
Published: Sung period (?)

6. The *Pen-ts'ao meng-ch'üan*

Pen-ts'ao meng-ch'üan
"Elimination of Ignorance in Pharmaceutics"
12 + 1 chapters / 742 drug descriptions
Author: Ch'en Chia-mo (1521–1603)
    tzu: T'ing-ts'ai
    hao: Yüeh-p'eng tzu
    from: Ch'i-men in Anhui
Written: 1559–1565
Published: 1565

ration of drugs. With each work consisting of one chapter, they are not particularly extensive. Only in the case of the *Hsiu-chih yao fa* do we know a little more about the author.

P'ang An-shih came from a medical family with a rich tradition. He himself was supposed to have been especially successful in treating illnesses caused by cold. In addition to the *Hsiu-chih yao fa*, he also wrote the *Pen-ts'ao pu-i* ("Supplement to Pharmaceutics"), a work in the secondary tradition.

Others were apparently also involved in the authorship of the work—the well-known writer Su Tung-p'o (1036–1101), whose medical interests are also reflected in the prescription work *Su Shen liang fang* (to which he contributed one formula), and Huang T'ing-chien, the alleged author of the *Chu-tou fa* ("Methods of Cooking Beans") section in Yao K'o-ch'eng's *Shih-wu pen-ts'ao*.[96]

The Sung bibliographies list a Chang Chi as author of the *Chin-shih chih-yao fa*. It is unclear whether this is a reference to the Han period Chang Chi, whose name concealed an anonymous author, or whether another author of the same name wrote the work during the Sung period.[97]

The contents of all these works have been lost.

In addition to the processing of raw drugs into refined drugs and the further refinement into medicinal forms, the art of storage and the preservation of drugs also belonged to pharmaceutical technology. The *Pen-ts'ao meng-ch'üan* by Ch'en Chia-mo is devoted mainly to those questions concerning the most suitable state of drugs for medicinal use. It is a pen-ts'ao work with comprehensive contents, and justifiably could have been discussed with the works in the eclectic pen-ts'ao tradition. I have included it here, however, because of its unusually careful pharmaceutical directions, which are particularly evident in the treatises of a preliminary chapter.

The author's priorities are presented in the preface, dated 1565:

> Numerous *pen-ts'ao* works have been printed since antiquity, such as the *Ta-kuan [pen-ts'ao]*. Its contents are of profound significance, but it deals with only a few important elements. Another example is the *[Pen-ts'ao] chi-yao;* its comments are sketchy and insufficient. Finally, Wang Shih-shan from Wu-i compiled the *[Pen-ts'ao] hui-pien*[98] in which, fortunately, detailed descriptions and outlines are in the correct proportion. It is therefore to be valued as an intelligent and thorough work. Unfortunately, however, he also adopted and quoted the statements of various other authors and, in the process, exhausted himself in aimless discussion. Thus, this work—as all the others—can be considered incomplete.
>
> For a time I lived in the prefectural city. . . . I thought that I wished to revise this *[pen-ts'ao]* book in order to instruct students and avoid the disadvantages of the three [works mentioned above]. So I carefully attempted to understand all older works and differentiated their contents. [For me], the most important criteria [for the description of drugs] were [thermo-]influence and taste, rising and descending [properties of drugs in the body], and [information] concerning the extent of medicinal strength. The next important criteria were [data concerning] the quality of drugs, with respect to their place of origin, and the [appropriate]

time for collection, whether early or late. I then selected [information] on the conduits penetrated [by drugs] as well as on all the incompatibilities [of drugs when used together], as well as on preparation and storage. In addition, I selected the appropriate criteria for the use [of drugs] in curative treatment, and I have listed from prescription works [that are attributed] to the exemplary men [of antiquity] all that should be effective. I have also consulted older secondary literature, and I have added my own unworthy opinions, in order to expand previously incomplete explanations. . . .

I began this work in the 38th year of the period *chia-ching* [1559]. In the course of seven years I revised the manuscript five times before the work was finally completed. I entitled it *Pen-ts'ao meng-ch'üan;* I would like to dedicate it to all students [of pharmaceutics]. It is commonly said: "If the teacher was outstanding and generous, the heart of his students will be full of kind thoughts!" Bearing this in mind, how can instruction then be limited to two or three students? It should be available to all men![99]

A second preface to the *Pen-ts'ao meng-ch'üan* was written by Hsü Kuo, a scholar who later became president of the Ministry of Rites; it is also dated 1565.

The preliminary chapter following the prefaces contains a total of eighteen general treatises on pharmacy. They include information on drug geography, times for collection, directions for preserving drugs from decay, differentiating genuine and fraudulent drugs, and information on the classification and cutting of roots, as well as on the processing of drugs with water and wine. Theoretical treatises deal with the utilization of thermo-influence and taste for the treatment of illnesses and with the separation of drug combinations into ruler and minister elements.

Additional subjects include:

1. The "seven affections" (*ch'i-ch'ing*) of drugs which had been mentioned in the *Pen-ching* for the first time.　　七情
2. The "seven prescription combinations" (*ch'i-fang*), including:　　七方
   (a) Large prescriptions—against strong evil influences and against several symptoms appearing simultaneously. There are five different kinds of prescriptions called "large prescriptions," namely those with strong medicinal strength, those with many ingredients, those with heavy weight, those with heavy weight to be taken in one dose, and those that cure serious ills and afflictions of the Lower Burner.
   (b) Small prescriptions—against evil influences that are weak and do not penetrate the body deeply, and against illnesses with only one symptom. There are three different kinds of "small prescriptions," namely those that treat weak and shallow evil influences, those that treat afflictions of the Upper Burner, have small doses of light weight, and are to be taken internally in many doses, and those with a small number of ingredients against single symptoms.
   (c) Fast prescriptions—against acute and serious illnesses. There are four kinds of "fast prescriptions," namely those acting fast against dangerous illnesses, those prepared as decoctions for

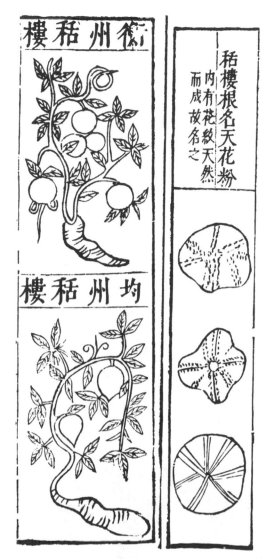

trichosanthes seeds and pericarp (*kua-lou:* left) and cross-sections of the root drug (*t'ien-hua-fen:* right)—*T'u-hsiang pen-ts'ao meng-ch'üan*

fast purging activity, those with drugs whose properties, that is, thermo-influence and taste, are strongly developed, and those that are employed to treat external manifestations of an acute illness.

(d) Slow prescriptions—against somatic deficiencies and chronic illnesses. There are six kinds of "slow prescriptions," namely those with many ingredients all of which restrain one another so that the actual strength of the individual ingredients is small, those with drugs without marked medicinal effectiveness for a slow elimination of the evil influences underlying the illness and avoidance of any harm to the proper influences, those with weakly developed taste, used in case one does not intend to achieve fast results, those with sweet, soothing drugs, which develop their effects slowly, those applied as pills that slowly attack the evil influences, and, finally, those that employ slow-acting drugs to treat the basis, that is, to slowly increase the resistance of the organism so that the illness leaves by itself.

(e) Uneven prescriptions—prescriptions with only one drug or with an uneven number of ingredients, against uncomplicated illnesses.

(f) Even prescriptions—prescriptions with two drugs or with an even number of ingredients, against complicated illnesses.

(g) Repetitive prescriptions—combinations of several prescriptions in one treatment, or additional ingredients added to a fixed formula, or prescriptions with an equal amount of all ingredients.

The seven prescription combinations were mentioned first by Ch'eng Wu-i in his *Shang-han min li-lun;* they were based in turn on statements in the treatise *Chih-chen-yao ta-lun* of the *Su-wen.*

3. The "ten kinds of prescriptions" (*shih-chi*), namely comprehensive 十 劑 prescriptions, penetrating prescriptions, filling prescriptions, draining prescriptions, light prescriptions, heavy prescriptions, smooth prescriptions, rough prescriptions, dry prescriptions, and moist prescriptions. The ten kinds of prescriptions were probably introduced by Ch'en Ts'ang-ch'i in his *Pen-ts'ao shih-i.*

4. The five uses of drugs in different medicinal forms
5. The various weights and measures
6. The taking of drugs before and after meals
7. The main curative drugs and guiding drugs for each conduit
8. Adopted from Li Kao: "Rules and Correspondences in the Use of Drugs."

Excerpts from four of these treatises are presented here as examples:

The selection [of drugs] according to their places of origin.
    All herbs, trees, and worms originate in places appropriate for them. Concerning [thermo-]influence, taste, and medicinal potency [of drugs], one must start from all their differences and find out what is normal. Among the people it is said: "As the climate at a specific place nourishes tens of thousands of people, so too does a specific area of land bring forth its corresponding drugs." Scholars who endeavor to nourish their

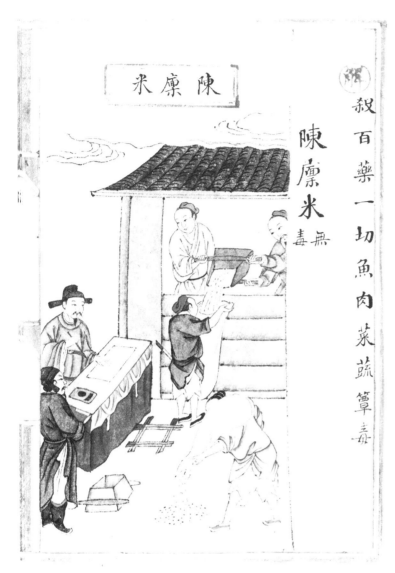

陳廩米
無毒

殺百藥一切魚肉菜蔬蕈毒

rice in a State warehouse *(ch'en-lin mi)*—Pen-ts'ao p'in-hui ching-yao

nocturnal preparation of yeast *(ch'ü)*—Pen-ts'ao p'in-hui ching-yao

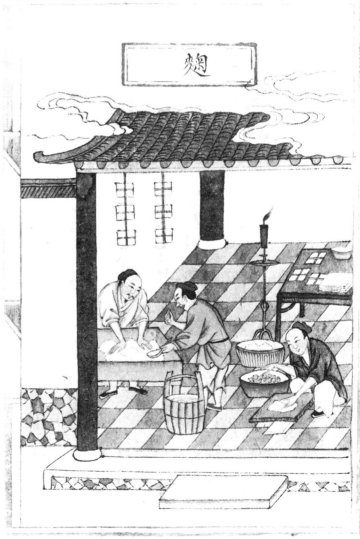

錫粉

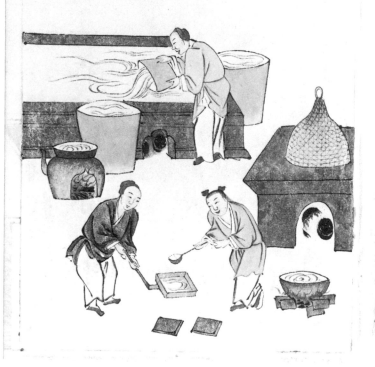

the preparation of alkaline lead carbonate *(fen-hsi)*—Pen-ts'ao p'in-hui ching-yao

the preparation of minium *(ch'ien-tan)*—Pen-ts'ao p'in-hui ching-yao

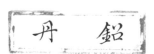

丹鉛

鉛丹出神農本經主吐逆胃反驚癇癲疾除熱以上朱宇神農

下氣鍊化還成九光久服通神明

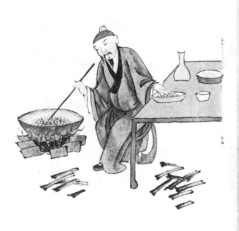

life by means of dietetic measures should always attempt to obtain genuine [drugs]. Often, however, they fear the hardship of long travel and restrict themselves to collecting drugs produced nearby as suitable substitutes [for distant, hard-to-find drugs]. They appear not to know that specimens of drugs growing both distant and nearby are sometimes interchangeable for [medicinal] application, but, in some cases must not be confused![100]

The collection [of original drug material] according to [specific] times.

Only the end of autumn and the beginning of spring are suitable times for the collection of root tips from herbs and trees. At the beginning of spring the [plant] saps begin to flow and do not yet fill branches and leaves. At the end of autumn the [plant] influences descend with the saps and return completely to the roots. According to actual experience, it appears most preferable if [the collection takes place] rather early in spring and rather late in autumn. Stems, leaves, blossoms, and fruits also follow the seasons in their suitability [for collection]. Thus, branches and stems should be picked before they grow old and when they are still abundantly permeated by sap. Blossoms are picked as buds—just before opening—since, at this point, they still completely possess their influences. Fruits are gathered when they have already matured; at this point their taste is most purely developed. Leaves should be picked when new; their power is then twice as strong [as later], and medicinal use is reliable and outstanding: therefore, they are especially suitable for the treatment of illnesses. Some things from the categories precious stones, minerals, fowl, quadrupeds, worms, and fish may be collected without regard for the season or age; with others, certain time periods must be taken into account. This has a profound basis and should not be dismissed as idle talk. In each case, follow the regulations; no action should be arbitrary and random![101]

Preventing the decay [of drugs] during storage.

During storage, precautions should be taken regularly [to prevent] the decay of drugs. [If drugs] have been dried in the shade, in the sun, or over fire without moisture being completely removed, the result will be insect infestation, discoloration, and putrefaction; damage [to the drug] then cannot be avoided during the coming spring and summer seasons. Much rain causes a [high] humidity [in the air], which penetrates [the drugs]. In the evenings, it sometimes happens that mice or worms gnaw [on the drugs]. Nevertheless, one must not be resigned—it is possible [to store drugs] over periods of months or years. During longer periods of rain, it is advisable to redry [drugs] over a fire. On clear, bright days, this must be carried out in the sun. For this process, coarse and rough [drugs] are spread out on a stand; small, soft [drugs] should be kept in an earthen jar. [The drug] *jen-shen* must be stored together with *hsi-hsin; ping-p'ien* should be stored with *teng-ts'ao.*

In the *Pen-ching* it is said that worm infestation is impossible if charred, glutinous rice is stored with *hsiang-ssu-tzu.* Musk should be wrapped in snake skin during storage; *p'eng-sha* must be stored together with *lü-tou. Sheng-chiang* must be stored in dry sand; *shan-yao,* once dried, is best preserved in a lime pit. *Ch'en-hsiang* and genuine *t'an-hsiang* are very aggressive and must be thickly wrapped in paper. Cocoon water and snow water from *la* day will be most efficacious if they are buried in a hole—a method that allows long storage times. The regulations for other drugs can be derived from these examples.[102]

The utilization of the [thermo-]influence and taste [of drugs] for curative treatment.

In treatment the emphasis rests on prescriptions, and drugs are combined to suitable prescriptions. Expert application of drugs [is achieved if thermo-]influence and taste are considered important. The [thermo-]influences are heaven. There are four such influences. Warm and hot correspond to the *yang* [influences] of heaven; cold and cool correspond to the *yin* [influences] of heaven. That which is *yang* rises; that which is *yin* descends. The tastes are earth. There are six tastes. Acrid, sweet, and neutral are the *yang* [influences] of earth; sour, bitter, and salty are the *yin* [influences] of earth. That which is *yang* floats; that which is *yin* dives. There are [drugs] that guide a [thermo-influence] [to the desired location]; others guide the taste; and there are drugs that guide both taste and [thermo-]influence. There are [drugs] that first guide the taste and then the [thermo-]influence; and others that guide in the reverse order. It is impossible to grasp all of them within one rule. It is also possible for one drug to have two, or even three tastes, or for one or two [thermo-]influences to be combined in one drug. If a strong hot [thermo-]influence and a weak cold [thermo-]influence are combined [in one drug], the cold [thermo-]influence will not take effect as such. If [on the other hand] a strong cold [thermo-]influence and a weak hot [thermo-]influence are combined, the hot influence will not be detected as such. If cold and hot [thermo-]influences are of equal proportions, the [thermo-influence of the drug] will appear warm. In some cases, the warm [thermo-]influence is so distinct it appears to be hot; in other cases, the cool [thermo-]influence is so strongly developed it appears to be cold. Careful distinctions must be made here. In addition, if cold and hot [thermo-]influences are of equal proportions, the hot portion may be dominant when [the drug] is taken during the day, and [the effect] will rise [in the body; if the same drug] is taken at night, the cold portion may dominate, and [the effect will] descend [in the body]. On clear, bright days, the hot [thermo-]influence is decisive; on dark days [the effects] follow the cold [thermo-]influence. Everything follows its correspondences; manifold variations occur.[103]

The individual monographs of the *Pen-ts'ao meng-ch'üan* are arranged according to the following pattern: herbs, trees, grains, vegetables, fruits, minerals, quadrupeds, fowl, worms, fish, and man. The text of the monographs relies heavily on the theories of the Chin-Yüan period; quotations from Li Kao, for example, are frequently included. In addition, the descriptions of individual drugs attach some importance to origin, preparation, and selection, without the information becoming very detailed. The first edition of the *Pen-ts'ao meng-ch'üan* was not illustrated.[104]

In 1628, an expanded edition of this work appeared under the title *T'u-hsiang pen-ts'ao meng-ch'üan* ("The Illustrated Abolition of Ignorance in Pharmaceutics"). It contained a third preface, whose author was given as Liu K'ung-tun. The expansion of this edition, with respect to the original, consists of a multitude of illustrations. Immediately following the table of contents are eight portraits of medical practitioners: Shun-yü I (ca. 180 B.C.), Chang Chi (142–222?), Hua T'o (110–207), Wang Shu-ho (210–285), Huang-fu Mi (215–282), Ko Hung (281–341), Sun Ssu-mo (581–682?), and Wei Tz'u-tsang (ca. 700).

A second section follows, entitled "Illustrations and Names of Famous Physicians in History" (*Li-tai ming-i t'u hsing shih*) and introduced by a preface from Hsiung Tsung-li, dated 1476.

Hsiung Tsung-li had written and published the *Li-tai ming-i t'u hsing shih* ("Illustrations and Names of Famous Physicians in His-

tory") as an independent work. As he wrote in the preface, his text
continued the tradition of the biographical works of the T'ang period
physician Kan Po-tsung, author of the *Li-tai ming-i hsing-shih* ("Names
of Famous Physicians in History"), and Hsü Shen-chai, the Sung author of the *Li-tai ming-i t'an-yüan pao-pen chih t'u* ("Illustrations
from Studies and Reports on the Origins of Renowned Physicians of
History").

Six sections from Hsiung Tsung-li's work were incorporated into
the *T'u-hsiang pen-ts'ao meng-ch'üan,* namely, one page of illustrations and one page of text devoted to each of the following more or
less legendary personalities: Fu Hsi, Shen-nung, Hsüan Yüan, Ch'i Po,
Lei-kung, and Pien Ch'io. It can be assumed that the eight illustrations
of physicians at the beginning of the *T'u-hsiang pen-ts'ao meng-ch'üan*
were taken from the *Li-tai ming-i t'u hsing-shih.*

Even more important than these historical portraits are the drug
illustrations added to the *T'u-hsiang pen-ts'ao meng-ch'üan.* Some
monographs are illustrated with two, or even three, pictures, each
according to differing specimens from several areas of origin. Usually,
the original plants or animals are presented; it is interesting, however,
that there are also illustrations of root cross-sections and of various
formations of root tubers, or differing bulbs.

The value of Ch'en Chia-mo's original work for pharmaceutical
practice was significantly enhanced by the drug illustrations. As a
result, the work received wide circulation.

Li Shih-chen, a contemporary of Ch'en Chia-mo, praised the *Pen-
ts'ao meng-ch'üan.* Four Ming editions and one from the Ch'ing period
have been preserved; the work was also well known in Japan.[105]

Like the *Pen-ts'ao meng-ch'üan,* the *Pen-ts'ao yüan-shih* belongs to
the pen-ts'ao works with comprehensive contents. It is discussed at
this point because its author, Li Chung-li, like Ch'en Chia-mo, was
particularly interested in pharmaceutical-technological instructions.

Little is known of Li Chung-li, except that he was the younger
brother of Li Chung-tzu (see p. 251) and passed the *chin-shih* exams
in 1595. The prefaces for the first edition were written by Lo Wen-
ying and Ma Ying-lung, a temporary minister in Ch'i and senior secretary of dietetics. The preface by Lo Wen-ying was dropped in later
editions.

The order of monographs was as follows: vegetables, herbs, trees,
fruits, worms/fish, fowl, quadrupeds, grain, metals/minerals, and man.
Already in the table of contents, at the beginning of the *Pen-ts'ao
yüan-shih,* there are general treatises following the individual drug
sections. For example, Li Chung-li wrote the following concerning the
fowl and quadruped section:

> All birds that have closed eyes following death, birds whose feet are
> not stretched out after death, white birds with dark heads, dark birds
> with white heads, birds with three feet, four claws, six toes, or four
> wings, birds of unusual appearance and abnormal color must not be
> eaten. Their consumption is fatal to man!

7. The *Pen-ts'ao yüan-shih ho Lei-kung p'ao-chih*

Pen-ts'ao yüan-shih ho Lei-kung p'ao-chih
"The Original Materia Medica Combined with
Lei-kung's [Methods] of [Drug] Preparation"
Short title: *Pen-ts'ao yüan-shih*
12 chapters / 550 drug descriptions
Author: Li Chung-li (ca. 1600)
    tzu: Shih-ch'iang
    hao: Cheng-shou
    from: Yung-ch'iu
Written: date unknown
Published: 1613

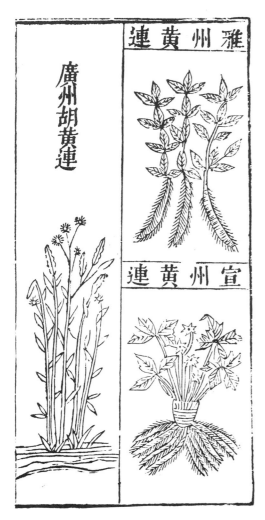

coptis rhizome (huang-lien)—T'u-hsiang pen-ts'ao meng-ch'üan

8. The P'ao-chih ta-fa

P'ao-chih ta-fa
"Highly Refined Method of Drug Preparation"
1 chapter / 439 drug descriptions
Author: Miu Hsi-yung (beginning of the seventeenth century)
    tzu: Chung-ch'un
    hao: Mu-t'ai
    from: Ch'ang-shu in Chiang-su
Written: ca. 1620
Published: date unknown

All black cows and sheep, those with a white head, only one liver or horn, the six domestic animals that are afflicted with epidemics or infested with boils, dead horses whose flesh is black beneath the saddle, the six domestic animals whose mouths are not closed after death, the meat of rabid dogs, all domestic animals whose flesh contains rice-like stars, all quadrupeds with a greenish liver, all quadrupeds that have died from poison, the six domestic animals whose flesh has spoiled and discolored—all of the above-mentioned [exceptions] must not be eaten. They either kill man or cause illness and produce toxic ulcers, swellings, and boils.[106]

The individual monographs of the Pen-ts'ao yüan-shih each begin with a descriptive text, devoted to, among other things, place of origin, collection times, and medicinally useful parts of the original source. In numerous quotations, the comments of earlier authors, beginning with the Pen-ching and Shuo-wen chieh-tzu, are repeated. Further information includes thermo-influence and taste, as well as the degree of medicinal potency.

Following these particular details in the monographs is a section, designated by large characters, entitled "Main Effects." In contrast to the Pen-ts'ao meng-ch'üan, it contains no references to the Chin-Yüan theories. Frequently, one, two, or even three illustrations, prepared by Li Chung-li, are added to the text. In addition to the sketches of drugs, the author included brief details on the quality standard of drugs, to enable a quick survey.

Also designated by large characters is a very extensive section entitled "Preparation," which has been added to most monographs. It contains, introduced by the words "Lei-kung wrote," several lines from the Lei-kung p'ao-chih lun. This method of dividing the drug monograph according to various technical aspects is reminiscent of the pattern used by the authors of the Pen-ts'ao p'in-hui ching-yao and by Li Shih-chen in the Pen-ts'ao kang mu (in a much more detailed manner, however) which appeared at approximately the same time as the Pen-ts'ao yüan-shih.

In 1754, the publisher Ts'ung-ch'eng t'ang brought out a new printing of the Pen-ts'ao yüan-shih. It is characterized by a small, pocketbook format; the eight volumes are each no larger than 15 by 10.5 centimeters. The ease of carrying this work, even on trips—which such a format guaranteed—like its practical contents, brought the Pen-ts'ao yüan-shih a certain popularity. Even today, in addition to the original Ming editions, seven printings from the Ch'ing period have been preserved. The 1844 edition of the Hsin-yüan t'ang publishing house, edited by Ko Miao, varies greatly from the original in the arrangement of the contents and contains additional revisions.[107]

The peak of interest in literature on the methods of drug preparation appears to have been in the last hundred years of the Ming period. At no other time was such detailed information given in so many different works within such a short period as in the decade around 1600. Although I have only discussed examples from the literature that are extensively devoted to such questions, it must not be overlooked that, for example, detailed descriptions of this type can also be found in the *Pen-ts'ao kang mu*.

Miu Hsi-yung, whom we have already encountered as the author of the *Shen-nung pen-ts'ao ching shu* (see C, V, 2.2), followed the interests of his time. Without informing his readers of his source, Miu copied the methods of drug preparation from the *Cheng-lei pen-ts'ao* and published them as an independent work. The entire text of this rather short book was divided into two major parts. The first part contains the monographs, ordered in various sections. They are very short—rarely exceeding two lines—and focus on the appearance of different kinds of one and the same drug, on the appropriate origin, on synergistic effects if specific drugs are consumed together, on age groups that may or may not eat a specific drug, and, of course, on methods of processing raw drugs into refined drugs. The structure of the monographs is not systematized; the information mentioned above is given only where appropriate. At the end of the monograph section, a paragraph was added by Chuang Chi-kuang. Here the reader is told that this book was compiled because contemporary practitioners relied on family traditions but were completely unaware of Shen-nung's Pen-ts'ao and of the writings on the preparation methods by exemplary people of former times. According to Chuang Chi-kuang, the text of the book was dictated to him by Miu Hsi-yung; Chuang Chi-kuang then edited it.[108]

The second part of the *P'ao-chih ta-fa* comprises a general survey of drug usage. The topics dealt with here include rules to be observed in the preparation of specific forms of medication, rules for the boiling of drugs, the timing of the intake of medications (including references to desirable amounts), incompatibilities with drugs and food, the intake of drugs during pregnancy, the seasoning of six specific drugs, as well as restrictions on the intake of specific drugs and foods at the time of a treatment with specific medications or at the time of specific illnesses.

The following list of seventeen different methods to prepare refined (or raw) drugs from the original materials, offered by the *P'ao-chih ta-fa*, may serve as an example of the kind of sophisticated pharmaceutical techniques that were advocated in the literature of the second millennium A.D.[109] How many of these techniques were actually employed in practice, though, cannot be determined now.

p'ao: The dry-heating of drugs directly over the fire or in a pan. A 炮 gap must be left between the fire and the object; the one must not come into direct contact with the other. The drugs should neither be moved nor turned. The operation is concluded when a particular smoke starts to rise.

lan: The heating of the drugs either in the fire or just over it until 爁 a certain degree of charring has been reached.

po: The dry-heating in a pan until the drugs grow brittle and begin 煿 to crack and burst.

chih: The heating of drugs in all the possible liquids or coatings such 炙 as wine, ginger juice, honey, and the like, until thoroughly cooked.

煨 *wei:* The cooking of drugs in hot ash until thoroughly cooked.

炒 *ch'ao:* The roasting of drugs in a pan until they begin to turn yellow-ish. During this preparation process, the drugs are often turned and moved about.

煅 *tuan:* The dry-heating in a pan or over the fire; used for mineral and horn drugs.

煉 *lien:* The heating of metals, including physical processes such as melting.

製 *chih:* The altering of the characteristics of drugs by means of prep-arations involving chemical processes such as the removal of poisons or the weakening of the drug's effects, through water, wine, and other methods.

度 *tu:* The precise measurement of the required size of the drugs.

飛 *fei:* The fine grinding of minerals. After being ground, they are put into a mortar, whereby the impurities collect on the surface and can be poured away. The heavy pure sediment is finally used for medicinal purposes.

伏 *fu:* The storing and preserving of drugs for lengthy periods before they are used.

鎊 *p'ang:* The fine shaving of bones and similar drugs.

搬 *sha:* The pounding of seed drugs, for instance, with the back of the hand.

晒 *shai:* The drying in the sun until the drugs contract and shrink.

曝 *p'u:* The drying in the sun for short periods.

露 *lu:* The exposing of drugs to the dew, in the evening or early morning.

Miu Hsi-yung's *P'ao-chih ta-fa* does not appear to have reached a wide circulation. Only three editions from the late Ming and Ch'ing dynasty are known in addition to the 1959 reprint in the People's Republic of China.

9. The *Lei-kung p'ao-chih yao-hsing chieh*

Lei-kung p'ao-chih yao-hsing chieh
"Elucidation of Drug Preparation and Drug Properties According to Lei-kung"
6 chapters / 269 drug descriptions
Author: unknown
Written: seventeenth century
Published: date unknown

To this day, at least on Taiwan, the *pen-ts'ao* work published by the well-known medical author Li Chung-tzu, the older brother of Li Chung-li, which specialized on pharmaceutical technology is the most frequently encountered among practitioners of traditional Chinese medicine. The work is comprised of monographs which are divided into a general section, closely associated with the eclectic tradition, and quotations, which are usually added to this section from the *Lei-kung p'ao-chih lun*. The list of the publications of Li Chung-li, included in the *Chiang-nan t'ung-chih*, did not mention the *Lei-kung p'ao-chih yao-hsing chieh*.[110] In a 1905 edition of the work, Li Kao is given as the author[111]—this, however, is just as improbable as the authorship of Li Chung-li. Under the title *Lei-kung p'ao-chih yao-hsing fu* ("Lei-kung's Song of Drug Preparation and Drug Properties") or *Lei-kung yao-hsing fu* ("Lei-kung's Song of Drug Properties"), several editions appeared in which the *Lei-kung p'ao-chih yao-hsing chieh* and the *Chen-chu nang chih-chang pu-i yao-hsing fu*, which we encountered among the Chin-Yüan works, were edited together.[112]

Several authors attempted to compose pharmaceutical works either completely or partially in verse. They combined with this stylistic method the goal of facilitating students' memorization of monographs. These works are thus characterized as specialized literature for beginning students.

Two different examples have already been presented in previous chapters. In the *Chiu-huang-yeh p'u* by Yao K'o-ch'eng (see D, I, 14 p. 225), one half of each monograph is a "drug poem." Here, the verse often did not describe the properties of the drugs in a very detailed manner; such information was reserved for the prose sections of the monographs. During times of need—for which the work was written—it was sufficient, if one did not have the book itself in hand, to remember the short, easily learned poems, in order to understand the applicability of drugs under certain conditions.

The second example I have already discussed was the *Chen-chu nang chih-chang pu-i yao-hsing fu* (see D, III, 9); at this point, however, we must return to its form. Extensive portions of the general comments and monographs, complete monographs, and, above all, the various "songs" of the first and second chapters of this work were composed in verse. Apparently, the author considered these sections particularly valuable for memorization. Four rhyme schemes are most common:

1. *a-a-b-a c-c-d-c e-e-f-e*, etc.
2. *a-b-c-b a-b-d-b c-b-f-b*, etc.
3. *a-b-c-b-d-b-e-b-*, etc., with differing line lengths
4. *a-a-b-b c-c-d-d*, etc.

This style appears to be quite meaningful and to have proved successful; the *Chen-chu nang chih-chang pu-i yao-hsing fu*, at least in the double edition with the *Lei-kung p'ao-chih yao-hsing chieh*, still enjoys great popularity and circulation.

Two additional representatives of this genre will be introduced here.

Like his father, Kung Hsin, Kung T'ing-hsien belonged to the so-called Ch'i-Huang school of medical practitioners in the seventeenth century. Both wrote several medical works and were, for a time, officials in the Imperial Medical Department. Kung T'ing-hsien's best-known work is the *Wan-ping hui-ch'un* ("Return to Spring from Ten Thousand Illnesses"). From this book, Kung adopted 240 drugs as the basis for his descriptions in the *Yao-hsing ko-k'uo*, adding 160 monographs of frequently used drugs.

The individual monographs are short and—with the exception of a commentary in small print—are completely in verse. Each consists of only one line with sixteen characters, divided into four verses of four characters, utilizing the rhyme scheme *a-b-a-b*. The goal of these monographs is informational value. Included are details on the taste and effects of the drugs.

1. The *Yao-hsing ko-k'uo*

Yao-hsing ko-k'uo
"Drug Properties in Verse"
1 chapter / 400 drug descriptions
Author: Kung T'ing-hsien (seventeenth century)
    tzu: Tzu-ts'ai
    hao: Yün-lin shan-jen
    from: Chin-hsi hsien in Chiang-hsi
Written: ca. 1615
Published: date unknown

The commentary in small print was also written by Kung T'ing-hsien and contains information on the preparation of drugs.

Two editions of this work have been preserved—a Korean edition with the shortened title *Yao-hsing ko* and a Chinese edition in the collection *Shou-shih pao-yüan* from the Ming period. Both are undated. Only the preface by Kung T'ing-hsien in the Chinese edition carries a date—1615.[113]

2. The *Hui-min chü pen-ts'ao shih-chien*

Hui-min chü pen-ts'ao shih-chien
"Materia Medica in the Form of an Annotated Poem, from the Office for the Charitable Distribution [of Medications] to the People"
Short title: *Pen-ts'ao shih-chien*
10 chapters / 810 drug descriptions
Author: Chu Lun (eighteenth century)
    tzu: Tung-ch'iao
    from: Wu-chün in Chiang-su
Written: date unknown
Published: 1739

The *Pen-ts'ao shih-chien* by Chu Lun is probably the most extensive of the drug works composed completely (with the exception of the commentary) in verse. The arrangement of its monographs follows the *Pen-ts'ao kang mu* exactly. A poem, in which, among other things, the properties and indications of the substances in question are discussed, is devoted to each drug.

The first three sections—waters, fires, and soils—are each discussed in one monograph containing a four-line strophe with seven characters per line. The remaining monographs each consist of eight lines with seven characters per line.

As in the *Yao-hsing ko-k'uo,* the author also added prose commentaries in small print in which he discussed the mistakes of earlier authors and other viewpoints.

The first edition of the *Pen-ts'ao shih-chien* contained a preface, written by a contemporary of Chu Lun named Huang Ho-ming. Huang Ho-ming discussed in detail the intention of the authors of this literary genre:

> At the beginning of his studies, when someone reads [the medical literature], must he not heave a deep sigh with the feeling of looking on an ocean, and must he not imagine himself as though on a ridge between two different directions? My own heart suffered from this for years. In [the year] *ting-i* [1737], I was transferred as prefect from Jung-chou to Ku-su. There I met Master Chu Tung-ch'iao, the administrator of the Office for Charitable Distribution [of Medicine] to the People [*hui-min chü*]. In [the district of] Wu, the teachings of Hsüan [Yüan] and Ch'i [Po] had already been practiced for generations in his family, with great skill. In the Office, Chu carried out medical treatments with serious devotion and achieved success regularly. I admired him greatly. One day I acquired his *Pen-ts'ao shih-chien.* I read it carefully several times. The subdivisions [in this work] are clearly arranged; the important elements are stressed, material that is puzzling is investigated, [the insignificant] has been eliminated, the mysterious is elucidated. The sentences are brilliant and the meaning is clear. The work can truly serve as a ferry if one has lost his way, and as a bright lamp in a dark room. Its value is not solely its facilitation of memorization and recitation of wonderful medical knowledge, but, in addition, it makes subtleties known and expands rare knowledge. In this manner, a powerful effect develops, bringing near the Golden Age of eternal life. The individual sections, in which waters, grains, vegetables, and foods are described, are comprehensive and excellently compiled. This is what the princely man needs [to be able] to carry out [medicine] as a sideline and to explore [health care] in detail. It is definitely impossible to reject this [work] on the basis of the writings of Ch'i [Po] and Huang-[ti].
> If one considers the incomparability of the rhyme scheme and the skilled realization of the pairings, the "*Pen-ts'ao shih-chien*" represents

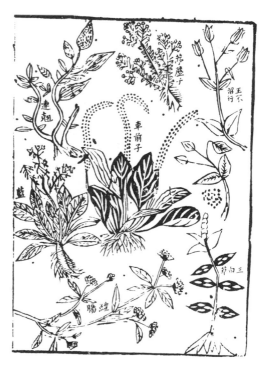

plantain (*ch'e-ch'ien-ts'ao:* middle)—illustrations from the *Pen-ts'ao hui-yen*

the outstanding work of a poet. Another work like this one will never
be written again![114]

In the second edition of the *Pen-ts'ao shih-chien*, which appeared
in 1762, additional prefaces by Wang Yu-tun (dated 1757), Chiang
P'u (dated 1756), and Wang Chin (dated 1745) were included. The
edition ends with an afterword by Hsü Yüeh-lien. A total of five
printings of the *Pen-ts'ao shih-chien* are known and have been preserved; the last of them was published in 1899.[115]

V. VARIOUS PEN-TS'AO WORKS WITH
SPECIALIZED CONTENTS

1. The *Chih-wu ming-shih-t'u k'ao*, a Pen-ts'ao Work Limited to Plants

Chih-wu ming-shih-t'u k'ao
"Treatise on [the Achievement of Consistency among] the Names, Facts, and Illustrations of Plants"
38 chapters / 1714 drug descriptions
Author: Wu Ch'i-chün (1789–1847)
    tzu: Yo-chai
    hao: Yü-lou-nung
    from: Ku-shih in Ho-nan
Written: ca. 1825–1847
Published: 1848

Chih-wu ming-shih-t'u k'ao ch'ang-pien
"Selected Materials for a Treatise on [the Achievement of Consistency among] the Names, Facts, and Illustrations of Plants"
22 chapters / 838 drug descriptions
Author: Wu Ch'i-chün (1789–1847)
    tzu: Yo-chai
    hao: Yü-lou-nung
    from: Ku-shih in Ho-nan
Written: ca. 1825–1847
Published: 1848

amomum fruit *(tou-k'ou)*—Chih-wu ming-shih t'u k'ao

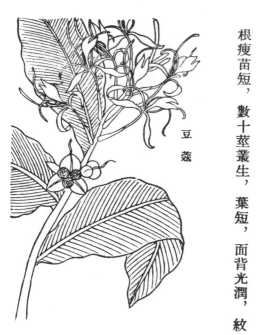

Wu Ch'i-chün wrote the best-known Chinese botanical work of the nineteenth century. In 1817, he passed the *chin-shih* exams with the best results. After a period at the Han-lin Academy, which he also left as the best student, his career as an official—provincial education inspector and vice-president of the War Ministry—took him to Hu-pei and Chiang-hsi. Later he held the positions of governor and of governor-general in the provinces of Hu-nan, Hu-pei, Yün-nan, Kuei-chou, Fu-chien, and Shan-hsi. This career is noteworthy because it was largely responsible for the creation of the *Chih-wu ming-shih-t'u k'ao*.

During his many travels through large regions, Wu Ch'i-chün kept his eyes open for the various plants along the way. In spite of his important position, he did not hesitate to speak with the simplest people. He mentions, in various monographs, that on this or that plant, erroneous views were widespread among the scholars, and that he had been able to find out the actual fact only by talking with the peasants.[116]

Apparently, Wu Ch'i-chün did not pursue his studies as a sporadic sideline, but rather in a serious and systematic manner. When he came to a region during a season that was unfavorable for botanical studies, he made every effort to return at a more suitable time. In the monograph on the *yu-t'ou* vegetable, he lamented that he had always been able to travel to the region concerned only in winter and the trips had, consequently, remained unsuccessful. Even then, at the time when he recorded the yu-t'ou monograph, he claimed he was still plagued by a certain uneasiness as a result. In another case, as well, Wu Ch'i-chün expressed his regrets concerning what was only a semisuccess:

> In Lu-shan, there is the bean-leaf plain. The [bean-leaf] vegetable grows there. When I passed the Lu Mountains, I took efforts to go there and to procure some of this [vegetable]. But we found no one along the way to prepare it. Therefore, I saw its appearance, but its taste remained unknown to me. Here the following saying seems appropriate: "To eat of the [horse-]meat, but not of the horse-liver!"[117]

Wu Ch'i-chün was able to inspect more than fifteen hundred plants during the course of the years. In the *Chih-wu min-shih-t'u k'ao*, he repeatedly criticized previous errors and reproached the authors for having relied on hearsay instead of trusting personal experience and observation.

Upon closer examination of the work, it appears that Wu Ch'i-chün died—at fifty-seven years old—before he was able to complete this sizable work. This assumption, which was expressed both by Na Ch'i and by the editors of the Peking edition of 1963, is supported by several peculiarities in the *Chih-wu ming-shih-t'u k'ao*, especially in the structure, which are not in accordance with Wu Ch'i-chün's great carefulness.

This is already apparent in the arrangement of the monographs. They follow the pattern: grains, vegetables, mountain herbs, swamp herbs, rock herbs, water herbs, bindweed herbs, aromatic herbs, poison herbs, aromatic herbs, flowers, fruits, and trees. The eleven monographs of aromatic herbs found between the groups of bindweed herbs and poison herbs are misplaced. There is no apparent reason why they should be separated from the main group of aromatic herbs which follows the poison herbs.

The length of the individual monographs varies greatly. Some extend over several pages; others are only a few lines long. In several cases, there is no text at all for an illustration and a plant name. Several monographs, in different places, have the same text. Some monographs do have the complete illustration and text part, but the plant name is missing. In some monographs, we find longer text passages which have no connection whatsoever to the monographs; they evidently belong in other sections.

The method of quotation is often inexact and wrong. Thus, the author always stated whether a drug had already been described in the *Pen-ching* or in the *Ming-i pieh-lu*, and into which class of drug it had been grouped there. Here, the drugs of the former upper class are recorded as coming from the lower, those which were taken from the *Pen-ching* are designated *Ming-i pieh-lu* and vice versa.[118]

Wu Ch'i-chün apparently had not found time for a final correction of his *Chih-wu ming-shih-t'u k'ao;* the inconsistencies and mistakes of the work, which have been mentioned as examples here, were scarcely his intention.

In the individual monographs, the author discussed the appearance and color, thermo-influence and taste, the origin of the plants and methods of their cultivation, the medicinally usable parts of the plants, and the medicinal value of the drugs. Again and again, Wu Ch'i-chün devoted himself to the problem that numerous drugs bearing the same names are actually different, and that, conversely, one drug is frequently known under several names. A systematization of the information in the monographs, in the manner of, for example, the *Pen-ts'ao kang mu,* is not discernible. Several monographs constitute complete quotations from earlier pen-ts'ao works; very often, Wu Ch'i-chün referred back to the *T'u-ching pen-ts'ao* and to the *Chiu-huang pen-ts'ao.* Occasionally, he digressed from the actual botanical topic in order to tell stories, in prose or in verse form, which are connected to the described drugs or plants, or in order to express personal views on political or ethical issues:

> *Huang-ch'i.* In the *Pen-ching, huang-ch'i* [had been grouped] in the upper class of drugs; there are several types. Those which come from Shan-hsi and from Mongolia are good. Yunnan products have a laxative effect and are not used.
>
> Yü-lou-nung says: *Huang-ch'i* is a product of the West. The following event is recorded in the annals of the administrative district of Ch'un-an: "At the time of the governmental period *chia-ching* [1522–1566] there was a rumor among the people that [the plant] *huang-ch'i* was growing in this area. Thereupon the authorities issued an order demanding delivery of this [plant]. But, in fact, there was no *huang-ch'i*

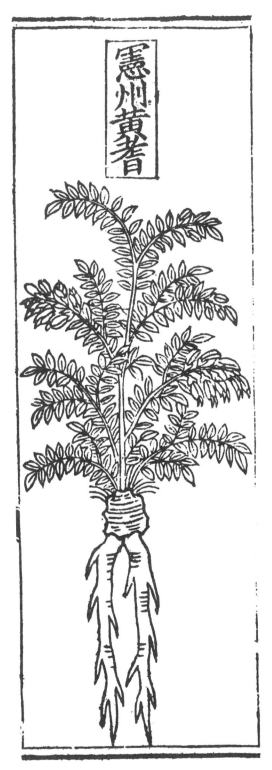

astragalus root *(huang-ch'i)—Ch'ung-hsiu cheng-ho pen-ts'ao*

and [another herb] commonly called *ma-shou* or *mu-su* [was chosen as a] substitute. The physician who was sent to deliver [the herb] was almost beaten to death. He was able to gain freedom only through a payment of thirty to forty [pieces of] gold. Alas! In former times the kings saw to it that there was a proper relation between the products [exacted] and the [size of the] land [where they grew]. Thus, they extended the benefit [of any region and its products] to posterity. Now, shall benefit be turned into harm? The administration of a particular region has to levy tributes [on behalf of the central government]; this has been so since the three eras of antiquity, and there is no way to change that. But the [official] demands [for the native products] are so numerous now and the solicitation of provisions is so extensive that one should think whether the people do not suffer because of this.

The elite of young girls from Lo-yang and the records about *li-chih* from P'u-t'ien are transported over thousands of miles. They permit happiness only for a short time and the exemplary men regret [that all these girls and fruits are taken away from their native land just to produce some short-lived joy somewhere else]. In former times, *li-chih* also existed in Yunnan by the Yüan-chiang River. The demand for it [by the authorities] was so great that, eventually, all trees were cut down. [Formerly], there were occasionally shrimp in the K'un-min Sea. The fishermen there feared the demands [of the authorities]. As soon as they caught such shrimp, they hid them and did not dare to sell them on the markets. Thus, the people fear the officials like devils! When I read the annals [of the individual administrative districts] with regard to items produced, they do not state 'poor region without any growth,' but 'existed formerly, no longer extant today,' because one fears that, otherwise, the high officials would immediately register their demands according to the annals. That is really very sad![119]

Ch'ien-li-chi ["Reaching-a-Goal-in-a-Thousand-Miles"]
Ch'ien-li-chi was first recorded in the *Pen-ts'ao shih-i*. The *T'u-ching [pen-ts'ao]* describes *ch'ien-li kuang* ["Thousand-miles-Brightness"] and *ch'ien-li-chi* as having the same appearance. Li Shih-chen combined [these two plants in one monograph]. That was correct. They have luxuriant yellow blossoms, but those that have dissimilar leaves are from different species, even though their blossoms are the same. Folk healers use [this plant] today to treat the eyes, and they call it *chiu-li ming* ["Nine-Miles-Brilliance"].

Yü-lou-nung says: The drugs have different names in different places. The name *ch'ien-li kuang* is common everywhere from Ling-ch'iao to Yü-chang, and from P'eng-li and the Tung-t'ing [Lake] to Yeh-lang and the Ts'ang-ko [River]. When one hears the name, one knows immediately that the drug must have an effect on the eyes. Its blossoms are yellow, like those of chrysanthemum. They reach their stage of full bloom in the fall and absorb the influence of metal.[120] Perhaps it is a kind of chrysanthemum? Old blossoms [of this plant] become fluffy and then resemble those of the dandelion. The physicians in Yunnan use this plant to wash out the poison from abscesses. I look at it and regret that it cannot serve me as a bright light! Even though there is such an excellent medicinal herb, how could it help me? So I composed a poem:

I climb [a mountain] above the Yunnan sea,
and there I stop because of unexpected sights.
As my eyes gaze far into the distance,
my thoughts wander over thousands of miles.

When I look to the left over a thousand miles,
there begin the rolling waves of the Tung-t'ing Lake.
The water roars like that of the rivers Chiang and Han;
how could anyone paddle his boat there?

When I glance to the right over a thousand miles,
the rivers Lan and Ts'ang appear like one line.
Red hair and golden teeth,[121]
are sent off to poverty and desolation.

When I peer ahead over a thousand miles,
I behold the Chiu-i and Ts'ang-wu Mountains.
Heavy clouds roll everywhere,
the waves of the sea and T'ien-wu.[122]

When I turn my eyes back over a thousand miles,
the Chin-sha and Min-chiang Rivers appear;
they flow eastward ceaselessly,
carrying along the ships from Wu.

Where is the jade metropolis?
It is 36,000 miles from here!
We are separated from it by white clouds,
the multitude of stars stuns the sky.

Spruces, cooled by dew;
mulberry trees, seized by frost.
How could I obtain such divine eyes
to behold the heavenly region?

Chüeh-kuang and *hsieh-hou*
are related to you [as plants].
I shall trust the words of the people
and wipe my eyes [with you].[123]

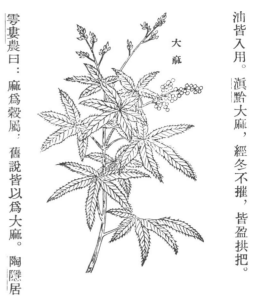

hemp *(ta-ma)—Chih-wu ming-shih t'u k'ao*

The illustrations added to the text are not based on models from previous pen-ts'ao works; they are of the highest quality. Clear sketches illustrate the characteristic traits of each plant.

The work as a whole is of value, as it represents the botanical knowledge accessible to a nineteenth-century scholar in China. Quoting lengthy excerpts from medical, pharmaceutical, botanical, agricultural, and etymological sources, the *Chih-wu ming-shih-t'u k'ao* is also an important work in that it provides ample data as a starting point for research on the history of specific plants in China.

While the descriptions of plants in the *Chih-wu ming-shih-t'u k'ao* contain many lengthy commentaries written by Wu Ch'i-chün himself, based on his personal studies and thoughts, the *Chih-wu ming-shih-t'u k'ao ch'ang-pien* comprises almost exclusively materials that Wu Ch'i-chün took from earlier works and which he had expanded by only a few commentaries.[124]

2.1. The *Hu pen-ts'ao*

Cheng Ch'ien was a scholar of the T'ang period. His poetry and landscape painting brought him fame. Unfortunately, his materia medica which dealt specifically with the medications of the Hu—that is, peoples neighboring the Chinese in the northwest—was lost very early. Li Shih-chen already wrote that he had not been able to see this work.[125] Only a number of quotations have been preserved. They are found, above all, in a work entitled *Pei-hu lu*, which was written around 875 by Tuan Kung-lu. On the basis of the *Pei-hu lu*, Berthold Laufer concluded, for example, that Cheng Ch'ien had probably been the first author in China to call attention to the wild walnut.[126]

2. Regionally Specialized Pen-ts'ao Works

Hu pen-ts'ao
"Materia Medica of the Hu Lands"
7 chapters / number of drug descriptions: unknown
Author: Cheng Ch'ien (eighth century)
    tzu: Jo-chai
    hao: Kuang-wen
    from: Jung-yang in Ho-nan
Written: date unknown
Published: date unknown

Nan-hai yao p'u
"The Book of Drugs from the South Sea"
Short title: *Hai-yao p'u*
1 chapter / number of drug descriptions: unknown
Author: unknown
Written: T'ang period (?)
Published: date unknown

2.2. The *Nan-hai yao-p'u*

The contents of the *Nan-hai yao-p'u* have also been almost entirely lost for a long time. Only six quotations were taken over by the authors of the *Chia-yu pen-ts'ao*. The list of works used as source material for the *Chia-yu pen-ts'ao* contains the following brief description of the text:

> [The *Nan-hai yao-p'u*] lists various drugs of the south. It describes the places of origin and the experiences one has had with their therapeutic effects. The contents are not structured in any special way, and the work was probably written by an author toward the end of the T'ang period.[127]

3. Lists of Secondary Names for Drugs

Chu-yao i-ming
"Secondary Names of All Drugs"
10 chapters
Author: Shih Hsing-chih
        from: Sha-men in Ho-nan
Written: ca. 600 or earlier
Published: date unknown

Yao-ming p'u
"The Book of Drug Names"
1 chapter
Author: Hou Ning-chi (tenth century)
Written: date unknown
Published: date unknown

Yao-ming shih
"The Poem of Drug Names"
1 chapter
Author: Ch'en Ya (Sung period)
    tzu: Ya-chih (?)
    from: Yang-chou (?)
Written: date unknown
Published: date unknown

Chu-yao pieh-ming lu
"Enumeration of the Secondary Names of All Drugs"
1 chapter
Author: unknown
Written: date unknown; an unpublished manuscript from the end of the Ch'ing period or the beginning of the republic has been preserved

Ku-chin yao-wu pieh-ming k'ao
"A study of the Secondary Names of Drugs from Old and New Times"
1 chapter / 716 primary drug names
Author: Liu Ya-nung (twentieth century)
Written: date unknown
Published: 1936

3.1. The *Chu-yao i-ming*

3.2. The *Yao-ming p'u*

3.3. The *Yao-ming shih*

3.4. The *Chu-yao pieh-ming lu*

3.5. The *Ku-chin yao-wu pieh-ming k'ao*

Although the list of special works on drug synonyms is fairly long—it extends from the sixth-seventh century into the time of the republic—not much can be said about the individual works.

The *Yao-ming p'u* has been preserved, at least in part. In the *Shuo-fu*, we find a list, so entitled, of 193 drug names used only regionally or rarely, together with their better-known equivalents.[128] Judging by its title, the *Yao-ming shih* seems to have been composed in verse, in order to facilitate memorization of the synonyms.[129]

The *Ku-chin yao-wu pieh-ming k'ao* is a modern work. The author, Liu Ya-nung, published it himself.[130] It contains a list of 716 names of traditional Chinese drugs, including a large number of secondary names for each. The work is preceded by 54 drug illustrations under the heading "Selected Important Illustrations of Medicinal Drugs." The *Ku-chin yao-wu pieh-ming k'ao* is, unfortunately, quite rare and is not indexed. Otherwise, it might enable the solution of a number of questions concerning rare drug names that appear in various literary genres.

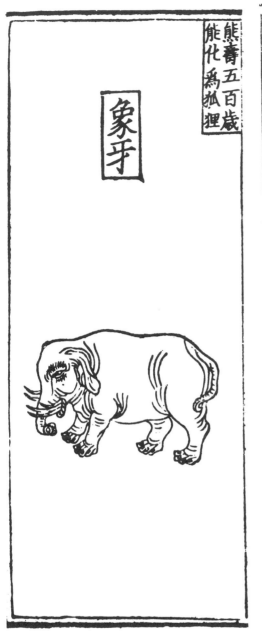

熊壽五百歲
能化爲狐狸

象牙

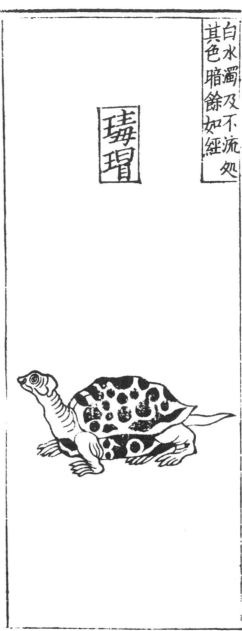

白水濁及不流処
其色暗餘如縕

瑇瑁

elephant tusks *(hsiang-ya)—Ch'ung-hsiu cheng-ho pen-ts'ao*

Tortoise carapace *(tai-mao)—Ch'ung-hsiu cheng-ho pen-ts'ao*

E. The Chinese Pharmacopoeias
of the Twentieth Century

I. THE PHARMACOPOEIAS OF THE
REPUBLIC OF CHINA

1. On the Historical Background of Medicine and Pharmacy in Early Twentieth-Century China

It is difficult to imagine the excitement with which China met the introduction of Western science and medicine in the late nineteenth and early twentieth century. The powerful military, technological, and ideological impact of Western culture on China occurred toward the end of an epoch in Chinese history that had left the "Middle Empire" so exhausted that neither its political structure nor its economic resources—and least of all its traditional sciences—provided any realistic chance for coping successfully with this new force from outside. China's historical situation at the moment of its clash with the Western nations engendered the enthusiasm with which an overwhelming majority of Chinese intellectuals welcomed a new method of expanding knowledge.[1]

There had been, during the last centuries of the imperial dynasties, an increasingly intensive search for ways to solve the problems of Chinese society. Beginning in the seventeenth century, numerous mutually contradictory philosophical approaches to ordering, restructuring, or even revolutionizing China's society were developed. The resulting increase in heterogeneity of the Chinese world view was paralleled in Chinese medicine. Reading through the Chinese medical literature from the twelfth century through the eighteenth and nineteenth centuries on, one is invariably left with an impression of a growing lack of unified theoretical orientation among Chinese intellectuals and practitioners concerned with health care principles. Conflicting exegeses of the traditional concepts of yinyang and of the Five Phases sought to integrate the personal experience of the individual with the classical theories from antiquity to achieve progress in day-to-day medical practice. None of these many attempts at reconciliation was sufficiently convincing to push the other competing doctrines aside and emerge as a generally recognized and dominating paradigm.[2]

Into this multifaceted internal struggle for the appropriate way out of confusion stepped unexpectedly and uninvitedly the civilization of the West. It opened various visions. At first the missionaries appeared to tell of Christianity. They failed, however, to achieve lasting success.[3] Then a magic word entered China which in the eyes of many influential thinkers soon became linked with the promise of a better future—the word was "science."[4] Within a few decades, this Western concept of

261

the dynamics of knowledge, of the methodological search for objectivity and reproducible truths became immensely attractive for all those who were concerned with reforming Chinese culture through adaptation to the changing realities of interior and international politics.

Modern Western medicine followed as an integrated part of this promising science. Viewed retrospectively, medicine from around the turn of the century still had far to go toward the diagnostic and therapeutic achievements of today. It seems, though, that there were mainly two aspects that led the Chinese reformers and revolutionaries to believe that a healing system based on science was superior to their own medical traditions. These aspects were, first, health politics and public health associated with Western medicine and, second, expectations of Western health care practice. As with the sciences, Western medicine was supported by a certainty of the fantastic possibilities that vigorous application of the scientific method would guarantee for the future. Traditional Chinese medicine, whose only progress was seen in the fact that for centuries an ever growing number of authors had competed for a correct exegesis of the classics of antiquity, was in no way able to offer such promising perspectives. It became identified as part of the value system of the old society and was condemned to vanish. Only a small number of conservatives supported the representatives of traditional Chinese healing.

Thus, when in 1914, a delegation of practitioners of traditional Chinese medicine approached Wang Ta-hsieh, the head of the Ministry of Education, asking him to register a "Peking Medical Society," he bluntly told them: "I have decided to abandon Chinese medicine from now on and not to make any use of Chinese pharmacy!"[5] Such was the general mood of the time. In the political arena, both the nationalists, organized in the Kuo-min-tang party, and the Marxists, saw, for the time being, no reason to exclude any specific aspect—such as traditional materia medica—from the cultural heritage they now considered an obstacle on China's long and difficult way into an era of renewed strength and international influence.[6]

It is only with this historical background in mind that one can understand the contents and structure of the pharmacopoeias of the Republic of China, especially so if one searches, in these works, for traces of traditional Chinese pharmaceutical knowledge and substances.

In the long history of pen-ts'ao literature, several drug compendia had been produced, by imperial order, by official committees including civil service personnel and government-appointed experts. Nevertheless, as I have pointed out earlier, none of these works could justly be called a pharmacopoeia in the modern sense of this term, simply because they were not designed to provide physicians or pharmacists with fixed standards of drug quality and drug usage, adherence to which was enforced by government authorities.

The first such pharmacopoeia—the Chinese chose the term yao-tien ("drug code")—was published in China in 1930. As we read in its preface, its authors were quite aware of China's pharmaceutical past; in fact, the preface itself reminds us in some respects of the prefaces quoted, in preceding chapters of this book, from previous

2. China's First Pharmacopoeia: the *Chung-hua yao-tien* of 1930

Chung-hua yao-tien, ti-i-pan
"Chinese Drug Code, First Edition"
Main text and appendixes / 676 drug descriptions
Editor-in-chief: Liu Jui-heng
Published: 1930

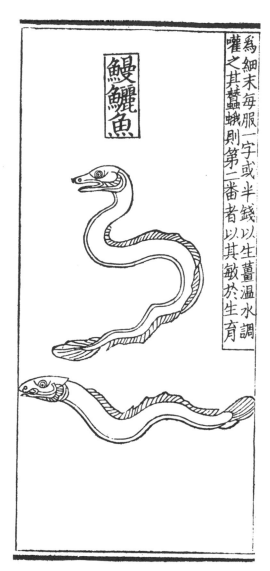

為細末每服一字或半錢以生薑溫水調
虁之其蠱蝨則第二番者以其敏於生育

eels *(man-li-yü)—Ch'ung-hsiu cheng-ho pen-ts'ao*

drug compendia. In contrast to the purpose of historical delineations of pen-ts'ao literature in the drug works of the main tradition, though, the author of the preface to the *Chung-hua yao-tien* did not intend to demonstrate continuity; he intended instead to point out a decisive break in the history of Chinese pharmaceutical literature. For him, the traditional pen-ts'ao works, although highly appreciated in the past, were nothing but "waste-paper" now. He saw the *Chung-hua yao-tien* as a late joining by China of a tradition that had been initiated many centuries ago in the West, by the government of the city of Nuremberg when it issued the *Dispensatorium* of Valerius Cordus as the first "drug code" of the world:

> When physicians [utilize] drugs it is quite difficult for them to distinguish their characteristics. Some prescriptions are produced through chemical processes. There are rules underlying therapeutic treatment. In efficacious decoctions the blending [of the ingredients] is most important and for the weighing [of these ingredients] one must pay attention to the different units with not even the slightest aberrations being permitted. When one calculates what is normal and when one takes hold of what is proper, there must be fixed standards. This is the purpose for which drug codes of all countries are compiled. The earliest drug code in the world was published by the Nuremberg government in 1542. This book generated a widespread impact; all the [other] countries followed in the footsteps of Nuremberg. Meritorious editors often produced official compilations. Although in our own country no book was created as a drug code, the old drugs were fully laid out in the *pen-ts'ao* [works]. In the distant past of precivilization, there are no indications of literary records [of pharmaceutical knowledge]. The correct [use of the] name *pen-ts'ao* appears, for the first time, in the records on [the emperor] Hsiao P'ing. Then, [pharmaceutical knowledge] was recited in ten thousand words and it was further transmitted by the scriptures of Lou Hu. [The authors of the bibliographical] section of the Sui [history] searched everywhere [for *pen-ts'ao* titles], and they recorded quite a number of such writings. And still, [most of] the private studies by individual authors were not mentioned in the official collections. Then, during the T'ang and Shu periods, two definitive books were published. During the Sung [dynasty], T'ang Shen-wei once again conducted a comprehensive examination of the entire literature and produced the work *Cheng-lei pen-ts'ao*. In the *cheng-ho* period, Mr. Ts'ao was ordered to compare [all materials extant]. When the *shao-hsing* era came up, [the emperor] handed this task over to the *chou-chien* office and a new book was printed. The significance [of all these scriptures] equaled that of drug codes. These documents were highly valued by the medical world. But if recent knowledge is not added [to these texts], it is rather difficult to discover the essence of the Creation; and if there are no mistakes [of former times] that can be eliminated, how can there be one-sided and useless prescriptions?[7] The [pen-ts'ao] books were bought heatedly, and they were valued like finest gold. They [were appreciated like] shining treasures and rich dresses, but today they are nothing but waste-paper. Since the end of the Ch'ing [government], when all trade restrictions were removed, the old teachings have deteriorated and a new medicine has risen instead. The selection [of modern substances] to enter our basket of drugs included a large number [of strong medications suitable] to confuse one's mind.[8] Even if pills of only the size of eggs of small birds were produced, one was not to commit the slightest inaccuracy. And still no codified standards existed concerning a differentiation of these drugs. All the poisons [one can think of] were brought together for medical treatments, and yet there

were no decisive rules [to use them]. When [I, Liu] Jui-heng began to participate in the government, I proposed to elaborate [such rules]. Subsequently an office was established in the capital [for research on this issue]. It contained books sending out an aroma which expelled all the evil. I called together experts from all over the country. These people exhausted their special expertise, and they put to effort all their skills. They burned the oil [of their lamps] to continue their task even at night. Once and again they revised their manuscripts and rearranged their data until, finally, after years had passed, they let their bamboo slabs dry [for final writing]. As a result of this, everybody who has to make a decision knows, from now on, what to look out for. A mound of nine fathoms has been erected;[9] the height of the cliff has luckily been reached! One should live in fear of posterity and, therefore, I hope that [this work] will be subjected to continuous improvement. This is my greatest desire. Together we shall strive for rapid progress, year after year!

Republic of China, 19th year, 5th month.
Written by Liu Jui-heng.[10]

The first Chinese drug code was printed in October 1930 and was enacted in August of the following year.

2.1. Structure and content of the first drug code of China

Following the preface we find a list of twenty-eight names of persons who contributed to this work, headed by Liu Jui-heng, then minister of health of the Republic of China, as editor-in-chief.

Next comes a section of twenty-eight general introductory statements, explaining the structure of the drug code and its most advantageous usage. From the first of these statements we learn that the individual monographs were ordered alphabetically according to the Latin designations of the drugs described as they were used in the English literature. The following statement explains the structure of the heading of each monograph. First the Chinese name of the respective substance or formula is given, then the English-style Latin designation and its abbreviation, followed by, if there was a difference, the German-style Latin designation. In case the substance described is a chemical drug, summary formula and molecular weight are added to the heading of the monograph. The third statement elucidates the structure of the individual monographs. Accordingly they are divided along the following criteria: (1) origin of the drug, (2) standard contents, (3) methods of preparation, (4) nature and appearance, (5) identification tests, (6) analysis, (7) determination of content or physiological analysis, (8) storage methods, (9) suitable forms of medication, and (10) dosage (minimum and maximum individual dosage; daily maximum dosage).

The remaining introductory statements refer to technical details such as the designation of chemical substances, and to units of measurement, selection of proper drugs, sizes of sieves, different degrees of fineness of powders, and to the tables of the appendix.

The monograph section, following these introductory statements, reflects the European materia medica of the time. If, in some rare instances, one finds a drug described that was known in China traditionally, it was incorporated only because it was part of European pharmacy. An example is *Oleum Tiglii*—that is, the oil of pa-tou—a drug whose description we have followed through the entire history of Chinese pen-ts'ao literature. Pa-tou itself was not included in the *Chung-hua yao-tien* of 1930; on the oil we read the following.

> *Pa-tou oil*
> *Oleum Tiglii*, Ol. Tiglii; *Oleum Crotonis*
> This article is a fat oil which is obtained from the seeds of *Croton Tiglium Linné* [*pa-tou*], a plant of the family *ta-chi* [*Euphorbiaceae*].
>
> *Attention:* This article easily causes measleslike pustules on contact with the skin or any membrane. When handling [this article] one must take care.
>
> *Nature and Appearance:* This article is a light yellow or yellowish-brown colored slightly sticky and thick, fluorescent liquid. It has a slight but quite characteristic odor. Its taste is pungent. Extreme caution is advisable when tasting this substance with one's mouth.
>
> This article dissolves in alcohol only very little. If one leaves it [in alcohol] for a little while, the degree of solution increases. It dissolves easily in ether, chloroform, fat oils, and volatile oils.
>
> *Identification and methods of analysis:* (1) Take 1 cc of this article, add water-free alcohol 2 cc, after mixing [the two components] add heat and a clear solution will result. Then let it become cold again and [the oil] will separate [from the alcohol] either completely or partially.
>
> (2) If this article is brought on enzyme test paper (moisten with alcohol for preparation), it will display an acid reaction.
>
> (3) The specific gravity of this article, at 25°C, is 0.935–0.950.
>
> (4) Take 2 cc of this article, add a mixture of 1 cc fuming nitric acid and 1 cc distilled water, stir for a few minutes, let sit for 24 hours. There must not be a partial or complete hardening (test for other oils).
>
> (5) The alkaline value of this article is 200–215.
>
> (6) The iodine value of this article is 104–110.
>
> *Storage methods:* Keep in tightly sealed, small brown-colored glass bottles; store in a cold, dark place.
>
> *Dosage:* Individual doses: 0.02–0.05cc
> daily doses: 0.15 cc[11]

The monographs, altogether numbering 676, are followed by the appendixes which offer the following information:

1. The necessary test-reagents (including indicator-liquids and volumetric solutions), from *Acetonum* to *Solutio Sodii Thiosulfatis volumetrica Decinormalis*.
2. Special reactions of individual substances in pure state.
3. General examination methods (e.g., to check for heavy metals, arsenic, or chlorides and iodides; to determine the iodine value; to determine the contents of alcohol in volatile oils; to determine the melting point; to determine the refractory index).
4. Tables
    (a) table of frequently prepared medications that ought to be kept in stock by all pharmacies permanently (127 substances from *Acacia* to *Zinci sulphas*)
    (b) table of poisonous medications that have to be kept locked and separate from the other drugs
    (c) table of strong medications that have to be kept separate from the other drugs

(d) dosage tables for adults

(e) table of atomic weights

(f) table of secondary names

(g) table of specific gravity of acids, bases, and alcohols.

The volume is concluded by one index each of the Chinese and Latin names.

2.2. The integration of Western terminology

In essence, the first drug code of China constituted a selection, and transfer into Chinese language, of a materia medica and related pharmaceutical procedures as they were described in the official pharmacopoeias of various European states (as well as in the *United States Pharmacopoeia*) of that time.

There were only a few instances where the terminology employed in the *Chung-hua yao-tien* adopted terms used in traditional Chinese pharmaceutical literature. Thus, the *Pilulae* were designated with the traditional Chinese term for pills, that is, *wan*. But most of the forms of medication referred to in the *Chung-hua yao-tien* were not known in China before and, consequently, new terms had to be introduced. In some instances obsolete, old characters were chosen which, because of their meaning and pronunciation, came close to what they were now meant to designate. For instance, to designate the Western term *elixir,* a character was selected that was used in Chinese antiquity to designate various kinds of wine, made from millet, rice, or other grains. It consisted of two parts; left a radical indicating the meaning of "wine," right a radical being pronounced "*e*". A similar character 酏 was chosen for *tinctura:* its left part indicated the meaning of "wine," 酊 while its right part was pronounced "*ting*." Other forms of medication were designated by combinations of Chinese characters in an attempt to reflect their actual character: *capsulae* were termed *chiao-nang* 膠囊 ("gelatin-containers"); *emplastrum* was termed *ying-kao* ("stiff paste"); 硬膏 *linimentum* was termed *ch'a-chi* ("preparation to rub"). 搽劑

In the case of the chemical elements, new characters were designed. Some Western names of medical substances were simply designated with Chinese characters reflecting the Western pronunciation of these names. Thus, *atropina* was designated with characters being read 阿託品 *a-t'o-p'in,* and *barbitalum* was designated with Chinese characters 巴比持魯 being read *pa-pi-t'e-lu.*

The terminology employed in the *Chung-hua yao-tien* was pointed out here in detail as only one indicator of the fact that the first drug code of China should be regarded as a totally alien body in Chinese culture. It was accessible only for those few who had received a modern Western-type pharmaceutical training, and it was entirely inaccessible for those hundreds of thousands who were knowledgeable in traditional Chinese materia medica and who continued to practice traditional Chinese pharmacy all over the country. The *Chung-hua yao-tien* resulted from a complete renunciation of Chinese traditions and from a complete turn towards Western therapeutic methods. It is not entirely without irony that as a consequence of this policy, a large number of medications found entrance to China, and were accepted officially, which were part of traditional European materia medica, while, at the same time, the indigenous heritage was disregarded. One reason for this, of course, lay in the fact that at that time a scientific basis had been elaborated already for a number of herbal drugs which had been handed down, in Europe, through the centuries. Such a legitimation was not yet available for traditional Chinese drugs.

A first unchanged reprint of the *Chung-hua yao-tien* was printed in 1936; it appeared in 1937. The publisher added to the title the designation "Second Edition." This rather misleading practice was continued until at least an eighth unchanged reprint appeared in Hong Kong in 1953, designated as "Eighth Edition." The official "Second Edition," that is, a completely revised version of the drug code of the Republic of China, appeared only in 1959.

3. The *Pharmacopoea Chinensis Editio II*

Chung-hua yao-tien, ti-erh-pan
"Chinese Drug Code, Second Edition"
Latin title: *Pharmacopoea Chinensis Editio II*
Main text and appendixes / 681 drug descriptions
Editor-in-chief: Liu Jui-heng
Published: 1959

In accordance with such customs in the West, the second edition of the drug code of the Republic of China was named, in addition to *Chung-hua yao-tien Second Edition, Pharmacopoea Chinensis Editio II*. Again I quote the preface in full length because it is rather informative:

Those who discussed medicine in ancient times often cultivated medicine and pharmacy together. Although in recent times medicine and pharmacy have been separated, each having its own respective disciplines, there is still a cooperation on the basis of a division of labor. And because [the practitioners of medicine and pharmacy] ever seek refinement in what they do, they are particularly able to achieve the effects of mutual assistance and mutual perfection. Now, any therapeutic effect is intimately related to the quality of drugs [employed], and each country has produced a drug code [providing information] on the examination of each single drug, on summary formulas and molecular weights, on preparation methods and origin, on nature and appearance, on ingredients and contents, on methods to identify and to analyze, on methods of storage and on dosage, and so on, [enabling the practitioner to know] how to conform to legal standards. Today's physics and chemistry are subject to continuous and rapid change, and the progress in the medical and pharmaceutical sciences is, as a result, miraculously fast. For this reason, each country's drug code is repeatedly published again in new editions. When the Chinese drug code was first published in the fifth month of the nineteenth year of the Republic, it was already suggested that it should be revised every ten years in order to correspond to the requirements [of pharmaceutical practice]. This was a very good idea. In the twenty-ninth year [of the Republic], the time for revision had come but just at this time the anti-Japanese war affairs had reached their climax, and there was no time to take up this task. After demobilization we were confronted with the seditious uprising of the bandit-communists which, again, led to years without peace, thus causing further delay and postponement of the project. Since the government was moved to Taiwan the people receive an education and no efforts are spared. Those who could be useful for a counterattack and for the restoration of the nation were all taken into service. None of them did not give all his strength to proceed toward [this goal]. In this respect, especially the drug code, which is related to the existence and welfare of the people, had to be adapted to the time by means of a further revision. This ministry, therefore, in the tenth month of the fortieth year of the Republic [1951] established a committee for the revision of

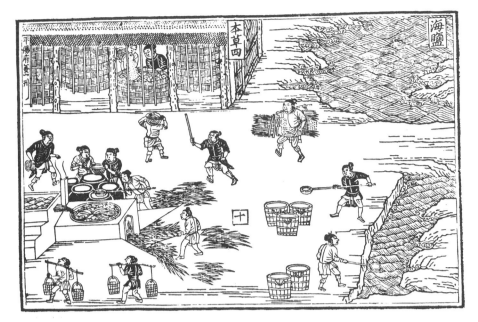

Sequences of illustrations from *Pen-ts'ao* works of various centuries depicting the production of salt which show both the close imitation of the original subject and stylistic changes dictated by contemporary requirements. The situation is similar for the continuity of themes in drug illustrations. The following scenes, with varying completeness, are generally included: the collection of salt water from the sea in buckets, the evaporation of salt water in basins over fire, the introduction of salt water from the sea into drying basins, the filling of sacks with dried salt, and the weighing of the product before representatives of the State salt monopoly.

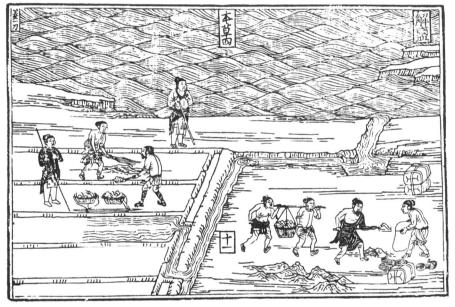

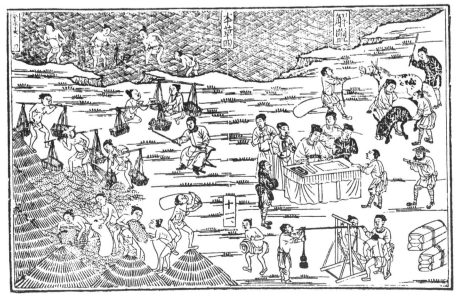

the production of salt—illustrations from the 1249 edition of the *Ch'ung-hsiu cheng-ho pen-ts'ao*

the Chinese drug code; calling together, as its committee members, all those scholars of this country who are experts in the medical and pharmaceutical sciences. Liu Jui-heng was asked to head the entire affair as an adviser. Within three years the first draft of the main text was completed. Subsequently a group for general arrangement was organized to gather [further] material, to uncover discrepancies, to supplement the main text, and to add appendixes. [This group] spent more than a year with careful reading and then completed a definite draft. From the first edition 297 articles were removed, 302 articles were added, bringing the total number to 681 articles [described in monographs]. Again a group was set up for renewed examination [of the draft], which carefully investigated [the work and did the final] editing. Now it will be handed over to the printer. I am pleased to see the completion [of this project], and it is therefore that I have linked a few words in order to fill the first [page] of this [book].

> T'ien Chiung-chin, recorded in Taipei
> Republic of China, 48th year, 11th month, 12th day[12]

3.1. Structure and content of the Drug Code of the Republic of China, second edition

The preface was written by T'ien Chiung-chin as head of the Ministry of Interior Affairs, which was responsible, at that time, for matters of health care. As he indicated, Liu Jui-heng, head of the Ministry of Health in 1930, was appointed editor-in-chief.

The legal character of the pharmacopoeia is displayed more openly in the second than in the first edition. The front page contains the information: "Law of the Ministry of Interior Affairs. T'ai (48) Interior/Hygiene No. 21370. Law to publish the Enactment of the Second Edition of the Drug Code of China. The Minister T'ien Chiung-chin. Republic of China, 48th year, 11th month, 12th day."

The preface is followed by a general table of contents, a list of contributors, a list of articles from the first edition that were not adopted by the second edition, and a list of articles adopted, for the first time, by the second edition. Next come the general introductory statements which, in comparison with the first edition, were largely newly formulated. Again, the legal character of the pharmocopoeia is brought out more strongly here than in the first edition. Thus, after the official Chinese and Latin names of the pharmacopoeia and after a survey of its contents we read the following statement:

> Legal drugs:
> (1) All legal drugs and products—simply called "drugs" below—recorded in the main text of this Drug Code, their deployment, purchase, and sale, as well as production, must conform to the legal specifications listed in this Drug Code with respect to norms of purity and contents, as well as to their standards of effectiveness, at the time when they are used for therapeutic purposes.[13]

The following statement of the introductory section informs the reader that the monographs in the second edition of the drug code once again are ordered according to the English-style Latin names of

the production of salt—illustrations from a Yüan edition of the *Hsin-pien lei-yao t'u-chu pen-ts'ao*

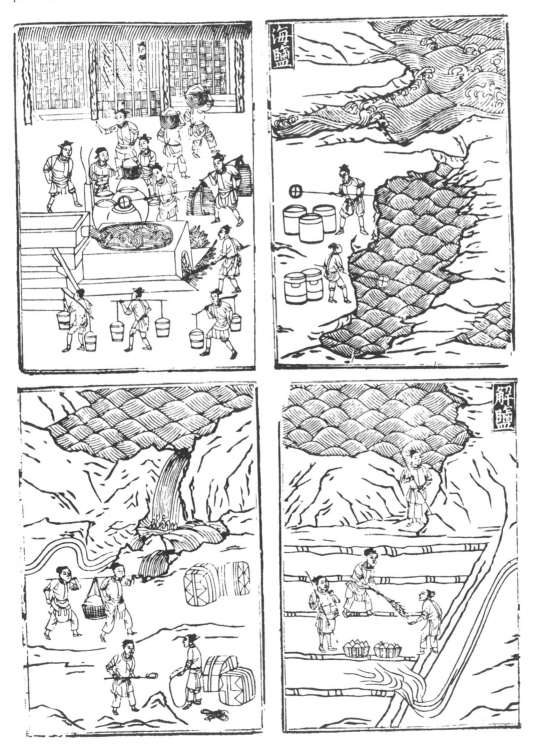

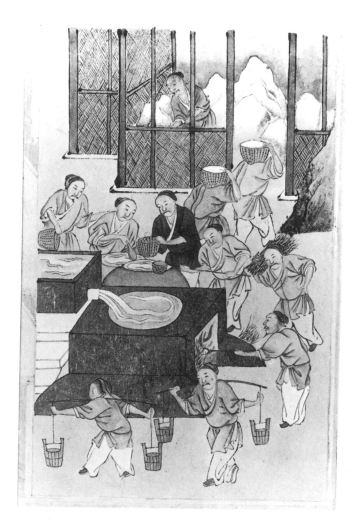

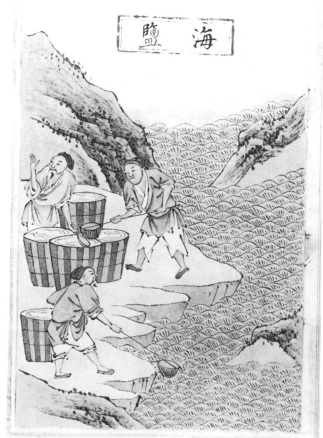

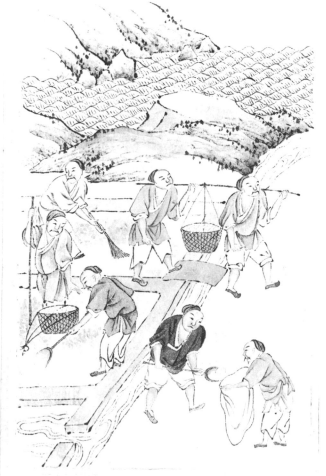

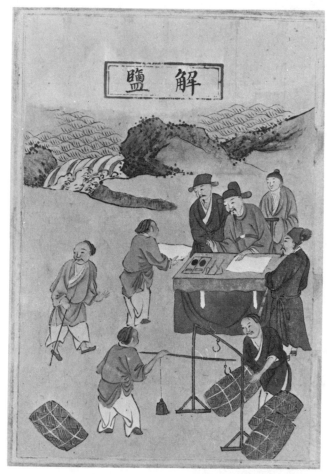

the production of salt—illustrations from an
18th century edition of the *Cheng-lei-pen-ts'ao*
in the collection *Szu-k'u ch'üan-shu*

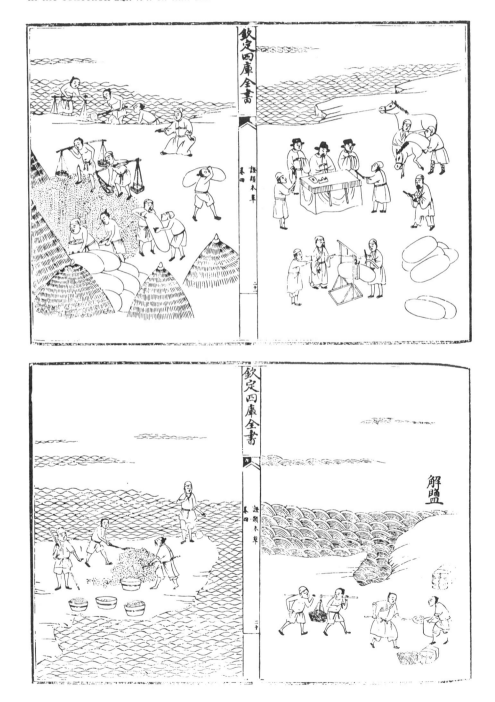

the substances and preparations described. The third statement lists the criteria according to which the medications are described in the individual monographs, namely (1) name, (2) Latin name and its abbreviation, (3) structural formula, summary formula, and molecular weight, if it is a chemical substance, (4) secondary names, (5) method of production or origin, (6) norms of contents and effectiveness (7) nature and appearance, (8) identification, (9) analysis of purity and general norms, (10) determination of contents and determination of effectiveness, (11) methods of storage, (12) labeling, and (13) dosage. The German-style Latin names of the drugs are only occasionally mentioned under the rubric of secondary names. Many of the old monographs adopted from the first edition were rearranged in the second edition, since the former chemical designations of substances were replaced by generic designations, resulting in a different alphabetical order. Most obvious among newly adopted forms of medication are injection-liquids, tablets, and vaccines.

The appendixes and tables do not have to be treated here in detail; they were modified in the second edition of the *Chung-hua yao-tien* corresponding to recent developments in Western pharmacy. Two indexes of Chinese and Latin names conclude the volume.

The second edition of *Chung-hua yao-tien* disregarded traditional Chinese materia medica, pharmaceutical procedures, and forms of medication to the same extent as did the first edition. This official policy is rather noteworthy in light of the fact that the government of the Republic of China, after its move to Taiwan, had eliminated virtually all restrictions placed upon the practice of traditional Chinese medicine and pharmacy by the Japanese who held administrative control over Taiwan from 1895 to 1945.[14] Despite a reality of ubiquitous coexistence of Western-type and traditional pharmacies on Taiwan, the government did not take any steps to widen the scope of its drug code to include—and thus standardize and control—the usage of traditional Chinese materia medica. Traditional Chinese pharmacy did not offer any objective criteria of its own that would have allowed a reliable evaluation of the properties of different wares. Taste and thermo-influence, color and smell were sufficient criteria for traditional practitioners, but they did not appeal to an administration that favored the objectivity and reproducible nature of scientific insights as the basis of all knowledge. A standardization of traditional materia medica would have been possible only by means of modern pharmacognostic and pharmacological research on the active ingredients of traditional Chinese drugs. This, however, implied the integration of traditional Chinese materia medica into modern Western-style pharmacy and would have had no impact on the practice of traditional pharmacy on Taiwan as long as the latter was permitted to continue along centuries-old lines. To completely outlaw the traditional way of Chinese pharmacy and remodel it in accordance with the example of Western-style pharmacy would have been politically unfeasible.

4. The *Pharmacopoea Chinensis Editio III*

The policy of neglecting traditional Chinese pharmacy was continued with the third revised edition of the drug code of the Republic of

China. It was issued by the Public Health Office of the government in March 1980, and it was enacted as law six months later.

The preface, written by the head of that office and editor-in-chief Wang Chin-mao, focused merely on organizational details of the compilation of this work and needs not be quoted here in translation. Two statements, though, deserve attention. First, from now on, a standing committee was entrusted with continuous work on the revision of the drug code and, second, the author of the preface took care to point out the adaptation of the contents of this work to the official pharmacopoeias of the Western world and Japan, and to the standards of drug usage as formulated in international conventions.[15]

The structure of the *Pharmacopoea Chinensis Editio III*, as the drug code was named officially, corresponds to the structure of the previous edition. One innovation is a comparative list, preceding the general introductory statements, of old and new, Chinese and Latin designations of medications, which had been exchanged in accordance with the most recent international standards.

The monographs contain a new rubric, that is, a reference to the therapeutic indication or general usage of the article described, as, for instance, "external disinfectant," "sleep-inducing substance," or "auxiliary material for the preparation of specific forms of medication."

The appendixes are very detailed and comprehensive; they contain elaborate descriptions of the most recent test-methods of Western pharmacy to examine, by means of physical, chemical, or biological procedures, identity, purity, contents, or other specific characteristics of the medications described in the monographs.

Thus, the latest edition of the drug code of the Republic of China, currently in force, constitutes a highly sophisticated compendium solely concerned with modern Western-type pharmacy. Like its predecessors, it completely neglects the reality of the continuing practice of traditional Chinese pharmacy all over the island. There are no signs in the *Pharmacopoea Chinensis Editio III* of any attempts to incorporate Chinese traditional drugs on the basis of modern scientific insights as to their active ingredients.

Taiwan's health care situation is marked by a therapeutic plurality. Besides pragmatic folk healers, Buddhist religious therapy and shamanistic practitioners have a large and trusting clientele. The same is true for practitioners of traditional acupuncture and for those who base their practice on traditional Chinese materia medica. All these groups live in a situation of what I have called elsewhere unstructured coexistence[16] with a Western-style medicine and pharmacy, with varying degrees of unstructured integration (when traditional pharmacies or traditional physicians sell or employ antibiotics with their herbal remedies), unstructured cooperation (when, for instance, traditional practitioners have their patients undergo modern diagnostic tests and then treat them with traditional remedies), or unstructured competition (when unchecked claims and counterclaims are published or disseminated concerning the superiority of one system over the other). While it is easy to point out the drawbacks of such a situation, it should not be overlooked that the only alternative would be a repressive policy where the viewpoints of one group in society are en-

Chung-hua yao-tien, ti-san-pan
"Chinese Drug Code, Third Edition"
Latin title: *Pharmacopoea Chinensis Editio III*
Main text and appendixes / 747 drug descriptions
Editor-in-chief: Wang Chin-mao
Published: 1980

forced as the standards of the entire population. Modern Western-style medicine and pharmacy are the only therapeutic systems that base large parts of their knowledge and practice on technical criteria, thus allowing for a high degree of standardization both of therapeutic procedures and of the means employed in therapy. If the insights of science are considered as nearest to truth, a policy might be advocated demanding the extension of scientific principles to competing systems of health care. As a consequence, some aspects of these competing systems (for instance, certain therapeutic techniques) could be recognized as "valuable" because their effectiveness can be verified with scientific methods; but the system as such would have to be eliminated because—and this may be a truism—no therapeutic system outside of modern scientific medicine can be completely legitimated by scientific principles. In the long run, if such a policy is pursued, the "valuable" aspects of competing systems will become adjuncts of modern Western medicine. If, in contrast, the issue of therapeutic plurality is seen from a viewpoint of social relativity which might entail the argument that a person's or a social group's understanding of the origins of illness and of the necessary measures to prevent or treat illness is generally socially conditioned and legitimate in its own right, there is no justification at all to force one segment of the population to resort to "alien" therapeutic means which are believed in by another segment of the population. Such a viewpoint might lead to a policy of unstructured or structured coexistence between differently conceptualized therapy systems in one society. In a situation of unstructured or loosely structured coexistence of various therapy systems a risk exists, of course, that people are cheated or even harmed by charlatans taking advantage of such liberalism. Yet, such a risk might be matched (or even offset) by the advantage of having the freedom to choose any therapy one desires which, in the long run, may result in better "health" than any forcibly introduced system with its accompanying frictions and problems of patient compliance.

We do not know whether such considerations or merely the requirements of political feasibility have led to the situation on Taiwan as described above. In this regard it might be of interest to point out the background of two persons who are listed at prominent places among the contributors to the latest edition of the drug code of the Republic of China. Right after the editor-in-chief Wang Chin-mao, one finds the name of Hsü Hung-yüan as one of three vice-editors-in-chief. Dr. Hsü was trained in Japan and operates, on Taiwan, a firm producing what are called "scientific Chinese drugs," that is, powder extracts from traditional Chinese herbs in various combinations. Dr. Hsü has also founded, in California, the Oriental Healing Arts Institute, with its own journal, "dedicated to introducing and furthering research and understanding of the centuries-old Chinese traditional system of medicine."[17] Also mentioned among the contributors, as first of the editors, is Dr. Na Ch'i, also trained in Japan and a former professor in the pharmaceutical section of Taipei Medical College. He is the best-known historian of traditional Chinese *pen-ts'ao* literature on Taiwan.

In the twenties and thirties, the Chinese Marxists were among the most ardent proponents within the quite heterogeneous reformist group that could see the future of medicine in China only on a path bound to science. They viewed traditional Chinese medicine as irreparably linked to the feudal society of imperial times, and because they themselves believed their own social theory, that is, Marxism, to be "science" and therefore a socially oriented equivalent of the natural sciences, they approved only of modern scientific medicine. Still in 1941, T'an Chuang, an eminent Marxist, called traditional Chinese medicine and pharmaceutics "millennia-old garbage,"[18] and it was only in 1958 that Mao Tse-tung made his famous remark, "Chinese medicine and pharmacy constitute a great treasure-house. Efforts should be undertaken to uncover it and to raise its standard!" Between 1941 and 1958 an obvious reevaluation of the traditional heritage had taken place for at least two reasons. On the one hand, there were simply not enough resources available after the revolution and establishment of the People's Republic in 1949 to provide a modern, science-oriented health care system for China in its entirety. On the other hand, in the forties, men such as T'an Chuang, besides ridiculing traditional Chinese medicine, began criticizing an uncritical transfer of Western medicine to China. They pointed out a "capitalistic, imperialistic, and colonialistic" context of Western medical practice in China. The goal was to develop a new medicine, based on scientific principles and taking into regard both Western and Chinese indigenous resources as far as they appeared suitable for health care in socialist China. In this regard, it is often overlooked that Mao Tse-tung, with his dictum quoted above, never issued a clearance certificate for traditional Chinese medicine. He emphasized that the treasure-house had to be "uncovered" and "raised in its standard." Despite repeated praises of the value of traditional heritage, there has—to my knowledge—never been voiced an unconditional appreciation of traditional Chinese medicine and pharmacy by any official authority in the government of the People's Republic of China down to this very day. Contents and structure of the two drug codes issued in the People's Republic so far provide ample evidence of that country's recent policy concerning the coexistence of traditional Chinese and modern Western pharmacy.

1.1. The preface

The first drug code of the People's Republic of China was published in 1953. The entire preface reads as follows:

1. The First Drug Code of the People's Republic of China

> Medicine and pharmacy in China have a long history of several thousand years, and during this time, our fine working people have already accumulated valuable experiences. The *Pen-ts'ao* in circulation today is one of the outstanding achievements of our ancestors; it is a great literary work which—in all respects—has the form of a drug code. Because China was subject to feudal rule over several thousand years

Chung-hua jen-min-kung-ho-kuo yao-tien, i-chiu-wu-san nien pan
"Drug Code of the People's Republic of China, Edition of the year 1953"
Short title: *Chung-kuo yao-tien, i-chiu-wu-san nien-pan*
        "Drug Code of China, Edition of the year 1953"
Main text and appendixes / 531 drug descriptions
Editor-in-chief: Li Te-ch'üan
Published: 1953

and to imperialist invasion over the past one hundred years, and, in addition, to exploitation and oppression by the false government of the Kuo-min-tang, which meant neglect of the people's welfare and of the scientific legacy of our fatherland, it was, of course, out of the question that [the *Pen-ts'ao*] was systematized and researched on the basis of science. As a consequence, many good pharmaceutical substances could not fully bring into play their utility of being able to cure illnesses and to safeguard the health of the broad masses of the people. Furthermore, ever since the introduction of medicine and pharmacy from the West, the material conditions of our country, the special characteristics of our nation, and the actual needs of the broad masses of the people were never taken into consideration. Medicine and pharmacy were blindly sucked up from abroad, and a drug code was compiled which appears to have been forcibly moved here in its entirety from capitalist countries: the *Chung-hua yao-tien*.

After the establishment of the People's Republic of China, under the correct leadership of the Chinese Communist Party, the first national conference on public health was convened in 1950, pointing out already—for public health work—the correct orientation for serving industry, agriculture, and the military. The present new Drug Code of China was compiled in complete accordance with the correct orientation pointed out at that conference. This drug code, basically speaking, must fulfill two conditions. First, it must be popular, that is to say, it must conform with the needs of the broad masses. Second, it must conform with our national conditions, that is to say, it must fully utilize pharmaceutical substances produced in this country. Since the Drug Code of the New China has fulfilled these two conditions, it is truly a national and popular drug code.

The compilation of this new drug code, involving some ten compilation committee members, took two years. Those pharmaceutical substances required in general therapy were included for the most part. Because of limitations owing to the current conditions, the contents [of this drug code] still have many deficiencies. But we are confident that, in the future, we will do analyses, conduct research, and carry out corrections on the basis of scientific methods, thus seeking continuous improvement in accordance with the requirements of medical therapy, with actual production and with empirical and research materials. We hope that all those active in medicine, pharmacy, and public health in the entire country will continuously provide us with the results of their experiences, and that all those active in scientific work in the entire country will continuously provide us with the results of their research, enabling us to revise this drug code step by step, to correct old mistakes, to incorporate new things, and to produce a drug code with perfect contents as an enrichment of the treasure-house of medicine and pharmacy of the New China.

Li Te-ch'üan, August 1953,
in the Public Health Ministry[19]

1.2. Structure and content of the first drug code of the People's Republic of China

The preface is followed by a list of contributors, headed by Li Te-ch'üan, the minister, himself. Among the persons named are some who had contributed—twenty-three years earlier—to the *Chung-hua yao-tien,* criticized here so severely.

The subsequent "General Introduction" calls attention, first of all, to the official designation of this drug code, that is, *Chung-hua jen-min-kung-ho-kuo yao-tien* ("Drug Code of the People's Republic of China") *Edition of the Year 1953,* and its abbreviation *Chung-kuo yao-tien* ("Drug Code for China") *Edition of the Year 1953.* With this formulation, the editors made it quite clear that they did not intend to continue the precedent set by the *Chung-hua yao-tien.* A Latin designation was not provided.

The entire volume is divided into a main text and appendixes. This is explained in the "General Introduction" as follows:

> The main text lists raw drugs, chemical drugs, biological products and preparations [from these] needed in medicine, pharmacy, and public health. The appendixes list general rules on preparations and biological products, general test methods, reagents and reagent liquids, indicators, volumetric solutions, and additional tables.
>
> The order of the monographs in the main text follows the number of strokes of [the first character of] their Chinese names. Each substance [listed] in the main text is described, if applicable, according to the following criteria:
>
> 1. Chinese and Latin name of the drug
> 2. Chemical structural formula
> 3. Summary formula and molecular weight
> 4. Preparation method or origin
> 5. Contents or effectivity
> 6. Nature and appearance
> 7. Identification
> 8. Analysis
> 9. Determination of content
> 10. Storage
> 11. Dosage
> 12. (Suitable) forms of medication.[20]

Further paragraphs of the general introduction refer to technical details, such as units of weight.

The general introduction is followed by a detailed table of contents and, then, by the main text with its 531 monographs, numbered in consecutive order.

Finally, the appendixes provide the following information:

1. General rules concerning the preparation of tablets, aromatic waters, injections, tinctures, infusions, extracts and liquid extracts, suppositories, ointments, ophthalmological ointments, decoctions, antitoxins, and vaccines.
2. General testing methods, for the determination of specific gravity, boiling point, melting point, and pH value, as well as for an analysis of raw drugs.
3. Biological determination methods and other special determination methods; for instance, for the biological determination of Digitalis and penicillin.
4. Special reactions of drugs
5. Sterilization methods

6. Reagents and reagent liquids
7. Additional tables
   (a) table of specific gravity of alcohols
   (b) table of poisonous drugs
   (c) table of strong drugs
   (d) table of frequently prepared drugs that should be kept in stock permanently
   (e) dosages and mode of application (oral, subcutaneous, etc.)
   (f) table of dosages in proportion to different age groups
   (g) table of atomic weights

The volume is concluded by two indexes of the Chinese and Latin names.

1.3. Western and traditional Chinese elements in the first drug code of the People's Republic of China

The preface contains the claim that the first drug code of the People's Republic, in contrast to the first drug code of the Republic, shall take into regard indigenous medications of China, and we may assume that this does not only refer to modern drugs manufactured in China, rather than imported from abroad, but also to drugs of traditional Chinese materia medica; after all, the government of the Republic was criticized for its neglect of the drugs described in the pen-ts'ao literature. The result of this regard, though, is not very impressive. According to my own count, among a total of 581 monographs, only about 20 were devoted to such raw drugs described in the traditional Chinese pharmaceutical literature already, with most of these articles being also part of Western pharmacy, for instance, *Mentha, Zingiber, Foeniculum, Rheum, Digitalis, Areca,* and *Aurantii Cortex.* All the remaining monographs are devoted to either chemical substances (from *Acetanilidum* to *Zinci sulphas*), various preparations (from *Unguentum Hydrargyri Aminochloridi* to *Injectio Acidi Ascorbici* to *Liquor Zinci Chloridi* and to *Vaccinum Typhosum et Paratyphosum*) or natural substances, and preparations made from them, such as *Ergota* and *Oleum Jecoris Piscis, Extractum Belladonnae* and *Tinctura Nucis vomicis,* to name just a few examples.

All these medications are ordered, as pointed out in the general introduction, in accordance with the number of strokes of the first character of their Chinese name. Thus monograph 331: *Oculentum Hydrargyri Oxidi Flavi* is followed by monographs 332: *Coptis,* 333: *Tinctura Coptidis,* 334: *Extractum Coptidis Liquidum,* and 335: *Vaccinum Typhosum.* As a result, the relatively small number of traditional Chinese raw drugs—and *Coptis (huang-lien)* is one of them—were fully integrated with all the other drugs. It must be pointed out, however, that this integration is in full accordance with the maxim referred to in the preface, namely, that scientific principles had to form the basis of their consideration. Consequently, except for the Chinese names, no aspect of the monographs reminds one of the fact that a traditional Chinese drug is described here; the criteria of these descriptions are purely modern-pharmacognostic, from the microscopic powder analysis to the determination of content.

2.1. The preface

In 1977 the second edition of the drug code of the People's Republic of China was issued, in two volumes, under the official title *Chung-hua jen-min-kung-ho-kuo yao-tien, Edition of the Year 1977*. Both volumes carried the same short preface:

> This edition of the Drug Code was compiled under the intimate and sincere concern of the Central Committee of the Party with the wise leader chairman Hua as its head, in accordance with the need to develop the public health cause of our country, in conformance with the policies of our great leader and teacher chairman Mao to be independent and to be self-reliant and to combine Chinese and Western medicine and pharmacy, and with the collective cooperation of the Ministry of Commerce, the Ministry of Fuel and Chemical Industry, the Ministry of Public Health, the Public Health Unit of the General Logistics Department of the Chinese People's Liberation Army, as well as other concerned units.
>
> This edition of the Drug Code lists 1,925 drugs in frequent use, as well as seventy-four general rules on preparation and test methods. For convenient use it is divided into two parts, both of which are ordered according to the number of strokes [of the first character] of the Chinese names of the pharmaceutical substances.
>
> We hope that every concerned unit that—in the course of practice—continuously accumulates experiences will offer its suggestions for improvement in order to make the Drug Code even better, to safeguard the health of the people, and to serve the socialist revolution and the establishment of socialism.
>
> > Drug Code Committee of the Ministry
> > of Public Health of the People's Republic of China
> > October 1977[21]

2.2. The monograph section of the first volume

In both volumes, the preface is followed by a General Introduction, though each of these supplies different information. After pointing out the official designation of this drug code, the general introduction explains the structure and contents of each volume. Accordingly, the first volume contains, in its main text, the monographs of

> Chinese herbal drugs [including drugs of ethnic minorities], pharmaceutical substances extracted from Chinese herbal drugs, plant oils as well as preparations on the basis of set prescriptions [including set prescriptions of ethnic minorities]; the appendixes list general rules to examine and determine Chinese herbal drugs, general rules for the preparation [of specific medications], general rules for the processing of drugs, microscopic methods to identify Chinese herbal drugs and set formulas, general examination methods and determination methods,

2. The Second Drug Code of the People's Republic of China (currently in force)

Chung-hua   jen-min-kung-ho-kuo   yao-tien, i-chiu-ch'i-ch'i nien pan
"Drug Code of the People's Republic of China, Edition of the year 1977"
Short title: *Chung-kuo yao-tien, i-chiu-ch'i-ch'i nien pan*
   "Drug Code of China, Edition of the year 1977"
Main text and appendixes / Vol. 1: 1,153 descriptions of traditional Chinese drugs and formulas
   Vol. 2: 777 descriptions of Western-type medications
Author: Drug Code Committee, Ministry of Public Health, The People's Republic of China

reagents, reagent liquids, indicators, volumetric solutions, additional tables as well as Chinese herbal drugs and items necessary for [their] processing as used for the preparation of set formulas, but not listed in this Drug Code.[22]

Further paragraphs in the general introduction offer the usual information on the selection, origin, and treatment of Chinese raw drugs and of preparations produced from these.

A detailed table of contents precedes the 856-page monograph section, which is followed by 93 pages of appendixes and, finally, three different indexes, one for the Chinese names in Chinese characters, one for the Chinese names in pinyin romanization, and one for the Latin names of all articles mentioned in the main text and in the appendixes.

The monograph section combines, for the first time in a Chinese drug code, several hundred of the most important traditional herbal, animal, and mineral drugs and drug preparations. Thus, also for the first time in the history of Chinese pharmacy, official guidelines are available for a standardized usage of traditional Chinese materia medica.

As an example I will present the monograph on *Fructus Crotonis*, that is pa-tou, a drug whose description in Chinese pharmaceutical literature we have followed now over a period of almost 2,000 years. Pa-tou, romanized in the People's Republic of China as *badou*, was not mentioned in the first edition of the drug code of the People's Republic of 1953; in 1977 it was described as follows.

Badou, Fructus Crotonis.

This article is the dried, mature fruit of the plant *Croton tiglium* L., *pa-tou*, of the family *ta-chi*. It is collected in fall when the fruits are ripe, piled up for two to three days, spread out, and dried.

Nature and Appearance: This article has a circular shape like an egg. In general, [the fruit] has three edges; it is 1.8 to 2.2 centimeters long and measures 1.4 to 2 centimeters in diameter. The outside is of a grey-yellow coloring, sometimes of a deep [color], rough, and has six lines. It is capped flat on its top and carries a fruit stalk mark at its bottom. If one breaks open the fruit shell one can see three chambers, with each chamber containing one seed. The seeds are of a slightly elliptic shape; their length is 1.2 to 1.5 centimeters, with a diameter of 0.7 to 0.9 centimeters. The outside is of brown or grey-brown color; at one end is a dotlike scar of the seed-navel and seed-mound. At the other end is a slightly concave dot, and in between is a swelling of the seed-spine. The external seed-skin is thin and fragile. The internal seed-skin is a white-colored, thin membrane. The seed-kernel is of yellowish-white color; it is oily, has no odor, and has a pungent taste.

The best samples are those that are filled [by the seeds] and whose seed-kernel has a yellow-white color.

Identification: Take about 5.0 grams of this article, grind, add 10 milliliters of ether, allow to soak for two hours and stir up frequently. Then filter, put the filtrate into a test tube and, after evaporation [of the liquid], add 0.5 milliliter of a saturated solution of hydroxylamine-hydrochloride in methanol, as well as 1 drop of a 1 percent thymol-phthalein indicator liquid. Add further a saturated solution of potassium hydroxide in methanol until a bright blue color appears, and then add a few more drops. Add heat until boiling, wait until it has cooled down, and add diluted hydrochloric acid until a pH value of about 2 to 3 is reached. Add 3 drops of 10 percent ferrumtrichloride solution and 1 milliliter of chloroform. Stir. The lower phase solution will display a bright purplish red color.

Determination of contents: Take 5 grams of this article, determine the precise weight, pulverize to a fine powder, put into a reflux condenser, dissolve in ether, add heat and allow to reflux until the entire oil has been extracted; evaporate the ether, dry for one hour at 100 degrees. Wait until it has cooled down. Determine the precise weight. This article should contain no less than 50 percent oil.

Processing: raw *pa-tou:* discard the skin and use the kernel. For eternal use.

Pa-tou pulp: Take clean *pa-tou* kernels, pulverize to a fine powder, or crush to pulp. Extract the oil through pressing until one gets a loose powder that does not stick together like a cake. Or one takes clean *pa-tou* kernels, pulverizes them to a fine powder and determines the content of oil according to the method described under the rubric "determination of contents," adds a suitable amount of starch and creates a thorough mixture with 18 to 20 percent oil.

Nature and Taste: acrid, hot; strong medicinal effectiveness.

Functions and Main Indications: [Pa-tou] forcefully moves downward through constipations; drives out water, eliminates swellings; it is used against obstructions caused by accumulations of cold, swellings and pains in chest and abdomen, edemas, wind[-affected] throat, closure of the throat; externally for treatments of scabs, warts, and moles.

Usage and Dosage: 0.1 to 0.3 grams *pa-tou* pulp are mostly prepared into pills or powders and are divided for intake in several portions. For external use, take a suitable amount of the fresh article, grind a powder to smear or crush a pulp to pack on the afflicted region, wrapped in thin silk.

Attention: Pregnant women must not eat this; it should not be used together with *ch'ien-niu-tzu.*

Storage: Store in a dark, cool, dry place.[23]

2.3. The appendixes of the first volume

The appendixes of the first volume clearly show the degree to which elements of traditional Chinese and contemporary Western pharmacy were combined in the latest issue of the drug code of the People's Republic of China. I will provide here, for this reason, a rather detailed survey of the individual sections of the appendixes, and I will present parts of them in literal translation.

   1. General Rules on Preparations. (These are detailed guidelines for the preparation of pills, powders, pastes, wines, gums, tablets, injections, tinctures, dry and liquid extracts, capsules, ointments, and ophthalmological ointments.)
   2. General Rules on the Determination of Chinese Herbal Drugs.
   The determination of Chinese herbal drugs includes [an examination] of "nature and appearance," "identity-tests," "analyses," and "determination of contents." In the determination of Chinese herbal drugs one should combine traditional experiences in the differentiation [of drugs] with contemporary scientific methods, and one should combine tests by experts with the quality control [as conducted] by the masses. Also, the quality of analytic work should continuously be raised in order to assure safety and effectiveness in the use of drugs by the people.

In carrying out determinations, attention should be paid to the following rules.

When picking a sample, pay attention to its representativeness. In general, before picking a sample one should see to it that name, origin, and standards of the article as well as the way it is packed conform to one another. One should examine also the intactness of the package and the degree of cleanliness and whether the [article is in] an abnormal state on account of residual moisture, mildew, or contamination with any other substance. All this should be carefully noted down. If a specific package has severely deteriorated to a degree that it cannot be supplied for medicinal use, it should be handled separately, and it should not be included in the [materials] from which a sample is drawn.

To conduct a proper determination, it is possible, when necessary, to use, for comparison, samples of Chinese herbal drugs corresponding to the regulations of this edition of the Drug Code.

If Chinese herbal drugs delivered for determination are already cut, they must correspond to all norms of each single analytic section, except for those specified in the rubric "nature and appearance."

"Nature and Appearance" refers to test methods based on one's sense organs, that is, the observation of the outer appearance of Chinese herbal drugs, of their size, color, external characteristics, constitution, and how they were made into smaller pieces—this includes whether they were broken or cut—and also their odor and taste. If necessary, one may use a magnifying glass to carry out the observations. (Six specifications follow as to how to proceed when testing appearance, size, color, external characteristics, odor and taste).

The "identification" includes identifications on the basis of experience, microidentification, physical identification, and chemical identification. (Short specifications on each of these methods follow.)

"Analysis" and "Determination of Contents" refer to methods using physical or chemical procedures in carrying out determinations of the quality of Chinese herbal drugs. (The following specifications include detailed references to):

(a) determination of moisture

(b) determination of ash-content

(c) determination of ash residues nonsoluble in acids

(d) determination of ingredients that can be extracted because of their water-solubility

(e) determination of ingredients that can be extracted because of their alcohol-solubility

(f) determination of volatile oils.[24]

3. General Rules for the Processing of Chinese Herbal Drugs.

The processing of Chinese herbal drugs refers to the methods of cleaning, cutting, and heat-processing carried out to produce processed articles of fixed standards which suit the demands of therapy and the requirements of prescription formulas and preparations, and which assure safety and effectiveness in the use of drugs. (Detailed specifications follow concerning cleaning, cutting and heat-processing, the latter including various ways of roasting, boiling, stewing, steaming, warming in wine, vinegar, brine, ginger-juice, and honey, as well as scalding, burning, and heating until red-hot. All these methods were adopted from traditional Chinese pharmaceutical technology.)

4. Methods for microidentification of Chinese herbal drugs and set prescription-formulas

5. List of Chinese herbal drugs and of articles required for processing from set prescription-formulas not recorded in this Drug Code.

6. Method to determine specific gravity

7. Method to determine the boiling point

8. Method to determine the melting point

9. Method to determine the coagulation point

10. Method to determine the optical rotation
11. Method to determine the refractive index
12. Spectrophotometric and colorimetric methods
13. Chromatographic methods
    (a) column chromatography
    (b) paper chromatography
    (c) thin-layer chromatography
    (d) gas chromatography
14. General identification tests
15. Methods to determine the pH value
16. Methods to test on chlorides
17. Methods to determine the loss through desiccation
18. Method to analyze the residue after burning
19. Method to test on iron salts
20. Method to test on heavy metals
21. Method to test on arsenic salts
22. Method to determine the ethanol content
23. Method to analyze fats and fat oils
24. Method to test on pyrogenes
25. Method to test on the absence of bacteria
26. Method to examine glass containers used for injection preparations
27. Methods of potentiometric and dead-stop titration
28. Method to determine the *Eucalyptus*-oil-essence content
29. Method for a biological determination of *Digitalis*
30. Reagents
31. Reagent liquids
32. Test-papers
33. Indicator preparations and indicator liquids
34. Buffer liquids
35. Standard colorimetric liquids
36. Volumetric liquids and molar liquids
37. Table of poisonous and strong drugs
38. Table for the calculation of dosages for younger and older people
39. Table of atomic weights
40. Infrared absorption spectrums

2.4. The second volume

In contrast to the first volume which contains exclusively traditional Chinese raw drugs and preparations made from these, the second volume is devoted solely to substances and medications as they are used in contemporary Western-style pharmacy.

The structure of the second volume corresponds to that of the first. A main text contains the monographs which include descriptions of chemical products, of natural substances isolated from plants, animals, or minerals, as well as preparations in various forms of medications (tablets, injections, etc.). The appendixes again provide information and guidelines on methods of determination and analysis. They coincide, in part, with those provided in the first volume; others appear solely in the second volume because they are relevant only for the kind of medications dealt with here.

The volume is concluded by three indexes, as is the first volume.

As the comparison of structure and content of the drug codes of the Republic of China and of the People's Republic of China has demonstrated, their main difference lies in their attitudes toward tra-

3. Concluding Remarks on the Chinese Drug Codes and on the Situation of Traditional Chinese Pharmaceutics in Contemporary China

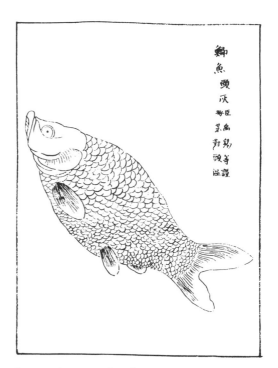

brace *(chi-yü)—Shao-hsing pen-ts'ao*

ditional Chinese pharmaceutics. While the most recent, third edition of the *Pharmacopoea Chinensis* from Taiwan does not take any aspect of traditional Chinese pharmacy into regard, approximately one half of the Drug Code of the People's Republic of China is devoted to remedies and accompanying pharmaceutical techniques from traditional Chinese pharmacy. While the traditional drugs had been integrated into the remaining materia medica, according to "alphabetical" principles, in the first edition of the drug code of the People's Republic of 1953, they were combined, and separated from the remaining medications, in one of two volumes of the edition of 1977. The reason for this new form may have been only to meaningfully divide one unhandy large volume into two convenient, small volumes, although this division into two separate volumes may also appear as a symbolic separation of traditional and modern pharmacy. In this regard we have to recall that the theoretical framework of the standardization and examination of the traditional drugs in the first volume is almost exclusively based on modern methods of Western pharmaceutical sciences.

The People's Republic of China has consistently pursued a course conceptualized, in its outlines, in the twenties and thirties of this century by early Marxist thinkers. In addition to the experiences of the people, modern science is recognized as the one and only basis of knowledge. As a consequence, traditional Chinese materia medica has been reevaluated over the past decades in accordance with contemporary scientific assumptions as to the active ingredients of, for instance, herbal substances and their most effective mode of application in therapy. All the traditional drugs incorporated into the Drug Code of the People's Republic of China should, therefore, be seen now as having been integrated into Western-style pharmacy. The respective monographs contain only a few allusions to the original frame of reference of the drugs, described in mentioning "Taste and Nature (i.e., thermo-influence)" and in listing the main indications and functions of the medications in traditional terminology. For many readers of these indications, the traditional terms employed may be of no greater significance than the use of ancient terms like *hysteria*, *stroke*, or *common cold* to anybody in the West.

No references can be found, though, to the ancient concepts of yinyang and the Five Phases. The latest edition of the Drug Code of the People's Republic of China was prepared during the political dominance of the so-called Gang of Four, that is, the radical leftist Shanghai faction of the Communist party, and it is well-known that during that period of time the old Chinese theories were most severely attacked as being "superstitions" from the past. In the meantime, the attitude has been somewhat liberalized, and it is possible for historians of science in China to conduct research on the contents and development of yinyang and Five Phases concepts. There are no signs, however, that there will be any official appreciation of this traditional Chinese world view as a legitimate alternative to modern science. Still, we know that significant segments of the population continue to adhere to these traditional thoughts.

Greater religious freedom during the past few years has obviously removed constraints from many people who once again openly resort to Buddhist temples, and there have also been widespread reports in the Chinese press, subsequent to the demise of the so-called Gang of Four, about a continued, albeit illegal, practice of demonological therapy in different regions of the entire country. We may conclude, then, that the ongoing plurality of therapeutic systems in the People's Republic of China is partially as unstructured as is therapeutic plurality on Taiwan. The major difference lies in the fact that in the People's Republic, a number of traditional therapeutic means, including acupuncture, materia medica, and bone-setting, have been selected for pragmatic or even conceptual integration into modern Western-style health care.

In addition, also in contrast to Taiwan, various attempts have been undertaken to integrate practitioners of traditional Chinese medicine (acupuncturists, herbalists, pharmacists, and bone-setters, but no shamans or priests) into the official health care delivery system. They may treat patients in private (after they have reached retirement age) or in public clinics, in hospitals specializing in traditional therapy as well as in hospitals dominated by Western-style medicine. In all these settings, practitioners of traditional Chinese medicine may rationalize their therapeutic recommendations on the basis of their traditional concepts. Ever since the founding of the People's Republic of China, numerous new interpretations of those ancient ideas that were defined as "Chinese medicine" in the twenties and thirties have been published, as have reprints of a wide range of works from the past.

Finally, as further contrast to Taiwan, it should be noted that in the People's Republic a large number of research institutes have been established where clinical and theoretical issues of traditional Chinese medicine are studied. One outstanding outcome of such research efforts is the *Chung-yao ta tz'u-tien* ("Comprehensive Dictionary of Chinese Pharmaceutics"), published by the Shanghai People's Press in 1977. It contains, in two of three volumes, 5,767 monographs on items used as drugs in traditional Chinese pharmacy. Where applicable, the *Chung-yao ta tz'u-tien* records for each drug its dominant name (which is not necessarily the oldest known designation) and secondary names (and the pen-ts'ao or other works where they were introduced), its nature (*hsing*, i.e., thermo-influence), taste, and medicinal potency (*tu*), main indications and contraindications, references to place of origin, time of gathering, and external appearance, conduit passage, modes of application, and dosage amounts, as well as pharmaceutical preparation and selected prescriptions—with all these data being quoted from traditional herbals and other relevant sources from remote antiquity to the early twentieth century. However, this traditional information comprises only about one-half of the individual monographs. In addition, data resulting from modern clinical, toxicological, pharmacological, and chemical-analytical research as well as modern botanical, mineralogical or zoological identifications are provided, not in a separate section but interspersed among the data quoted from traditional sources.

The third volume combines various indexes, including a list of all chemical components identified in Chinese drugs (with their structure

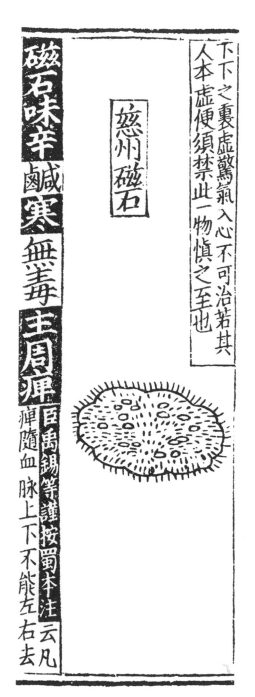

磁石味辛鹵鹹寒無毒主周痺

慈州磁石

下下之裏虛驚氣入心不可治若其
人本虛便須禁此一物慎之至也

痺隨血脉上下不能左右去

臣禹錫等謹按蜀本注云凡

magnetite *(tz'u-shih)—Ch'ung-hsiu cheng-ho pen-ts'ao*

formulas), a list of clinical syndromes and diseases with numbers referring to the monographs of drugs considered to be effective against these syndromes and diseases (continuing a tradition initiated by T'ao Hung-ching), and, finally, a comprehensive list of international references to analytical, pharmacological, and clinical research on the drugs described in the first two volumes. The *Chung-yao ta tz'u-tien* could be called a timely successor to the works of T'ao Hung-ching and Li Shih-chen; it is an invaluable tool for both traditional and Western-style practitioners and scholars. It represents, so far, the most advanced synthesis of traditional pragmatic pen-ts'ao knowledge and modern science.

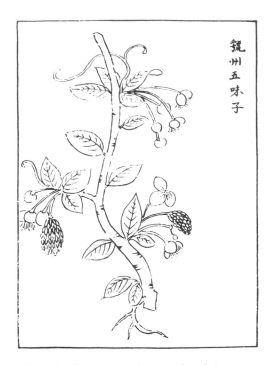

schisandra fruit (*wu-wei-tzu*)—*Shao-hsing pen-ts'ao*

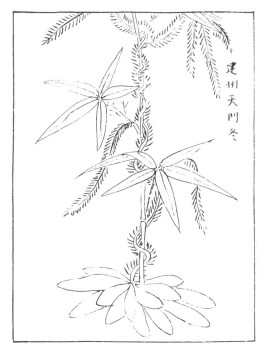

asparagus species (*t'ien-men tung*)—*Shao-hsing pen-ts'ao*

liquidamber tree resin (*feng-hsiang-chih*)—*Shao-hsing pen-ts'ao*

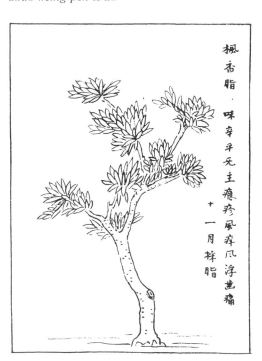

birthwort root (*ch'ing-mu-hsiang*)—*Shao-hsing pen-ts'ao*

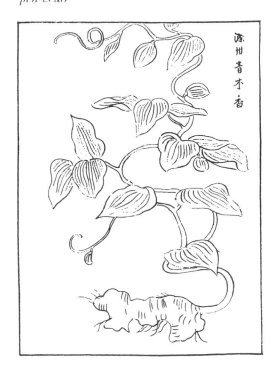

Notes

ABBREVIATIONS FOR FREQUENTLY CITED WORKS:

CKICK   Tamba Mototane. *Chung-kuo i-chi k'ao*. Peking, 1956.
CYTTT   *Chung-yao ta tz'u-tien*. Shanghai 1977.
HTPTSL   Lung Po-chien. *Hsien-ts'un pen-ts'ao shu-lu*. Peking, 1957.
MCHI   Unschuld, Paul U. *Medicine in China, A History of Ideas* (references are to chapters and sections).
SICICK   Okanishi Tameto. *Sung-i-ch'ien i-chi k'ao*. Taipei, 1967.

A: INTRODUCTION

1. Unschuld (1979).
2. Needham (1970), pp. 379–395.
3. Wu Te-to (1979), p. 472; Na Ch'i (1974), p. 48.
4. Goltz (1969); Goltz (1970).
5. Schmauderer (1970), p. 1.

B: SHEN-NUNG, PEN-TS'AO AND THE ORIGINS OF PHARMACEUTICAL LITERATURE IN CHINA

1. The term *tu*, in general, carries the meaning "poison." In the early pharmaceutical literature, though, it was used to designate the degree of medical effectiveness of drugs. See also p. 165. For a detailed etymology of the term *tu*, see P. Unschuld (1975).

2. *Huai-nan tzu*, "Hsiu-wu hsün," SPPY, chap. 19, p. 1a.

3. Na Ch'i (1970b), p. 101.

4. *Pen-ts'ao ching chi-chu* (1972), p. 1C–1D (references are to quarters of each page, as p. 1A, 1B, 1C, 1D).

5. *Erh-shih ssu-shih, Han-shu*, PNP, pp. 1539b–1540a.

6. Ibid., p. 1352a; SICICK, p. 1168.

7. Ibid., p. 2361a; SICICK, p. 1168.

8. SICICK, p. 1168.

9. *Shuo-wen chieh-tzu* (1970), p. 27.

10. SICICK, p. 1168.

11. Ibid.

12. MCHI: 1.

13. Hu Hou-hsüan (1944); Yen I-p'ing (1951); MCHI: 1.2.–1.5.

14. Ma Chi-hsing (1979); *Wu-shih-erh ping fang* (1979); Shuai Hsüeh-chung et al. (1980); Chung I-yen and Ling Hsiang (1975); T'ang Lan (1975); "Ma-wang-tui Han-mu ch'u-t'u i-shu shih-wen" (1975); Akahori Akira (1978c, 1979); P. Unschuld (1983).

15. *Wu-shih-erh ping-fang* (1979); P. Unschuld (1982); Harper (1982).

16. Ma Chi-hsing (1979).

17. Chavannes (1913), pp. 113–116.

18. *Wu-wei Han-tai i-chien* (1975); see also the articles in *Wen-wu* (1973), nr. 12, pp. 18–31; Akahori Akira (1978d).

19. *Wu-wei Han-tai i-chien* (1975), pp. 22b–23b.

C: THE PEN-TS'AO LITERATURE WITH
COMPREHENSIVE CONTENTS

1. These include the *Yang-sheng lun,* the *Po-wu chih,* and the *Pao-p'u tzu,* as well as the T'ang period encyclopedia *I-wen lei-chü* by Ou-yang Hsün, and the Sung encyclopedia *T'ai-p'ing yü-lan* by Li Fang.

2. Okanishi Tameto (1967), p. 172; see also Akahori (1978c) for relations between recently unearthed manuscripts and the contents of the earliest herbals still extant.

3. *Ch'ung-chi hsin-hsiu pen-ts'ao* (1964), pp. 27–28.

4. Ibid., p. 29.

5. Ibid., p. 30.

6. Ibid., p. 31.

7. Ibid.

8. The body's depots include the liver, the heart, the spleen, the lung, and the kidneys; cf. MCHI: 3.1.4.2.

9. The body's palaces include the stomach, the gall, the bladder, the large intestine, the small intestine, and the Triple Burner; cf. MCHI: 3.1.4.2.

10. *Ch'ung-chi hsin-hsiu pen-ts'ao* (1964), pp. 32–34.

11. Ibid., p. 34.

12. Cf. MCHI: 2.4.

13. *Ch'ung-chi hsin-hsiu pen-ts'ao* (1964), p. 34.

14. Ibid., pp. 34–35.

15. On the identification of the Chinese term as "malaria," see Miyashita Saburo (1979).

16. *Ch'ung-chi hsin-hsiu pen-ts'ao* (1964), p. 35.

17. See below, p. 27.

18. See below, pp. 94–95.

19. *Ch'ung-chi hsin-hsiu pen-ts'ao* (1964), p. 313.

20. *Pen-ts'ao ching chi-chu* (1972), p. 88C.

21. Ibid., p. 20D.

22. MCHI: 2.2.

23. *Pen-ts'ao ching chi-chu* (1972), p. 43B.

24. Ibid., p. 42B.

25. Ibid., p. 120C.

26. Okanishi (1967), p. 176.

27. A designation for the fossils of bones and teeth of various origins. Oracle bones, which in ancient times had been inscribed with characters and which later were utilized as medical drugs, were also grouped in this category.

28. CYTTT, monograph 3046.

29. MCHI: 4.5.

30. Ibid., 2, 3.1.1.

31. Ibid., 3.1.2.

32. Cf. Harper (1982).

33. *Ch'ung-chi hsin-hsiu pen-ts'ao* (1964), p. 409.

34. Na Ch'i (1974), pp. 106–107.

35. Ibid.

36. Ibid.

37. Ibid., p. 105.

38. Biographical details on T'ao Hung-ching are given in Strickmann (1979); Akahori (1978a); *Erh-shih-ssu-shih, Nan-shih,* "Lieh-ch'uan" 66, PNP, pp. 12810a–12812a.

39. Strickmann (1979), p. 190.

40. Ibid., p. 137.

41. Ibid., pp. 167–168.

42. SICICK, pp. 1193–1194.

43. A legendary minister. He was consulted by the Yellow Emperor on the secrets of medicine.

44. See the biography of Pien Ch'io in the *Shih-chi* for the story of Prince Huan. He disregarded Pien Ch'io's advice for early therapeutic intervention until it was too late.

45. A famous healer whose biography, together with case histories, is also recorded in the *Shih-chi*.

46. This may be, as Watanabe Kōzo has pointed out, an allusion to a statement in chap. 13 ("Chi-yen") of Ko Hung's *Pao-p'u tzu, Nei-p'ien*. According to Ko Hung, the hibiscus and the willow are very sturdy, and even cuttings from them will grow again if planted correctly. Once they are really harmed, though, even the best soil and the best watering will not be sufficient to keep them from dying. In contrast, man is easily vulnerable, and no breathing exercise or medication will, in the long run, prevent his death if he does not care for his constitution in the vigor of youth. It is man's inner condition that invites or repels the illness-causing agents attacking him from the outside. Cf. Watanabe Kōzo (1953a), nr. 6, p. 2; Ware (1966), pp. 220–225; *Pao-p'u tzu* (1969), p. 59.

47. The story of Li Tzu-yü, presumably the first man to use drugs against demonic illnesses, is recorded in the *Sou-shen hou-chi* from the 3rd or 4th century. Cf. DeGroot (1892–1910), vol. 6, pp. 1078–1082; MCHI: 2.3.

48. See Legge (1960), vol. 5: *Tso-chuan*, bk. VIII, Duke Ch'eng, 10th year, for this story. *Kao* designates a region below the throat, and *huang* designates a region above the heart.

49. *Ch'ung-chi hsin-hsiu pen-ts'ao* (1964), pp. 28–36.

50. *Pen-ts'ao ching chi-chu* (1972), p. 6C.

51. Ibid., p. 6D.

52. Ibid., p. 7B.

53. Ibid., p. 7C.

54. Ibid., p. 7D.

55. Ibid., pp. 7D–8B.

56. Ibid., p. 9D.

57. *Ch'ung-chi hsin-hsiu pen-ts'ao* (1964), p. 313.

58. Lo Chen-yü (1968), pp. 7375–7443.

59. *Pen-ts'ao ching chi-chu* (1955), afterword by Fan Hsing-chun.

60. *Ch'ung-chi hsin-hsiu pen-ts'ao* (1964), p. 119.

61. Ibid., p. 138.

62. Lü Shang-chih (1971), p. 93.

63. *Ch'ung-chi hsin-hsiu pen-ts'ao* (1964), p. 119.

64. *Pen-ts'ao ching chi-chu* (1972), p. 68B.

65. Ibid., p. 49A.

66. CYTTT, monograph 3305.

67. *Ch'ung-chi hsin-hsiu pen-ts'ao* (1964), pp. 52–53; *Pen-ts'ao ching chi-chu* (1955), p. 51.

68. *Pen-ts'ao ching chi-chu* (1955), afterword by Fan Hsing-chun, p. 3.

69. *Ch'ung-chi hsin-hsiu pen-ts'ao* (1964), pp. 19–21.

70. *Hsin-hsiu pen-ts'ao* (1955), afterword by Fan Hsing-chun, pp. 1–7.

71. These are the *Yü-chih pen-ts'ao p'in-hui ching-yao* and the *Pen-ts'ao p'in-hui ching-yao hsü-chi*; see below pp. 128–145.

72. *Ch'ung-chi hsin-hsiu pen-ts'ao* (1964), afterword by Okanishi Tameto, pp. 7–10; *Hsin-hsiu pen-ts'ao* (1955), afterword by Fan Hsing-chun, pp. 1–7.

73. *Ch'ung-chi hsin-hsiu pen-ts'ao* (1964), p. 339.

74. See chap. A, Introduction, n. 3.

75. Okanishi Tameto (1959a, 1954a).

76. These are the chapters 4, 5, 12, 13, 14, 15, 17, 18, 19, 20.

77. *Ch'ung-chi hsin-hsiu pen-ts'ao* (1964), preface by Okanishi Tameto, pp. 6–12; ibid., afterword by Okanishi Tameto, pp. 11–16.

78. Ibid., preface, p. 3.

79. SICICK, pp. 1207–1208.

80. Ibid., p. 1207; *Ching-shih cheng-lei ta-kuan pen-ts'ao* (1970), pp. 416–417.

81. Needham (1970), p. 311.

82. Needham (1962), p. 100.

83. Ibid., p. 106.

84. *Ching-shih cheng-lei ta-kuan pen-ts'ao* (1970), p. 83.

85. Needham (1959), p. 674.

86. *Ching-shih cheng-lei ta-kuan pen-ts'ao* (1970), pp. 99–100.

87. Needham (1970), p. 369; *Pen-ts'ao kang mu* (1933), vol. 3, p. 3.

88. *Ching-shih cheng-lei ta-kuan pen-ts'ao* (1970), p. 388.

89. Needham (1961), p. 199.

90. *Erh-shih-ssu-shih, Wu-tai shih-chi*, PNP, chap. 64, p. 18909.

91. *Ching-shih cheng-lei ta-kuan pen-ts'ao* (1970), p. 476.

92. Ibid., p. 551; Okanishi Tameto (1942), pp. 2–3.

93. Bauer (1976), pp. 206–207.

94. Kracke, Jr. (1954–1955).

95. SICICK, p. 1209.

96. Okanishi (1967), pp. 180–181.

97. Ibid.

98. *Ching-shih cheng-lei ta-kuan pen-ts'ao* (1970), pp. 22–23.

99. Okanishi (1967), p. 182.

100. *Ching-shih cheng-lei ta-kuan pen-ts'ao* (1970), pp. 22–23.

101. SICICK, pp. 1214–1215.

102. *Ching-shih cheng-lei ta-kuan pen-ts'ao* (1970), pp. 23–24.

103. SICICK, pp. 1214, 1217.

104. *Pen-ts'ao kang mu* (1933), "Hsü-li shang," chap. 1, p. 6.

105. SICICK, pp. 1228–1229.

106. Watanabe Kōzo (1953c), p. 163.

107. Ibid., p. 162.

108. Okanishi (1959b), p. 1086.

109. SICICK, pp. 1229–1230.

110. Watanabe (1953c), pp. 161ff.

111. Okanishi Tameto (1951), p. 66.

112. *Ching-shih cheng-lei ta-kuan pen-ts'ao* (1970), pp. 1–2.

113. SICICK, pp. 1236–1244.

114. Okanishi (1967), pp. 183–186.

115. *Shao-hsing chiao-ting ching-shih cheng-lei pei-chi pen-ts'ao* (1971), annotations by Okanishi Tameto, pp. 48–49.

116. Ibid., p. 32.

117. SICICK, pp. 1277–1278.

118. *Shao-hsing chiao-ting ching-shih cheng-lei pei-chi pen-ts'ao* (1971), annotations by Okanishi Tameto, p. 33.

118a. Hummel (1941).

119. Watanabe (1953c), p. 165; Okanishi (1951), pp. 69–70; CKICK, pp. 146–147.

120. SICICK, pp. 1281–1282.

121. Okanishi (1967), p. 186.

122. *Pen-ts'ao yen-i* (1957), "Hsü-li shang," chap. 1, p. 1.

123. Ibid., pp. 3–4.

124. Ibid., pp. 4–5.

125. Ibid.

126. Ibid.

127. Ibid., p. 6.

128. Ibid., pp. 6–7.

129. Ibid., p. 7.

130. Ibid.

131. Ibid., p. 8

132. *Huang-ti nei-ching su-wen ling-shu ho-pien* (1968), p. 193.

133. Ibid., p. 195.

134. MCHI: 2.2.

135. *Huang-ti nei-ching su-wen ling-shu ho-pien* (1968), p. 52.

136. *Pen-ts'ao yen-i* (1957), "Hsü-li shang," chap. 1, p. 7.

137. Ibid., pp. 12–13.

138. Ibid., p. 93.

139. Ibid., p. 102.

140. MCHI: 7.2.3.

141. *Pen-ts'ao kang mu* (1933), "Hsü-li shang," chap. 1, p. 7.

142. *Erh-shih-szu-shih, Chin-shih,* PNP, chap. 131, p. 26000a.

143. *Chi-sheng pa-ts'ui* (1970).

144. MCHI: 7.2.2.4.

145. *Erh-shih-ssu-shih, Yüan-shih,* PNP, chap. 203, pp. 28865b–28866b.

146. HTPTSL, p. 119.

147. Ibid.

148. *Chen-chu nang chih-chang pu-i yao-hsing fu* (1965), pp. 4–21.

149. On the "Chang Chi renaissance" during the Chin-Yüan period, see MCHI: 7.2.1.1.

150. Probably a reference to the *Shang-han lun.*

151. Probably a reference to the *Ping-chi ch'i-i pao-ming chi.*

152. *T'ang-yeh pen-ts'ao* (1956), pp. 1–2.

153. Ibid., p. 4.

154. P. Unschuld (1973a), pp. 38–42, 46; U. Unschuld (1977), pp. 242–244.

155. *T'ang-yeh pen-ts'ao* (1956), p. 9; U. Unschuld (1972), p. 79.

156. Okanishi (1967), p. 201.

157. *Huang-ti nei-ching su-wen ling-shu ho-pien* (1968), p. 663.

158. Rall (1970), p. 72.

159. *Pen-ts'ao fa-hui,* n.d., p. 109.

160. Okanishi Tameto (1970), p. 148; HTPTSL, pp. 38–39.

161. CKICK, p. 183.

162. *Pen-ts'ao chi-yao;* Okanishi (1970), pp. 148–149; HTPTSL, pp. 41–42; CKICK, p. 183.

163. *Pen-ts'ao hui;* Okanishi (1970), p. 159; HTPTSL, p. 64; CKICK, pp. 206–208.

164. *Pen-ts'ao shu* (1876), preliminary chap., pp. 1a–2a.

165. Okanishi (1970), p. 158; HTPTSL, p. 62.

166. *Pen-ts'ao shu kou-yüan* (1958), p. 3.

167. Okanishi (1970), p. 163.

168. P. Unschuld (1973a), pp. 44–46, 112–113.

169. Li Chin-hua (1932), p. 56; *Ming shih-lu* (1967), chap. 202, p. 4a.

170. Li Chin-hua (1932), p. 56; *Ming shih-lu* (1967), chap. 202, p. 4b.

171. *Ming shih-lu* (1967), chap. 202, pp. 3b–4b.

172. Okanishi Tameto (1952).

173. A somewhat liberally condensed version of the story; Chang Yü-hsi and his colleagues wrote the *Chia-yu pen-ts'ao,* versions of which later appeared as the *Cheng-lei pen-ts'ao* and the *Cheng-ho pen-ts'ao.*

174. *Pen-ts'ao p'in-hui ching-yao* (1964), pp. 11–14.

175. *Huang-chi ching-shih shu,* SPPY, vol. 4, chap. 6, pp. 22a ff.

176. *Pen-ts'ao p'in-hui ching-yao* (1964), pp. 15–16.

177. Ibid., p. 16.

178. Okanishi (1952), pp. 158–159.

179. Bertuccioli (1956a), p. 63.

180. For a detailed analysis of structure and contents of the *Pen-ts'ao p'in-hui ching-yao,* see also Liu Cheng-hsiung (1977).

181. Okanishi (1952), p. 87.

182. Okanishi Tameto (1969), p. 21; Bertuccioli (1956a), p. 64.

183. Bertuccioli (1956a), p. 63.

184. Wang Chung-min (1936).

185. Fuchs (1966), pp. 62–63.

186. P. Unschuld (1973b), pp. 24–27.

187. Ōtsuka Yasuō (1978).

188. Li Ch'ing-chih, n.d.

189. The following discussion is based on biographical material from the following sources: *Erh-shih-ssu-shih*, *Ming-shih*, PNP, chap. 299, pp. 32226a–b; Lu Gwei-djen (1966); Chang Hui-chien (1955); Lü Shang-chih (1971); Ch'en Pang-hsien (1956); Watanabe Kōzo (1953b).

190. These are the following works: *P'in-hu mai-hsüeh*, *Ch'i-ching pa-mai k'ao*, and *Mai-chüeh k'ao-cheng*. See below p. 161.

191. Watanabe (1953b), p. 7.

192. Lu Gwei-djen (1966), pp. 386–387.

193. Ibid.

194. Watanabe (1953b), p. 6; Chang Hui-chien (1955), p. 5.

195. *Erh-shih-ssu-shih*, *Ming-shih*, PNP, chap. 299, pp. 32226a–b.

196. Watanabe (1953b), p. 7.

197. *Pen-ts'ao kang mu* (1933), "Fan-li," p. 30.

198. Ibid., chap. 35, p. 63.

199. For further details, see Spence (1972).

200. *Pen-ts'ao kang mu* (1933), chap. 23, pp. 87–88.

201. Lu Gwei-djen (1966), p. 388.

202. HTPTSL, pp. 44–47.

203. Wang Chi-min (1954), pp. 3–8.

204. Watanabe (1953b), p. 8.

205. *Pen-ts'ao kang mu* (1933), "Hsü-li shang," p. 8.

206. HTPTSL, p. 48.

207. *Pen-ts'ao kang mu shih-i* (1971), p. 12.

208. Ibid., p. 237.

209. Purportedly a black shining mineral mined in Spain. It is supposed to hang as an amulet on the breast of children to protect them from fright and evil influences. The stone itself is said to absorb these hazards and destroy them.

210. Chao Hsüeh-min was unable to provide any further description of this stone. Among other things, it was said to be suitable for the prevention of difficult childbirth. For this purpose it is soaked overnight in sesame oil, and the resulting mixture is then applied to the abdomen and face of the woman in labor.

211. Taoist designation for an area of the body located below the navel. In men it is the location of the "chamber of essence (or: semen)" (*ching-shih*) and in woman it refers to the "womb palace" (*pao-kung*). In both cases it is the site for the formation of the *nei-tan*, the essence for the creation and preservation of life.

室宮丹
精胞內

212. *Pen-ts'ao kang mu shih-i* (1971), pp. 34–35.

213. P. Unschuld (1978).

214. Okanishi (1970), p. 162; *Pen-ts'ao kang mu shih-i* (1971), afterword by Chang Ying-ch'ang, p. 1.

215. P. Unschuld (1973a), p. 53.

216. CKICK, p. 198.

217. Okanishi (1970), p. 156.

218. Ibid.; HTPTSL, p. 56.

219. Okanishi (1970), p. 158; HTPTSL, pp. 63–64.

220. *I-fang chi-chieh* (1970), "Fan-li," p. 1.

221. *Pen-ts'ao pei-yao* (1967), "Fan-li," p. 3.

222. CKICK, pp. 219–220.

223. HTPTSL, pp. 68–69.

224. Ibid., pp. 73–74.

225. CKICK, pp. 219–220.

226. *Pen-ts'ao ch'iu-chen*, n.d., "Fan-li," p. 6.

227. Ibid., p. 265.

228. For a discussion of the meaning of *ming-men*, see MCHI: 8.2.2.1.

229. Ibid., 8.2.1.

230. Bauer (1976), pp. 251–252.

231. Ibid., p. 251.

232. Hummel (1970), pp. 421–425.

233. Bauer (1976), p. 252.

234. Hummel (1970), p. 913.

235. HTPTSL, p. 1.

236. Okanishi Tameto (1974), p. 310.

237. CKICK, p. 157.

238. HTPTSL, p. 53.

239. *Pen-ts'ao ching shu* (1891), chap. 14, p. 1b.

240. Ibid., p. 2a.

241. See also Okanishi (1970), pp. 156–158.

242. CKICK, p. 201.

243. HTPTSL, pp. 55–56.

244. CKICK, pp. 204–205.

245. *Ch'ing-shih* (1961), chap. 501, p. 5447.

246. Ibid.

247. Okanishi (1970), pp. 158–159.

248. Ch'en Pang-hsien (1956), p. 140.

249. A reference to Chang Chi of the Han era.

250. A reference to Sun Ssu-mo.

251. *Pen-ching feng-yüan* (1957), pp. 1a–2b.

252. Ibid., chap. 3, pp. 113–114.

253. Okanishi (1970), pp. 160–161.

254. Hummel (1970), p. 322.

255. *Hsü Ling-t'ai i-shu ch'üan-chi* (1969), "I-hsüeh yüan-liu lun," pp. 85–86.

256. CKICK, p. 159.

257. *Hsü Ling-t'ai i-shu ch'üan-chi* (1969), "Shen-nung pen-ts'ao ching pai-chung lu," pp. 132–133.

258. A Taoist work compiled in the 2nd century A.D. with commentaries as late as the Sung dynasty.

259. *Hsü Ling-t'ai i-shu ch'üan-chi* (1969), "Shen-nung pen-ts'ao ching pai-chung lu," p. 152.

260. Hummel (1970), p. 676.

261. Okanishi Tameto (1954b), pp. 10–12.

262. SICICK, pp. 1175–1181; HTPTSL, pp. 2–3; Okanishi (1970), p. 163.

263. *Ch'ing-shih* (1961), chap. 501, p. 5451.

264. Okanishi (1970), p. 163.

265. Tsou Shu's biography in the Ch'ing history and Okanishi refer to this work as *Pen-ts'ao ching shu*. In order to avoid a mix-up with Miu Hsi-yung's work of the same title, I follow the HTPTSL which mentions the title *Pen-ching shu-cheng*. This title was adopted also for the 1969 edition of this work in Taipei.

266. *Pen-ching shu cheng* (1969), p. 1.

267. Okanishi (1970), p. 163; HTPTSL, pp. 9–10.

268. SICICK, p. 1182; HTPTSL, p. 3.

269. *Ch'ing-shih* (1961), chap. 506, p. 5499.

270. SICICK, pp. 1181–1182; HTPTSL, pp. 3–4.

271. *Ch'ing-shih* (1961), chap. 481, p. 5217; SICICK, pp. 1182–1183; HTPTSL, p. 4.

272. SICICK, pp. 1183–1184; HTPTSL, p. 4.

273. Ch'en Pang-hsien (1920), p. 101b.

274. Ibid., pp. 101b–102b; MCHI: 8.2., 8.3.

275. MCHI: 9.2.3., 9.3.

D: THE PEN-TS'AO LITERATURE WITH SPECIALIZED CONTENTS

1. *Chou-li chu-shu chi pu-cheng* (1969), chap. 5, pp. 1a–b; Biot (1851), vol. 1, pp. 92 ff.

2. Shinoda Osamu (1970), p. 309.

3. *Huang-ti nei-ching su-wen ling-shu ho-pien* (1968), p. 541.

4. SICICK, pp. 1330–1331.

5. Shinoda (1970), p. 309.

6. A metaphor for exemplary reverential behavior towards parents. Chi Lu was a disciple of Confucius. He had distinguished himself carrying sacks of rice from a great distance for his parents during a time of need.

7. CKICK, p. 223.

8. Nakao Manzō (1930), p. 26.

9. *Erh-shih-szu-shih, Chiu-T'ang-shu*, PNP, chap. 141, p. 15706.

10. *Pei-chi ch'ien-chin yao-fang* (1965), p. 464.

11. Ibid., p. 465.

12. Ibid., p. 471.

13. Ibid., p. 472.

14. Nakao Manzō (1930), p. 58.

15. Ibid., p. 99.

16. Ibid., pp. 107–108.

17. Ibid., pp. 13–14.

18. Ibid., p. 6.

19. Ibid., p. 5; SICICK, p. 1338; *Tun-huang shih-shih ku pen-ts'ao* (1931), preface by Chao Yüan-huang; see also *Shih-liao pen-ts'ao* (1931) and Shinoda Osamu (1963).

20. Nakao Manzō (1930), p. 104.

21. *Ch'ung-hsiu cheng-ho ching-shih cheng-lei pei-yung pen-ts'ao* (1957), p. 356.

22. SICICK, p. 1343.

23. SICICK, p. 1345.

24. Ibid.

25. Ibid.

26. Quoted from the *Huang-ti nei-ching su-wen;* cf. note D. 3.

27. Shinoda Osamu and Tanaka Seiichi (1972), pp. 177–178.

28. Bauer (1976), p. 212.

29. *Yin-shan cheng-yao* (1972), pp. 176–177.

30. This paragraph is copied from a section of the *Ch'ien-chin fang*, a work by Sun Ssu-mo (full title: *Pei-chi ch'ien-chin yao-fang;* see above p. 198).

31. Shinoda and Tanaka (1972), p. 185.

32. Ibid., pp. 222–223; copied from a section of the *Cheng-lei pen-ts'ao;* cf. Shinoda Osamu (1972), p. 602.

33. Shinoda and Tanaka (1972), p. 223.

34. Ishida Mikinosuke (1959), p. 44.

35. Ibid., p. 57.

36. Ibid., pp. 47–48.

37. Shinoda (1972), p. 600.

38. Lao Yan-Shuan (1969), pp. 402–406.

39. Ibid., p. 408; Miyashita Saburo (1965), pp. 939–940.

40. Franke (1970).

41. Shinoda (1972), p. 594.

42. Ishida (1959), pp. 56–57.

43. CKICK, p. 228.

44. HTPTSL, pp. 103–104.

45. *Pen-ts'ao kang mu* (1933), "Hsü-li shang," p. 8; HTPTSL, pp. 105–106.

46. Na Ch'i (1971b), p. 282; Okanishi (1970), p. 148.

47. CKICK, p. 915.

48. *Pen-ts'ao yüeh-yen* (1660), chap. 3, p. 56a.

49. Ibid., p. 49a.

50. Ibid., p. 63a.

51. HTPTSL, pp. 104–107.

52. Okanishi (1970), p. 151; CKICK, p. 188.

53. CKICK, p. 995.

54. *Pen-ts'ao yüeh-yen* (1660), chap 2, p. 15a.

55. HTPTSL, pp. 42–43.

56. Shinoda Osamu (1970), p. 352; HTPTSL, pp. 104–105.

57. Na Ch'i (1971b), p. 289; CKICK, pp. 229–230.

58. *Pei-k'ao shih-wu pen-ts'ao kang mu*, n.d., "Chiu-huang yeh-p'u," chap. 1, p. 25a.

59. Literally, "herb in front of the carriage."

60. Literally, "beside the path" and "carriage wheel."

61. *Pei-k'ao shih-wu pen-ts'ao kang mu*, n.d., "Chiu-huang yeh-p'u," chap. 1, p. 44a.

62. *Pei-k'ao shih-wu pen-ts'ao kang mu*, n.d., chap. 2, p. 23b.

63. *T'ien-i* is a term for a star in Chinese astrology which is viewed, according to its changing brightness, as a favorable or inauspicious omen for future events, including illnesses. The mention of the term *t'ien-i sheng* ("engendered by *t'ien-i*") was able to simulate to the dreamer the proper name "Physician T'ien" (T'ien *i-sheng*).

64. *Pei-k'ao shih-wu pen-ts'ao kang mu*, n.d., chap. 3, pp. 27b–28a.

65. Ibid., chap. 9, p. 45b.

66. *Erh-shih-ssu-shih, Sui-shu*, PNP, chap 34, p. 11625b.

67. *Ch'ung-chi hsin-hsiu pen-ts'ao* (1964), pp. 145–147.

68. *Pen-ts'ao kang mu* (1933), chap. 28, p. 20.

69. *Erh-shih-ssu-shih, Sung-shih*, PNP, chap. 207, p. 21420a.

70. SICICK, p. 1301.

71. *Pen-ts'ao kang mu* (1933), chap 28, p. 20–21.

72. SICICK, p. 1312.

73. An herbalist (legendary?) from the Ch'in dynasty who was known for his knowledge of miraculous drugs. It is unclear whether the following quotation has a real source.

74. *Li Wen kung chi* (1929), pp. 151a–153a.

75. P. Unschuld (1973a), p. 69.

76. *Erh-shih-ssu-shih, Sung-shih*, PNP, chap. 207, p. 21420a; SICICK, p. 1323.

77. MCHI: 7.2.1.2.

78. *Pen-ts'ao kang mu* (1933), chap. 12, p. 91.

79. Chang Hui-chien (1955), p. 2.

80. HTPTSL, p. 98.

81. *Jen-shen k'ao* (1830).

82. HTPTSL, pp. 98–99.

83. Such a multitude of indications could also be achieved by variations in the liquid with which a specific drug was to be consumed. As an example, see the range of indications associated with the intake of opium pills with varying liquids in the *Pen-ts'ao kang mu*, as quoted above, chap. C, sec. III.2.2.2.

84. Needham (1970), pp. 313–315.

85. *Pen-ts'ao kang mu* (1933), "Hsü-li shang," p. 2.

86. Ibid.

87. *Ching-shih cheng-lei ta-kuan pen-ts'ao* (1970), chap. 3, p. 73.

88. SICICK, pp. 1293–1295.

89. HTPTSL, p. 116.

90. SICICK, p. 1294.

91. *Lei-kung p'ao-chih yao-hsing chieh* (1965), p. 29.

92. Ibid., p. 18.

93. Ibid., p. 30.

94. Ibid., p. 52.

95. Ibid., p. 63.

96. SICICK, pp. 1317–1318; Ch'en Pang-hsien (1956), p. 241; *Erh-shih-ssu-shih, Sung-shih*, PNP, chap. 462, p. 24481b.

97. SICICK, p. 1324.

98. Okanishi (1970), p. 151.

99. CKICK, p. 189.

100. *T'u-hsiang pen-ts'ao meng-ch'üan*, n.d., p. 1a.

101. Ibid., p. 1b.

102. Ibid., p. 1b–2a.

103. Ibid., p. 3b.

104. Ting Fu-pao and Chou Yün-ch'ing (1955), pp. 457b–458a.

105. HTPTSL, pp. 43–44; Okanishi (1970), p. 152; Na Ch'i (1971b), pp. 293–294.

106. *Pen-ts'ao yüan-shih* (1754), table of contents.

107. HTPTSL, pp. 50–52; Okanishi (1970), p. 155.

108. *P'ao-chih ta-fa* (1959), pp. 83–84; the HTPTSL (p. 117) refers to Chuang Chi-kuang as Chuang Chi-hsien.

109. *P'ao-chih ta-fa* (1959), pp. 85–104.

110. CKICK, pp. 43, 200; HTPTSL, p. 117.

111. Ting Fu-pao and Chou Yün-ch'ing (1955), p. 461.

112. HTPTSL, p. 120.

113. Ibid., pp. 121–122; Kuroda Genji (1971), p. 276; Okanishi Tameto (1971), p. 144.

114. *Hui-min-chü pen-ts'ao shih-chien* (1899), pp. 2b–4b.

115. HTPTSL, p. 122; Na Ch'i (1971a), pp. 317–318.

116. Na Ch'i (1969b), pp. 188, 192, with detailed biographical data on Wu Ch'i-chün's civil service career; see also *Chih-wu ming-shih-t'u k'ao* (1963), pp. 1–2.

117. *Chih-wu ming-shih-t'u k'ao* (1963), p. 3.

118. Ibid., pp. 4–7; a list of orthographic mistakes, transpositions, repetitions, and similar deficiencies, as well as an index, arranged according to the number of strokes, of all drug names in both works of Wu Ch'i-chün is provided in Na Ch'i (1970c).

119. *Chih-wu ming-shih-t'u k'ao* (1963), pp. 150–151.

120. Reminiscent of the Five Phases theory; the autumn season is associated with the phase "metal."

121. Possibly an allusion to Europeans or Americans.

122. T'ien-wu is a name for the spirit of the ocean.

123. *Chih-wu ming-shih-t'u k'ao* (1963), pp. 484–485.

124. HTPTSL, p. 81; Okanishi (1970), pp. 164–165; Na Ch'i (1970c), p. 186.

125. *Pen-ts'ao kang mu* (1933), "Hsü-li shang," p. 4; SICICK, p. 1307.

126. Laufer (1967), p. 268.

127. SICICK, pp. 1308–1309.

128. *Shuo-fu* (1927), chap. 61, pp. 25b–28a; SICICK, p. 1312; HTPTSL, p. 20.

129. SICICK, p. 1316.

130. HTPTSL, p. 131.

E: THE CHINESE PHARMACOPOEIAS OF
THE TWENTIETH CENTURY

1. MCHI: 9.1.

2. Ibid., 8.2.2.

3. Ibid., 9.2.2.

4. Ibid., 9.2.3.

5. Ch'en Pang-hsien (1920), p. 137b.

6. See also Croizier (1968).

7. These are probably allusions to the opposition of conservative forces, first, to analyze the therapeutic value of Chinese drugs with modern scientific methods and, second, to reject at least some of the older knowledge as wrong. Conservatives in defense of "Chinese medicine" were quite divided as to their strategies in the conflict with Western medicine; some of them maintained (and still do so) that traditional Chinese pharmaceutics was developed thou-

sands of years ago while Western medicine is a recent phenomenon. Why, they ask, should the latter have surpassed the former? See also MCHI: 9.3.

8. An allusion to a statement in the *Shu-ching,* an ancient historical work, parts of which may have been written during the first millennium B.C. In pt. IV, bk. VIII, Pt. i:8, it says: "If a drug does not confuse one's mind, his illness will not be cured." Legge (1960), vol. 3, p. 252.

9. Also an allusion to a statement in the *Shu-ching.* In pt. V, bk. VII, p. 9, it says that "in raising a mound of nine fathoms the work is unfinished for want of one basket of earth." Legge (1960), vol. 3, p. 350.

10. *Chung-hua yao-tien* (1953), preface, n.p.

11. Ibid., pp. 481–482.

12. *Chung-hua yao-tien, Second Edition* (1959), preface, n.p.

13. Ibid., p. xxix.

14. P. Unschuld (1973a), pp. 30–33; Croizier (1968), pp. 211–212.

15. *Chung-hua yao-tien, Third Edition* (1980), p. ii.

16. P. Unschuld (1976).

17. *Bulletin of the Oriental Healing Arts Institute of U.S.A.* (1980), vol. 5, no. 5, preface "From the Publisher."

18. Croizier (1968), p. 155.

19. *Chung-hua jen-min-kung-ho-kuo yao-tien* (1954), preface, n.p.

20. Ibid., p. i.

21. *Chung-hua jen-min-kung-ho-kuo yao-tien* (1977), vol. 1, preface, n.p.

22. Ibid., p. ii.

23. Ibid., pp. 123–124.

24. Ibid., appendix, pp. 13–17.

Bibliography

Chinese Primary Sources (dates and places refer to editions used;
for Chinese characters see Indexes of Book Titles and Persons)

Chen-chu nang
    1970   by Chang Yüan-su. Fragment in *Chi-sheng pa-ts'ui*. Taipei.
Chen-chu nang chih-chang pu-i yao-hsing fu
    1965   by Chang Yüan-su (?), Li Kao (?); revised by P'u Li-i. Taipei.
Chi-sheng pa-ts'ui
    1970   by Wang Yün-wu, ed. Taipei.
Chih-wu ming-shih-t'u k'ao
    1963   by Wu Ch'i-chün. Peking.
Chih-wu ming-shih-t'u k'ao ch'ang-pien
    1963   by Wu Ch'i-chün. Peking.
Ch'ing-shih
    1961   by Kuo-fang yen-chiu-yüan. Taipei.
Ching-shih cheng-lei ta-kuan pen-ts'ao
    1970   by T'ang Shen-wei; ed. by Kimura Koiti. Tokyo.
Chiu-huang pen-ts'ao
    ca. 1725   by Chu Hsiao. Japanese edition, n.p.
周禮注疏及補正　楊家駱　*Chou-li chu-shu chi pu-cheng*
    1969   by Yang Chia-lo. Taipei.
Ch'ung-chi hsin-hsiu pen-ts'ao
    1964   by Okanishi Tameto, ed.
Ch'ung-hsiu cheng-ho ching-shih cheng-lei pei-yung pen-ts'ao
    1957   by Chang Ts'un-hui. Peking.
Chung-hua jen-min-kung-ho-kuo yao-tien, Edition of the year 1953
    1954   by Li Te-ch'üan, ed.-in-chief. Peking.
Chung-hua jen-min-kung-ho-kuo yao-tien, Edition of the year 1977
    1977   by a collective. Peking.
Chung-hua yao-tien, First Edition
    1953   by Liu Jui-heng, ed.-in-chief. Hong Kong.
Chung-hua yao-tien, Second Edition
    1959   by Liu Jui-heng, ed.-in-chief. Taipei.
Chung-hua yao-tien, Third Edition
    1980   by Wang Chin-mao, ed.-in-chief. Taipei.
二十四史　*Erh-shih-ssu-shih*
    n.d.   ed. Po-na-pen.
Hsin-hsiu pen-ts'ao
    1955   by Su Ching et al. Shanghai.

Hsin-pien lei-yao t'u-chu pen-ts'ao
        by Liu Hsin-fu, Yüan edition in the Library of the Imperial
        Household, Tokyo.

徐靈胎醫書全集

Hsü Ling-t'ai i-shu ch'üan-chi
  1969   by Hsü Ta-ch'un. Taipei.

Huai-nan tzu
  n.d.   by Liu An, ed. SPPY.

Huang-chi ching-shih shu
  n.d.   by Shao Yung, ed. SPPY.

黃帝內經素問靈樞合編
馬元臺　張隱庵

Huang-ti nei-ching su-wen ling-shu ho-pien
  1968   edited and annotated by Ma Yüan-t'ai and Chang Yin-an.
        Taipei.

Hui-min-chü pen-ts'ao shih-chien
  1899   by Chu Lun. Shanghai.

Hui-t'u pen-ts'ao kang mu hui-yen
        by Ni Chu-mo. Ch'ing edition in the Library of the Ryugoku
        University, Kyoto.

I-fang chi-chieh
  1970   by Wang Ang. Taipei.

Ishinpō
  1955   by Tamba Yasuyori. Peking.

Jen-shen k'ao
  1830   by T'ang Ping-chün. Japanese edition.

Ku-chin yao-wu pieh-ming k'ao
  1936   by Liu Ya-nung, n.p.

Lei-kung p'ao-chih yao-hsing chieh
  1965   by Li Chung-tzu (?) Taipei.

Lei-pien t'u-ching chi-chu yen-i pen-ts'ao
        by Hui Ch'ang. Yüan edition in the Library of the Imperial
        Household, Tokyo.

李文公集
明實錄

Li Wen kung chi
  1929   by Li Ao. SPTK I, 149, 1.2. Shanghai.

Ming shih-lu
  1967   Taipei.

P'ao-chih ta-fa
  1959   by Miu Hsi-yung. Peking.

Pao-p'u tzu
  1969   by Ko Hung. Taipei.

Pei-chi ch'ien-chin yao-fang
  1965   by Sun Ssu-mo. Taipei.

Pei-k'ao shih-wu pen-ts'ao kang mu
        by Yao K'o-ch'eng. Ch'ing edition in the Library of the Par-
        liament, Tokyo.

Pen-ching feng-yüan
  1957   by Chang Lu, n.p.

Pen-ching shu-cheng
  1969   by Tsou Shu. Taipei.

Pen-ts'ao chi-yao
        by Wang Lun. Ch'ing edition in the Library of Ryugoku Uni-
        versity, Kyoto.

Pen-ts'ao ching chi-chu
1955   by T'ao Hung-ching. Shanghai.

Pen-ts'ao ching chi-chu
1972   by T'ao Hung-ching; ed. by Mori Risshi and Okanishi Tameto. Osaka.

Pen-ts'ao ching shu
1891   by Miu Hsi-yung, n.p.

Pen-ts'ao ch'iu-chen
n.d.   by Huang Kung-hsiu. Hong Kong.

Pen-ts'ao fa-hui
n.d.   by Hsü Yung. MS. in the Library of the Parliament, Tokyo.

Pen-ts'ao hui
by Kuo P'ei-lan. Ch'ing edition in the Library of the Botanical Garden, Kyoto.

Pen-ts'ao hui-yao chien-chu
by Ku Yüan-chiao. Ch'ing edition in the Cabinet Library, Tokyo.

Pen-ts'ao kang mu
1933   by Li Shih-chen. Shanghai.

Pen-ts'ao kang mu shih-i
1971   by Chao Hsüeh-min. Hong Kong.

Pen-ts'ao pei-yao
1967   by Wang Ang. Taipei.

Pen-ts'ao p'in-hui ching-yao
ca. 1770   by Liu Wen-t'ai et al. MS. in the Staatsbibliothek Preussischer Kulturbesitz, Berlin.

Pen-ts'ao p'in-hui ching-yao
1964   by Liu Wen-t'ai et al. Peking.

Pen-ts'ao p'in-hui ching-yao hsü-chi
1964   by Wang Tao-ch'un and Chiang Chao-yüan. Peking.

Pen-ts'ao shu
1876   by Liu Jo-chin, n.p.

Pen-ts'ao shu kou-yüan
1958   by Yang Shih-t'ai. Shanghai.

Pen-ts'ao ts'ung-hsin
1968   by Wu I-lo. Taipei.

Pen-ts'ao yen-i
1957   by K'ou Tsung-shih. Shanghai.

Pen-ts'ao yen-i pu-i
1969   by Chu Chen-heng. Ed. in *Tan-hsi hsin-fa*, Taipei.

Pen-ts'ao yüan-shih
1754   by Li Chung-li, n.p.

Pen-ts'ao yüeh-yen
1660   by Hsüeh Chi. Japanese edition, n.p.

Shao-hsing chiao-ting ching-shih cheng-lei pei-chi pen-ts'ao
1971   by Wang Chi-hsien; ed. by Okanishi Tameto. Tokyo.

Shen-nung pen-ching
1743   by Lu Fu. Japanese edition, n.p.

Shen-nung pen-ts'ao ching
1969   by Sun Hsing-yen and Sun P'ing-i. Taipei.

Shen-p'u
 1808 by Huang Shu-ts'an. Ed. in *Chieh-yüeh shan-fang hui-ch'ao*, n.p.

Shih-liao pen-ts'ao
 1931 by Meng Shen. Ed. in *Tun-huang shih-shih ku pen-ts'ao*, Shanghai.

Shih-wu pen-ts'ao
 1620 by Wang Ying, n.p.

Shuo-fu
 1927 by T'ao Tsung-i. Shanghai.

Shuo-wen chieh-tzu
 1970 by Hsü Shen. Taipei.

Su Shen liang-fang
 1776 by Shen Kua, n.p.

丹 溪 心 法   *Tan-hsi hsin-fa*
 1969 by Chu Chen-heng. Taipei.

T'ang-yeh pen-ts'ao
 1956 by Wang Hao-ku. Peking.

T'u-hsiang pen-ts'ao meng-ch'üan
    by Ch'en Chia-mo. Ming edition in the Library of Ryugoku University, Kyoto.

敦 煌 石 室 古 本 草   *Tun-huang shih-shih ku pen-ts'ao*
 1931 by Nakaō Manzō. Shanghai.

東 垣 十 種 醫 書   *Tung-yüan shih-chung i-shu*
 1969 by Li Kao. Taipei.

Wan-fang chen-hsien
 1968 by Ts'ai Lieh-hsien. Ed. in *Pen-ts'ao kang mu*, Taipei.

Wu-shih-erh ping fang
 1979 by a collective (ed.). Peking.

Yao-hsing ko-k'uo
    by Kung T'ing-hsien. Ed. in *Shou-shih pao-yüan*. Ch'ing edition in Takeda Library, Osaka.

Yao-ming p'u
 1927 by Hou Ning-chi. Ed. in *Shuo-fu*, Shanghai.

中 國 食 經 叢 書   *Yin-shan cheng-yao*
 1972 by Hu Ssu-hui. Ed. in *Chugoku Shokukei Sōsho*, Tokyo.

Chinese and Japanese Secondary Sources

Akahori Akira　赤堀 昭
>　1978*a*　"Tō Kō-Kei to 'Shū-chū-honzō'." *Chūgoku no kagaku to kagakusha* (Yamada Keiji, ed.), Kyoto, pp. 309–367.
>　陶弘景と《集注本草》中國の科学と科学者
>
>　1978*b*　"Shinnō Honzōkei ni kisai sareta yakkō." *Nihon Ishigaku Zasshi* 24:1–13.
>　神農本草系に紀載された藥効
>　日本医史学雑誌
>
>　1978*c*　"Shin shutsudo shiryo ni yoru Chūgoku iyaku koten no minaoshi." *Kanpō no rinsō* 25:1–16.
>　新出土資料による中國医藥古典の見貞し
>　漢方の臨牀
>
>　1978*d*　"Mu-i Kandai iken ni tsuite." *Tōhō gakuhō* 50:75–107.
>　武威漢代医簡について
>　東方学報
>
>　1979　"Medical Manuscripts Found in Han Tomb no. 3 at Ma-wang-tui." *Sudhoffs Archiv* 63:297–301.

Chang Chuo-fu　張拙夫
>　1970　*Chung-kuo pen-ts'ao hsüeh.* Taipei.
>　中國本草學

Chang Hui-chien　張慧劍
>　1955　*Li Shih-chen.* Shanghai.
>　李時珍

Chang Tzu-kao　張子高
>　1962　"Chao Hsüeh-min 'Pen-ts'ao kang mu shih-i' chu-shu nien-tai chien lun wo-kuo shou-tz'u yung ch'iang-shui k'e t'ung-pan shih." *K'o-hsüeh-shih chi-k'an* 4:106–109.
>　趙学敏《本草綱目拾遺》著述年代
>　兼論我國首次用強水刻銅版事
>　科学史集刊

Chen Chan-yuen　陳存仁
>　1958　*Chung-kuo i-hsüeh yüan-liu.* Hong Kong.
>　中國醫學源流

Ch'en Pang-hsien 陳邦賢
1920 *Chung-kuo i-hsüeh shih*. Shanghai.
中國醫學史

1956 *Chung-kuo i-hsüeh jen-ming-chih*. Peking.
中國醫學人名誌

1969 *Chung-kuo i-hsüeh shih*. Taipei.
中國醫學史

Chung I-yen and Ling Hsiang 钟益研 凌襄
1975 "Wo-kuo hsien-i fa-hsien-ti tsui-ku i-fang—po-shu 'Wu-shih-erh ping fang'." *Wen-wu*, nr. 9, pp. 49–60.
我国现已发现的最古医方—帛书《五十二病方》 文物

Chung Ching-wen 鐘敬文
1931 "Wo-kuo ku-tai min-ch'ung kuan-yü i-yao ti chih-shih." *Shan-hai ching ti wen-hua-shih-ti yen-chiu*, n.p.
我國古代民眾關於醫藥的智識
山海經的文化史的研究

Goto Shiro and Nagasawa Motoo 後藤志朗 長沢元夫
1975 "Studies on the Laws of Combination of Drugs in 'Lei-gong Yao-dui'." *Yakushi Zasshi* 10:22–33.
藥史学雜誌

Hu Hou-hsüan 胡厚宣
1944 "Yin-jen chi-ping k'ao." *Chia-ku-hsüeh Shang-shih lun-ts'ung*. Ch'eng-tu.
殷人疾病考 甲骨學商史論叢

Ishida Mikinosuke 石田幹之助
1959 "Inzen Seiyō ni tsuite." *Shisen* 15:40–58.
《飲膳正要》について 史泉

Kitamura Shiro 北村四郎
1969 "Inzen Seiyō no Shokubutsu." *Acta Phytotax. Geobot.* 24:65–76.
《飲膳正要》の植物

K'uei Ching-feng 葵景峯
1964 "Shih-lun Li Shih-chen chi ch'i tsai k'o-hsüeh shang ti ch'eng-chiu." *K'o-hsüeh-shih chi-k'an* 7:63–80.
試論李時珍及其在科學上的成就
科學史集刊

Kuroda Genji 黑田源次
1971   *Chung-kuo i-hsüeh shu-mu.* Reprint of 1931 edition. Taipei.
中國醫學書目

Li Chin-hua 李晉華
1932   *Ming-tai ch'ih-chuan shu k'ao.* Peking.
明代勅撰書考

Li Ch'ing-chih 李清志
n.d.   "Chin shih k'un ch'ung ts'ao chuang, erh-shih-ch'i ch'üan." *Kuo-li chung-yang t'u-shu-kuan shan-pen shu-chih,* new vol. 12, no. 1, pp. 91–94. Taipei.
金石昆蟲草木林二十七卷
國立中央圖書館善本書志

Liu Cheng-hsiung 劉正雄
1977   "Ming Ch'ing liang-tai wei-i ch'ih-chuan pen-ts'ao—Pen-ts'ao p'in-hui ching-yao chi Hsü-chi chih k'ao-ch'a." Master of Pharmacy thesis. Graduate Institute of Chinese Pharmaceutical Sciences, China Medical College, Taipei.
明清兩代惟一勅撰本草　本草品彙
精要及續集之考察

Lo Chen-yü 羅振玉
1968   "K'ai-yüan hsieh-pen Pen-ts'ao chi-chu hsü-lu ts'an-ch'üan." *Lo Hsüeh-t'ang hsien-sheng ch'üan-chi ch'u-pien.* Taipei.
開元寫本本草集注序錄殘巷
羅雪堂先生全集初編

Lü Shang-chih 呂尚志
1971   *Chung-kuo ku-tai ti i-hsüeh ti fa-ming ho ch'uang-tsao.* Hong Kong.
中國古代醫學家的發明和創造

Ma Chi-hsing 马继兴
1979   "Ma-wang-tui ku i-shu chung yu kuan yao-wu chih-chi ti wen-hsien k'ao-ch'a." *Yao-hsüeh t'ung-pao* 14:423–425.
马王堆古医书中有关药物制剂的文
献考察　药学通报

Miyashita Saburo 宮下三郎
1965   "On the Diffusion of Syrup to China and Japan." *Igakushi Kenkyū* 17:939.
医学史研究
1979   "Malaria (yao) in Chinese Medicine during the Chin and Yüan Periods." *Acta Asiatica* 36:90–112.

Mori Shikazō 森鹿三

1954   "Shinnō Honkei shōsai yakuhin ni tsuite." *Tōhō Gakuhō* 25:
        658–673.
        神農本經所載藥品について
        京都人文科学研究所

Morimura Ken-ichi 森村謙一

1970   "Honzō Kōmoku no shokubutsu kisai." *Minshin-jidai no ka-
        gaku gijutsushi*, ed. Yabuuchi and Yoshida. Kyoto. Pp. 257–
        325.
        本草綱目の植物記載   明清時代の
        科学技術史

1974   "Honzō Kōmoku ni okeru Ri Ji-chin no kindai shokubutsugaku-
        teki kiyo." *Kagakushi Kenkyu* 112:163–165.
        本草綱目における李時珍の近代植物
        学的寄与   科学史研究

1979   "Tōzai honzō hikaku ni okeru shizen chiriteki kanten ni tsuite."
        Nihon kagakushi gakkai, pp. 25–26.
        東西本草比較における自然地理的観
        点について   日本科学史学会

Na Ch'i 那琦

1969   "Yü-chih pen-ts'ao p'in-hui ching-yao." *Chung-kuo i-yao* 8:
        1–2.
        御製本草品彙精要   中國醫藥

1970a   "Pen-ts'ao fang-tu chi." *China Medical College Annual Bulletin*
        1, I, pp. 99–108; II, pp. 109–116.
        本草訪讀記

1970b   "Pen-ts'ao chung chih pi-hui wen-t'i." *China Medical College
        Annual Bulletin* 1:117–124.
        本草中之避諱問題

1970c   "Chih-wu ming-shih-t'u k'ao ch'ang-pien chi Chih-wu ming-
        shih-t'u k'ao chih k'ao-ch'a." *China Medical College Annual
        Bulletin* 1:185–199.
        植物名實圖考長編及植物名實圖考之
        考察

1971a   "Mei-kuo P'u-lin-ssu-tun ta-hsüeh Ko-ssu-te tung-fang t'u-shu-
        kuan suo ts'ang *pen-ts'ao* chih k'ao-ch'a." *China Medical Col-
        lege Annual Bulletin* 2:299–326.
        美國普林斯頓大學葛思德東方圖書館
        所藏本草之考察

1971b   "Mei-kuo kuo-hui t'u-shu-kuan suo ts'ang *pen-ts'ao* chih k'ao-
        ch'a." *China Medical College Annual Bulletin* 2:273–297.
        美國國會圖書館所藏本草之考察

1974   *Pen-ts'ao hsüeh*. Taipei.
        本草學

Nakao Manzō   中尾万三

1930   "Shokuryo Honzō no kōsatsu." *Shanghai tzu-jan k'o-hsüeh yen-chiu suo hui-pao* 1:5–214.

食療本草の考察　上海自然科學研究
所彙報

1933   "Shōkō Kōtei Keishi Shōrui Bikyu Honzō no kōsatsu." *Shanghai tzu-jan k'o-hsüeh yen-chiu suo hsin-pao* 2.

紹興校定經史證類備急本草の考察

Okanishi Tameto   岡西為人

1942   "Iwayuru Shokuhon Zukei no kōsatsu." *Nihon Ishigaku Zasshi* 104:1–6.

所謂蜀本圖經の考察　日本医史学雑誌

1951   "Shōrui Honzō ni kansuru nisan no chiken." *Annual Reports of Shionogi Research Laboratory* 1:64–71.

證類本草に関する二三の知見

1952   "Gosan Honzō Hin-i Seiyō." *Annual Reports of Shionogi Research Laboratory* 2:82–87.

御纂本草品彙精要

1954a   "Shinshu Honzō oyobi Shōrui Honzō no yakuhin-su." *Annual Reports of Shionogi Research Laboratory* 4:465–469.

新修本草及心證類本草の藥品數

1954b   "Shinnō Honzōkei shōsai no yakuhin ni tsuite." *Kanpō no rinshō* 6:9–28.

神農本草經所載の藥品について

漢方の臨床

1959a   "Shinshu Honzō no kōsei." *Journal of the Pharmacognostical Society of Japan* 13:1–6.

新修本草の構成

1959b   "The Main Current of the Chinese *Pen-ts'ao*." *Annual Reports of Shionogi Research Laboratory* 9:1079–1086.

1965   "Sōdai no ishohokan ni kansuru nisan no chiken." *Seikatsu-bunka kenkyu* 13:277–282.

宋代の臣書校勘に関する二三知見

生活文化研究

1967   "Chūgoku honzō no dentō to kingen no honzō." *Sōgen jidai no kagaku gijutsushi*, ed. Yabuuchi Kiyoshi. Tokyo. Pp. 171–210.

中國本草の伝統と銃の本草　宋元
時代の科学技術史

1969   "Gosei Honzō Hin-i Seiyō ni tsuite." *Idan* 39:20–24.

御製本草品彙精要について　医譚

1970   "Minshin no honzō." *Minshin jidai no kagaku gijutsushi*, ed. Yabuuchi and Yoshida. Kyoto. Pp. 147–182.

明清の本草　明清時代の科学技術史

1971   *Hsü Chung-kuo i-hsüeh shu-mu*. Taipei.

續中國醫學書目

1974   *Chugoku Isho Honzō-ko*. Osaka.
        中國醫書本草考
1977   *Honzō gaisetsu*. Osaka.
        本草概説

Ōtsuka Yasuō   大塚恭男
1978   "Honzō Hin-i Seiyō no ichi mihappyō hon ni tsuite." *Nihon Ishigaku Zasshi* 24:198–200.
        本草品彙精要の一未発表本について
        日本医史学雑誌

Shinoda Osamu   篠田統
1963   "Shokukei-kō." *Chūgoku chusei kagaku gijutsushi no kenkyū*, ed. Yabuuchi Kiyoshi. Tokyo. Pp. 307–320.
        食經考   中國中世科学技術史の研究
1967   "Inzen Seiyō ni tsuite." *Sōgen jidai no kagaku gijutsushi*, ed. Yabuuchi Kiyoshi. Tokyo. Pp. 329–340.
        飲膳正要について   宋元時代の科
        学技術史
1970   "Kinsei Shokukei-kō." *Minshin jidai no kagaku gijutsushi*, ed. Yabuuchi and Yoshida. Kyoto. Pp. 327–410.
        近世食經史   明清時代の科学技
        術史
1972   "Inzen Seiyō ni tsuite." *Chūgoku shokukei sōsho*, ed. Shinoda and Tanaka. Tokyo. Pp. 329–340.
        飲膳正要について   中國食經叢書

Shinoda Osamu and Tanaka Seiichi, eds.   篠田統   田中静一
1972   *Chugoku shokukei sōsho*. Tokyo.
        中國食經叢書

Shuai Hsüeh-chung et al.   帥学忠
1980   *Ma-wang-tui i-shu chuan-k'an*. Ch'ang-sha.
        马王堆医书专刊

T'ang Lan   唐兰
1975   "Ma-wang-tui po-shu 'Ch'üeh-ku shih-ch'i p'ien' k'ao." *Wen-wu*, no. 6, pp. 14–15.
        马王堆帛书《却谷食氣篇考》

Ting Fu-pao and Chou Yün-ch'ing   丁福保   周雲青
1955   *Ssu-pu tsung-lu i-yao pien*. Shanghai.
        四部總錄醫藥編

Wang Chia-yin　王嘉蔭
1957　*Pen-ts'ao kang mu ti kuang-wu shih-liao*. Peking.
本草綱目的礦物史料

Wang Chi-min　王吉民
1954　*Li Shih-chen wen-hsien chan-lan-hui t'e-k'an*. Shanghai.
李時珍文獻展覽會特刊

Wang Chung-min　王重民
1936　"Lo-ma fang-shu chi." *Chung-kuo t'u-shu chi-k'an* 3:238.
羅馬訪書記　中國圖書集刊

Watanabe Kōzo　渡邊幸三
1953a　"Honzō Shūchū joroku no yakuchū." *Kanpo* 2, no. 2:36–41;
no. 3:1–5; no. 4:1–3; no. 6:1–5; no. 8:1–8.
本草集注序錄の訳注　　漢方
1953b　"Ri Ji-chin no Honzō Kōmoku to sono hampon." *Toyoshi Kenkyu*
12:1–25.
李時珍の本草綱目とその版本
東洋史研究
1953c　"Tō Shinbi no Keishi Shōrui Bikyū Honzō no keitō to sono
hampon." *Tōhō Gakuhō* 21:160–206.
唐慎微の經史證類備急本草の系統
とその版本　　東方學報
1951　"Tō Kō-Kei no honzō ni taisuru bunkengakuteki kōsatsu." *Tōhō
Gakuhō* 20:195–222.
陶弘景の本草に對ちる文獻學的考察
東方學報

Wu Te-to　吳德鐸
1979　"Ts'ung 'Hsin-hsiu pen-ts'ao' k'an chung-jih liang kuo ti hsüeh-
shu chiao-liu." *Chung-hua wen-shih lun-ts'ung* 2:471–489.
从《新修本草》看中日两国的学术
交流　中华文史论丛

Yen I-p'ing　嚴一萍
1951　"Chung-kuo i-hsüeh chih ch'i-yüan chi k'ao-lüeh." *Ta-lu tsa-
chih* 2, no. 8:20–22; no. 9:14–17.
中國醫學之起源及攷畧　大陸雜誌
Publications by collectives:
1975　"Ma-wang-tui Han-mu ch'u-t'u i-shu shih-wen." *Wen-wu*, (1)
no. 6, pp. 1–5; (2) no. 9, pp. 35–48.
马王堆汉墓出土医书释文　　文物

1975   "Ma-wang-tui po-shu ssu-chung ku i-hsüeh i-shu chien-chieh."
        Wen-wu, no. 6, pp. 16–19.

马王堆帛书四種古医学佚书简介

文物

1975   "Ma-wang-tui san-hao Han-mu po-hua tao-yin-t'u ti ch'u-pu
        yen-chiu." *Wen-wu*, no. 6, pp. 6–13.

马王堆三号汉墓帛画导引图的初步研

究   文物

1975   *Wu-wei Han-tai i-chien*. Peking.

武威汉代医简

1979   *Chung-yao ta-tz'u-tien*. Shanghai.

中药大辞典

Western Secondary Sources

Bauer, Wolfgang
    1976   *China and the Search for Happiness.* New York.

Bertuccioli, Giulano
    1954   "Nota sul *Pen-ts'ao p'in-hui ching-yao.*" *Rivista degli Studi Orientali* 29:247–251.
    1956a   "A Note on Two Ming Manuscripts of the *Pen-ts'ao p'in-hui ching-yao.*" *Journal of Oriental Studies* 3:63–68.
    1956b   "Nuova nota sul *Pen-ts'ao p'in-hui ching-yao.*" *Rivista degli Studi Orientali* 31:179–181.

Biot, Edouard
    1851   *Le Tcheou-li.* Vol 1. Paris.

Chavannes, Edouard
    1913   *Les Documents Chinois decouverts par Aurel Stein.* Oxford.

Costantini, Vilma, and Sebastiana Papa
    1973   *Pen ts'ao p'in hui ching yao. Antico codice cinese di Farmacologia.* Milano.

Croizier, Ralph
    1968   *Traditional Medicine in Modern China.* Cambridge, Mass.

De Groot, J. J. M.
    1892–   *The Religious System of China.* Leyden.
    1910

Franke, Herbert
    1970   "Additional Notes on Non-Chinese Terms in the Yüan-Imperial Dietary Compendium *Yin-shan cheng-yao.*" *Zentralasiatische Studien des Seminars für Sprach- und Kulturwissenschaft Zentralasiens der Universität Bonn* 4:7–16.

Fuchs, Walter
    1966   *Chinesische und Mandjurische Handschriften und seltene Drucke.* Wiesbaden.

Goltz, Dietlinde
    1969   "Zur Entwicklungsgeschichte der Arzneibücher, Form-Inhalt-Problematik." *Pharmazeutische Zeitung* 114:1819–1827, 2009–2014.
    1970   "Grundzüge der Entwicklung einer pharmazeutischen Literatur." *Veröffentlichungen der Internationalen Gesellschaft für Geschichte der Pharmazie,* N.F., 36:59–64.

Harper, Donald
    1982   *The Wu-shih-erh ping fang.* Translation and Prolegomena. Ph.D. thesis. Berkeley.

Hummel, Arthur W.
    1941   "The Printed Herbal of A.D. 1249." *Isis* 33:439–442.
    1970   *Eminent Chinese of the Ch'ing Period.* Taipei.

Kracke, E. A., Jr.
    1954–   "Sung Society: Change Within Tradition." *Far Eastern Quarterly* 14.
    1955

Lao Yan-Shuan
    1969   "Notes on Non-Chinese Terms in the Yüan-Imperial Dietary Compendium *Yin-shan cheng-yao.*" *The Bulletin of the Institute of History and Philology Academia Sinica* 39:399–416.

Laufer, Berthold
    1967   *Sino-Iranica.* Taipei.

Legge, James
    1960   *The Chinese Classics.* 5 Vols. Hong Kong.

Lu Gwei-djen
    1966   "China's Greatest Naturalist; A Brief Biography of Li Shih-chen." *Physis* 8:383–392.

Needham, Joseph
    1959   *Science and Civilization in China.* Vol. 3. Cambridge.
    1961   *Science and Civilization in China.* Vol. 1. Cambridge.
    1962   *Science and Civilization in China.* Vol. 4:1. Cambridge.
    1970   *Clerks and Craftsmen in China and the West.* Cambridge.

Needham, Joseph and Lu Gwei-djen
    1951   "A Contribution to the History of Chinese Dietetics." *Isis* 42:13–20.

Rall, Jutta
    1970   *Die vier Grossen Medizinschulen der Mongolenzeit.* Wiesbaden.

Schmauderer, Eberhard
    1970   "Entwicklungsformen der Pharmakopöen." *Veröffentlichungen des Forschungsinstitutes des Deutschen Museums für die Geschichte der Naturwissenschaften und der Technik,* series A, 57.

Spence, Jonathan
    1972   "Das Opiumrauchen im China der Ch'ing-Zeit." *Saeculum* 23:397–425.

Strickmann, Michel
    1979   "On the Alchemy of T'ao Hung-ching." *Facets of Taoism,* ed. Holmes Welch and Anna Seidel. New Haven. Pp. 123–192.

Unschuld, Paul U.
    1973*a*   *Die Praxis des traditionellen chinesischen Heilsystems.* Wiesbaden.
    1973*b*   *Das Pen-ts'ao p'in-hui ching-yao. Ein Arzneibuch aus dem China der Kaiserzeit.* München.
    1975   "Zur Bedeutung des Terminus *tu* in der traditionellen medizinisch-pharmazeutischen Literatur Chinas." *Sudhoffs Archiv* 57:165–183.
    1976   "Western Medicine and Traditional Healing Systems: Competition, Cooperation or Integration?" *Ethics in Science and Medicine* 3:1–20.
    1978   "Das *Ch'uan-ya* und die Praxis chinesischer Landärzte im 18. Jahrhundert." *Sudhoffs Archiv* 62:378–407.
    1979   *Medical Ethics in Imperial China. A Study in Historical Anthropology.* Berkeley, Los Angeles and London.
    1982   "Ma-wang-tui *Materia Medica.* A Comparative Analysis of Early Chinese Pharmaceutical Knowledge." *Zinbun: Memoirs of the Research Institute for Humanistic Studies. Kyoto University* 18:11–63.
    1983   "Die Bedeutung der Ma-wang-tui-Funde für die chinesische Medizin- und Pharmaziegeschichte." *Aspekte der Pharmaziegeschichte,* ed. Peter Dilg. Graz. Pp. 389–416.

Unschuld, Ulrike
    1972   *Das T'ang-yeh pen-ts'ao und die Übertragung der klassischen chinesischen Medizintheorie auf die Praxis der Drogenanwendung.* Ph.D. dissertation, Munich.
    1977   "Traditional Chinese Pharmacology: An Analysis of its Development in the Thirteenth Century." *Isis* 68:224–248.

Ware, James R., trans.
    1966   *Alchemy, Medicine, Religion in the China of* A.D. *320.* Cambridge, Mass.

Index of Persons

何孟春　子元　Ho Meng-ch'un, *tzu:* Tzu-yüan, 165
　　　　　　(15th century)

赫世亨　Ho Shih-heng, 142
　　　　　(ca. 1700), civil servant

何首烏　田兒 能嗣　Ho Shou-wu, T'ien-erh, Neng-ssu, 230

和思輝　Ho Ssu-hui. *See* Hu Ssu-hui

后稷　Hou Chi, 12
　　　legendary director of agriculture under emperor Yao

侯寧極　Hou Ning-chi, 259
　　　　　(10th century), medical author

夏良心　宗堯　Hsia Liang-hsin, *tzu:* Tsung-yao, 160
　　　　　　(ca. 1603), publisher, civil servant

蕭敬　克恭 梅東　Hsiao Ching, *tzu:* K'e-kung, *hao:* Mei-tung, 129
　　　　　　(1438–1528), eunuch

孝平 劉衍　Hsiao P'ing, Liu K'an, 263
　　　　　(8 B.C.–A.D. 6), Han-emperor

孝宗 朱祐樘　Hsiao-tsung, Chu Yu-t'ang, 129, 143, 148
　　　　　(1470–1505), Ming-emperor

謝肇淛　Hsieh Chao-chi, 14
　　　　　(Ming-era)

獻帝 劉協　Hsien-ti, Liu Hsieh, 31
　　　　　(181–234), Han-emperor

憲王　Hsien-wang, son of Chu Hsiao, 221
　　　　(ca. 1400)

熊宗立 道軒　Hsiung Tsung-li, *tzu:* Tao-hsüan, 247, 248
　　　　　(15th century), physician, medical author

徐鍇　Hsü Chieh, 212
　　　　(9th century)

徐之才 士茂　Hsü Chih-ts'ai, *tzu:* Shih-mao, 75, 149, 154
　　　　　(ca. 510–590), medical author

許敬宗　Hsü Ching-tsung, 46
　　　　　(592–672), historiographer

徐福　Hsü Fu, 13
　　　　(3d century B.C.)

許孝崇　Hsü Hsiao-ch'ung, 44
　　　　　(ca. 650), civil servant

王世昌　歷山　　Wang Shih-ch'ang, *tzu:* Li-shan, 130

（ca. 1503), painter

王世貞　元美鳳州　Wang Shih-chen, *tzu:* Yüan-mei, *hao:* Feng-chou, 148, 160

(1526–1593), civil servant, poet

汪石山　　　Wang Shih-shan. *See* Wang Chi

王守仁　伯安陽明　Wang Shou-jen, *tzu:* Po-an, *hao:* Yang-ming, 181, 182

(1472–1528), civil servant, philosopher

王叔和　　　Wang Shu-ho. *See* Wang Hsi

王太僕　　　Wang T'ai-p'u. *See* Wang T'ing

王道純　　　Wang Tao-ch'un, 142, 143

(ca. 1701), medical official

王大燮　　　Wang Ta-hsieh, 262

(ca. 1914), minister of education

王綖　太僕開塘　Wang T'ing, *tzu:* T'ai-p'u, *hao:* K'ai-t'ang, 156

(Ming-era), physician, medical author

汪穎　　　Wang Ying, 224, 225

(ca. 1600), medical author

王祐　景叔　Wang Yu, *tzu:* Ching-shu, 58, 61, 132

(ca. 980), civil servant, writer

王玉　　　Wang Yü, 133

(ca. 1503), civil servant

汪由敦　師茗　謹堂松泉　Wang Yu-tun, *tzu:* Shih-ming, *hao:* Chin-t'ang, Sung-ch'üan, 254

(1692–1758), civil servant

渡邊幸三　　　Watanabe Kozo, 71, 147, 162

韋訊逍　慈藏　Wei Hsün-tao, *hao:* Tz'u-tsang, 247

(ca. 700), physician

韋慈藏　　　Wei Tz'u-tsang. *See* Wei Hsün-tao

文潞公　　　Wen Lu-kung. *See* Wen Yen-po

文俶　　　Wen Shu, 145

(1594–1634), painter, daughter of Wen Ts'ung-hsien

文從簡　彥可　Wen Ts'ung-chien, *tzu:* Yen-k'o, 145

(1574–1648), painter, father of Wen Shu

文王　昌　周　Wen Wang, Ch'ang, duke of Chou, 216

(1231–1135 B.C.)

文彥博　寬夫　Wen Yen-po, *tzu:* K'uan-fu, 109

(1006–1097), medical author

Index of Book Titles

Index of Drugs

The identification of ancient Chinese drugs in terms of modern botany, zoology, or chemistry/mineralogy is often rather problematic. The following data should be regarded with caution; they were taken, for the most part, from what appears to be the most reliable source available, the *Chung-yao ta tz'u-tien*. Numbers referring to the listing of the drugs in the *Chung-yao ta tz'u-tien* have been added, in parentheses, to the scientific designations. Following the parentheses, page numbers in italics refer to illustrations; all others to references in the text.

陳皮	*ch'en-p'i*	dried peels of Citrus tangerina Hort. (5535), 112, 134
雞	*chi*	chickens, *218*
雞腸	*chi-ch'ang*	entire herb of Trigonotis peduncularis (Trev.) Benth. (2415), 44, 59
及己	*chi-chi*	root of Chloranthus serratus (Thunb.) Roem. et Schult. (0460), 44
奇功石	*ch'i-kung-shih*	"wonderfully effective stone," 166
薺苨	*chi-ni*	root of Adenophora trachelioides Maxim. (3327), 64
鯽魚	*chi-yü*	brace, *285*
薑	*chiang*	See *sheng-chiang*
醬豉	*chiang-ch'ih*	soy sauce, 154
羌活	*ch'iang-huo*	rhizome of Notopterygium incisum Ting (2386), 65, 134, 159
交莖	*chiao-ching*	synonym for *ho-shou-wu*, 231
鉛粉	*ch'ien-fen*	lead-carbonate, 2 PbCO$_3$• Pb (OH)$_2$ (3847), 165, 176
千里及	*ch'ien-li-chi*	entire herb of Senecio scandens Buch.-Ham. (0443), 257
千里光	*ch'ien-li-kuang*	synonym for *ch'ien-li-chi*, 257
牽牛子	*ch'ien-niu (tzu)*	seeds of Pharbitis nil (L.) Choisy (3365), 155, 282
鉛丹	*ch'ien-tan*	minium, Pb$_3$O$_4$ (3845), 245
芝	*chih*	entire trunk of Ganoderma japonicum (Fr.) Lloyd (2395), 27, 228
赤箭	*ch'ih-chien*	synonym for *t'ien-ma-ken*, 66
赤小豆	*ch'ih-hsiao-tou*	beans of Phaseolus calcaratus Roxb. (2222), *189*
赤鬚子	*ch'ih-hsü-tzu*	"red whisker seeds" of uncertain identity, 240
陟釐	*chih-li*	identity uncertain, 44
枳實	*chih-shih*	young fruit of Poncirus trifoliata (L.) Raf. (3140), 39, 224
卮子	*chih-tzu*	fruit of Gardenia jasminoides Ellis. (4084), 160
金雞勒	*chin-chi-lei*	bark of Cinchona succirubra Pav. (2874), 166
青木香	*ch'ing-mu-hsiang*	root of Aristolochia debilis Sieb. et Zucc. (2496), 134, 159, 160, 288
青皮	*ch'ing-p'i*	unripe peels or young fruit of Citrus tangerina Hort. et Tanaka (2485), 134
荊三稜	*ching-san-leng*	stem tubers of Scirpus flaviatilis (Torr.) A. Gray (0097), *16*

井底沙 *ching-ti-sha*   sand from the bottom of wells, 200

荊子 *ching-tzu*   fruit of Vitex rotundifolia L. (5309), 44

九里明 *chiu-li-ming*   synonym for *ch'ien-li-chi*, 257

橘 *chü*   short for *chü-p'i*, 59

麹 *ch'ü*   yeast, 244

蒟醬 *chü-chiang*   leaves of Piper betle L. (5122), 222

蒟蒻 *chü-jo*   stem tubers of Amorphophallus rivieri Durieu (5121), 176

橘皮 *chü-p'i*   peels of Citrus tangerina Hort. et Tanaka (5532), 39

朱砂 *chu-sha*   cinnabar (1834), 74

犬 *ch'üan*   dog, 101

川芎 *ch'uan-hsiung*   rhizome of Ligusticum wallichii Franch. (0452), 112, 159

川楝 *ch'uan-lien*   fruit of Melia toosendan Sieb. et Zucc. (0459), 160

船底苔 *ch'uan-ti-t'ai*   moss from the bottom of boats, 114

英光 *chüeh-kuang*   mature fruit of Cassia tora L. (1906), 258

蓴(茶) *ch'un (ts'ai)*   vegetables of uncertain identity, 36

蘩蔞 *fan-lou*   stem and leaves of Stellaria media (L.) Cyr. (5628), 44, 59

礬石 *fan-shih*   alunite (1383), 63

防己 *fang-chi*   root of Stephania tetrandra S. Moore (1984), 33, 44, 104

防風 *fang-feng*   root of Saposhnikovia divaricata (Turcz.) Schischk. (1985), 104

防葵 *fang-k'uei*   identity uncertain, 44

飛廉 *fei-lien*   root or entire herb of Carduus crispus L. (0567), 44

棐子 *fei-tzu*   seeds of Torreya grandis Fort. (5273), 201, 211

粉錫 *fen-hsi*   synonym for *ch'ien-fen*, 165, 166, 245

粉霜 *fen-shuang*   purified calomel, Hg_2Cl_2 (4010), 115

楓香脂 *feng-hsiang-chih*   resin of Liquidambar taiwaniana Hance (5177), 288

鳳仙子 *feng-hsien-tzu*   seeds of Impatiens balsamina L. (0988), 176

扶移 *fu-i*   bark of Amelanchier sinica (Schneid.) Chun (2264), 63

芙蓉 *fu-jung*   Hibiscus mutalidis L. (0741), 158

茯苓 *fu-ling*   Poria cocos Wolf (3314), 66, 67

扶留 *fu-liu*   synonym for *chü-chiang*, 222

伏龍肝 *fu-lung-kan*   clay from the floor of a fireplace, 141

附子 *fu-tzu* rhizome of Aconitum carmichaeli Debx. (2414), 37, *39, 171,* 212

附子花 *fu-tzu-hua* flowers of Aconitum carmichaeli Debx. *171*

海松 *hai-sung* seeds of Pinus koraiensis Sieb. et Zucc. (3985), 154

海帶 *hai-tai* entire herb of Zostera marina L. (3969), 63

海藻 *hai-tsao* entire herb of Sargassum fusiforme (Harvey) Setch. (3978), 63

何首烏 *ho-shou-wu* root tubers of Polygonum multiflorum Thunb. (2310), *153, 225, 226, 230, 231*

厚朴 *hou-p'o* tree bark or root bark of Magnolia officinalis Rehd. et Wils. (3366), 66, *84*

細辛 *hsi-hsin* entire herb with root of Asarum heterotropoides Fr. Schmidt var. mandshuricum (Maximowicz) Kitagawa (3082), *33,* 112, 246

錫灰 *hsi-hui* "tin ashes," 131

奚毒 *hsi-tu* synonym for *wu-t'ou,* 66

相思子 *hsiang-ssu-tzu* seeds of Abrus precatorius L. (3129), 246

象牙 *hsiang-ya* elephant tusks, *184, 260*

消石 *hsiao-shih* niter, KNO$_3$ (3959), 42

蠍 *hsieh* scorpion, 162

邂逅 *hsieh-hou* identity uncertain, 258

蝤蛑 *hsiu-mou* crabs, 62, *193*

雄鵲 *hsiung-ch'iao* male magpie, 79

熊脂 *hsiung-chih* bear fat, *100*

雄黃 *hsiung-huang* realgar, AsS (4853), 90

萱草 *hsüan-ts'ao* root of Hemerophyllis fulva L. (4832), *126*

虎杖 *hu-chang* rhizome of Polygonum cuspidatum Sieb. et Zucc. (2743), *103*

葫蘆巴 *hu-lu-pa* seeds of Trigonella foenum graecum L. (3221), 63, 219

胡麻油 *hu-ma-yu* oil from the seeds of Sesamum indicum DC. (4613), *179*

胡桃 *hu-t'ao* seed-kernels of Juglans regia L. (3224), 207

胡同律 *hu-t'ung-lü* resin dropped on the earth from Populus diversifolia Schrenk (3223), 59

黃耆 *huang-ch'i* dried root of Astragalus membranaceus (Fisch.) Bge. (4153), *120, 256,* 256

鈎吻	kou-wen	entire herb of Gelsemium elegans Benth. (3434), 37, 44, 176
菰筍	ku-sun	galls generated by the sting of Ustilago esculenta Henn. on Zizania caduciflora (Turcz.) Hand.-Mazz. (3333), 154
栝樓	kua-lou	fruit of Trichosanthes kirilowii Maxim. (3653), 33, 242
款冬花	k'uan-tung-hua	flower buds of Tussilago farfara L. (4782), 18, 159
廣木香	kuang-mu-hsiang	root of Saussurea lappa Clarke (0703), 134
光鹽	kuang-yen	natural table salt (1766), 59
桂	kuei	synonym for jou-kuei, 95, 113, 235
鬼皂莢	kuei-tsao-chia	fruit of Gleditsia sinensis Lam. (2326), 52
昆布	k'un-pu	Laminaria japonica Aresch. (2799), 204
缸中膏	kung-chung-kao	axle grease, 131
臘雪	la-hsüeh	snow of the twelfth month, 136
莨菪	lang-tang	seeds of Hyoscyamus niger L. (0649), 22
狼毒	lang-tu	root of Euphorbia fischeriana Steud. (3907), 37, 39, 44, 155
狼牙	lang-ya	entire herb of Agrimonia pilosa Ledeb. var. japonica (Miq.) Nakai (1372), 176
老陽子	lao-yang-tzu	synonym for pa-tou, 153
藜蘆	li-lu	rhizome of Veratrum nigrum L. (5652), 40, 104, 154
粱米	liang-mi	seed-kernels of sorghum vulgare Pers. (3929), 43, 44
梁上塵	liang-shang-ch'en	rafter dust, 179
靈砂	ling-sha	"spiritual sand," artificial cinnabar, 115
羚羊角	ling-yang-chiao	antelope horn, 8
絡石	lo-shih	stalk and leaves of Trachelospermum jasminoides (Lindl.) Lem. (3604), 44
綠礬	lü-fan	melanterite, FeSO$_4$ · 7 H$_2$0 (4715), 63
爐甘石	lu-kan-shih	smithsonite (3013), 134
蘆筍	lu-sun	young sprouts of Phragmites communis Trin. (2192), 154
菉豆	lü-tou	seeds of Phaseolus radiatus L. (4713), 246
鸕鷀	lu-tz'u	cormorant, 54
陸英	lu-ying	entire herb and root of Sambucus javanica Reinw. (5124), 59, 61, 66

豆林	*tou-lin*	identity uncertain, 159
蒼朮	*ts'ang-shu*	rhizome of Atractylodes lancea (Thunb.) DC. (2174), 134, 215
草果	*ts'ao-kuo*	synonym for *pai-tou-k'ou*, 134
草烏	*ts'ao-wu*	root tubers of Aconitum carmichaeli Dbx. (3287), 176
澤瀉	*tse-hsieh*	stem tubers of Alisma plantago-aquatica L. var. orientale Samuels. (3046), 22, 104
蚱蟬	*tse-shan*	cicada, 53, 99
突屈白	*t'u-ch'ü-pai*	identity uncertain, 59
土茯苓	*t'u-fu-ling*	rhizome of Smilax glabra Roxb. (0166), *153*
杜蘅	*tu-heng*	root or entire herb of Asarum forbesii Maxim. (2094), 44
獨活	*tu-huo*	rhizome of Angelica pubescens Maxim. (3510), 134, 159
土硫黃	*t'u-liu-huang*	"earth" sulphur (1260), *187*
菟絲	*t'u-ssu*	entire herb or seeds of Cuscuta chinensis Lam. (4123), 66
冬灰	*tung-hui*	ashes from *tzu-ts'ao*, 87
東壁土	*tung-pi-t'u*	soil scraped from a wall pointing east, 87, *178*
通脫	*t'ung-t'o*	synonum for *t'ung-ts'ao*, 67
通草	*t'ung-ts'ao*	stem marrow of Tetrapanax papyriferus (Hook.) K. Koch (4050), 63
紫鑛	*tzu-k'uang*	gumlike substance secreted on trees branches by Laccifer lacca Kerr. (4892), 59
磁石	*tz'u-shih*	magnetite (5320), 287
紫草	*tzu-ts'ao*	root of Lithospermum erythrorhizon Sieb. et Zucc. (4863), 175
鼃	*wa*	aquatic frog, *104*
五靈脂	*wu-ling-chih*	dried droppings of bats (0770), 160
吳茱萸	*wu-shu-yu*	unripe fruit of Evodia rutaecarpa (Juss.) Benth. (2280), 39
烏頭	*wu-t'ou*	synonym for *ts'ao-wu*, 172
烏賊魚	*wu-tse-yü*	cuttlefish, *45*
五味子	*wu-wei-tzu*	fruit of Schisandra chinensis (Turcz.) Baill. (0772), 234, 288

鴉片	ya-p'ien	synonym for *a-fu-jung*, 158, 159
野豬	yeh-chu	wild boar, *219*
夜合	yeh-ho	synonym for *ho-shou-wu*, 231
野苗	yeh-miao	synonym for *ho-shou-wu*, 231
燕覆草	yen-fu	stem of Akebia trifoliata (Thunb.) Koidz. (0706), 63
鶯薅草	yen-ju-ts'ao	"swallow's nest herb," *178*
烟草	yen-ts'ao	leaves of Nicotiana tabacum L. (3944), 166
茵蔯蒿	yin-ch'en-hao	stalk and leaves of Artemisia capillaris Thunb. (3305), 42
銀膏	yin-kao	silver amalgam, *201*
櫻桃	ying-t'ao	fruit of Prunus pseudocerasus Lindl. (5425), 78
罌子粟	ying-tzu-su	seeds of Papaver somniferum L. (5342), *158, 167*
柚	yu	ripe fruit of Citrus grandis (L.) Osbeck (3132), 44, 59
玉泉	yü-ch'üan	identity uncertain, 66, 87
玉屑	yü-hsieh	nephrite (1158), 66
榆仁	yü jen	fruit and seeds of Ulmus pumila L. (5089), 44
由跋	yu-pa	stem tubers of Arisaema ringens (Thunb.) Schott (1346), 44
油頭	yu-t'ou	identity uncertain, 255
遠志	yüan-chih	root of Polygala tenuifolia Willd. (2087), 33
芫花	yüan-hua	flower buds of Daphne genkwa Sieb. et Zucc. (2135), *37*, 40, 104, 154
垣衣	yüan-i	mosses growing on roofs and walls, 63
鳶尾	yüan-wei	rhizome of Iris tectorum Maxim. (2729), 44
雲實	yün-shih	seeds of Caesalpinia sepiaria Roxb. (0693), 44
擁劍	yung-chien	crabs, 62, 193

General Index

(Page numbers in italics refer to illustrations)

Comparative Studies of Health Systems and Medical Care

General Editor
CHARLES LESLIE

Editorial Board
FRED DUNN, M.D., University of California, San Francisco
RENEE FOX, University of Pennsylvania
ELIOT FREIDSON, New York University
YASUO OTSUKA, M.D., Yokohama City University Medical School
MAGDALENA SOKOLOWSKA, Polish Academy of Sciences
CARL E. TAYLOR, M.D., The Johns Hopkins University
K. N. UDUPA, M.S., F.R.C.S., Banaras Hindu University
PAUL U. UNSCHULD, University of Munich
FRANCIS ZIMMERMANN, Ecole des Hautes Etudes en
Sciences Sociales, Paris